T
M

# THE FABER POCKET
# MEDICAL DICTIONARY

BY
P. A. Riley MB, BS, PhD

AND
P. J. Cunningham BA, SRN, SCM, HVCert

REVISED BY
Elizabeth Forsythe MRCS, LRCP, DPH

*faber and faber*
LONDON·BOSTON

*First edition 1966*
*Second edition 1974*
*Revised Reprint 1977*
*Third edition 1979*
*Reprinted 1985*
*Published by Faber and Faber Limited*
*3 Queen Square, London WC1*
*Printed in Great Britain by*
*Richard Clay (The Chaucer Press) Ltd,*
*Bungay, Suffolk*
*All rights reserved*

**British Library Cataloguing in Publication Data**

Riley, Patrick Anthony
The Faber pocket medical dictionary – 3rd ed.
1. Medicine – Dictionaries
I. Title   II. Cunningham, Phyllis Jean
III. Forsythe, Elizabeth
610'.3     R121
ISBN 0–571–04999–0

# PREFACE TO THE THIRD EDITION

This dictionary is intended for medical students, trained nurses, paramedical workers, medical auxiliaries and the interested layman. It is designed to provide a ready-to-hand and simple guide to medical terminology. To this end, the number of entries has been reduced, the text brought up to date and measurements converted to the metric system although some of the imperial alternatives are still included.

The appendices have been extensively revised and that on diet has been considerably enlarged and the principles underlying sound diet in health and disease have been brought into line with current thinking. The appendix on groups of drugs has been rewritten and enlarged and the list of drugs has been omitted because it is impossible to keep this section up to date or make it applicable to all the countries where this dictionary is in use. The appendix on first aid has been rewritten to conform with the present thinking of medical authorities on this rapidly evolving subject.

My thanks are due to all those who have helped with specific specialities and particularly to Patricia Downie, Editor, Nursing and Medical Books, Faber and Faber, for her patience and her unlimited encouragement.

E.F.
1979

# CONTENTS

# ABBREVIATIONS OF SOME TERMS USED IN PRESCRIPTIONS

(The use of abbreviations in prescriptions is a dangerous practice and contrary to the policy of the DHSS)

| Abbreviation | Latin | |
|---|---|---|
| a.c. | ante cibos | before meals |
| ad. | adde | up to |
| ad. lib. | ad libitum | up to the desired amount |
| alt. die. | alternis diebus | every other day |
| aq. | aqua | water |
| aq. dest. | aqua destillata | distilled water |
| aurist. | auristillae | ear drops |
| b.d. <br> b.i.d. | bis in die | twice a day |
| B.N.F. | — | British National Formulary |
| B.P. | — | British Pharmacopoeia |
| c. | cum | with |
| comp. | compositus | compounded of |
| crem. | cremor | cream |
| dil. | dilue | dilute |
| ext. | extractum | extract |
| gutt. | guttae | drops |
| haust. | haustus | a draught |
| in d. | in dies | daily |
| inj. | injectio | injection |
| lot. | lotio | lotion |
| mist. | mistura | mixture |
| mit. | mitte | send |

| Abbreviation | Latin | |
|---|---|---|
| noct. | nocte | at night |
| oc. | oculentum | eye ointment |
| o.d. | omnes dies | every day |
| o.m. | omni mane | every morning |
| o.n. | omni nocte | every night |
| p.c. | post cibos | after meals |
| pig. | pigmentum | paint |
| p.r. | per rectum | by the rectum |
| p.r.n. | pro re nata | as the occasion arises |
| pulv. | pulvis | powder |
| p.v. | per vaginam | by the vagina |
| q.d. q.d.s. | quater in die | four times a day |
| q.s. | quantum sufficit | as much as required |
| R. | recipe | 'take thou'—instruction to the Pharmacist preceding the prescription |
| rep. | repetatur | let it be repeated |
| sig. | signetur | let it be labelled |
| s.o.s. | si opus sit | if circumstances require |
| stat. | statim | immediately |
| syr. | syrupus | syrup |
| t.d. t.d.s. | ter in die | three times a day |
| tinct. tr. | tinctura | tincture |
| ung. | unguentum | ointment |

# COMPARATIVE WEIGHTS AND MEASURES

## WEIGHT

*Metric System*

| | |
|---|---|
| 1 kilogram (kg) | = 1,000 grams |
| 1 gram (g) | = 1,000 milligrams |
| 1 milligram (mg) | = 1,000 micrograms |
| 1 microgram (μg) | = 1,000 nanograms |
| 1 nanogram (ng) | = 1,000 picograms (pg) |

**Conversions**

| *Imperial System* | *Metric System* |
|---|---|
| 1 pound (lb) | = 435·59 grams |
| 1 ounce (oz) | = 28·34 grams |

| *Metric System* | *Imperial System* |
|---|---|
| 1 kilogram (kg) | = 2·2046 pounds or 35·274 ounces |

## VOLUME

*Metric System*

| | |
|---|---|
| 1 litre (1) | = 1,000 millilitres |
| 1 millilitre (ml) | = 1·000028 cubic centimetres (cm³) |

(The millilitre and cubic centimetre are usually treated as identical.)

**Conversions**

| *Imperial System* | *Metric System* |
|---|---|
| 1 pint (pt) | = 568·25 millilitres |
| 1 fluid ounce (fl oz) | = 28·412 millilitres |
| 1 minim (m) | = 0·059192 millilitres |

*Metric System*    *Imperial System*
1 litre          = 1·7598 pints or 35·196 fluid ounces
1 millilitre (ml)   = 16·894 minims


A 1 per cent w/v solution means:
1 gram solute dissolved in solvent to make 100 ml. (1 oz in 5 pints is approximately 1%)

## LENGTH

*Metric System*
1 metre (m)       = 100 centimetres
1 centimetre (cm)  = 10 millimetres
1 millimetre (mm)  = 1,000 micrometres
1 micrometre ($\mu$m) = 1,000 nanometres (nm)

*British System*
1 mile = 1,760 yards
1 yard = 3 feet
1 foot = 12 inches

**Conversions**

*Metric System*    *British System*
1 metre (m)       = 39·370 inches
1 centimetre (cm)  = 0·39370 inches
1 millimetre (mm)  = 0·039370 inches
1 micrometre ($\mu$m) = 0·000039370 inches

*British System*    *Metric System*
1 mile = 1609·344 metres
1 yard = 91·44 centimetres
1 foot = 30·48 centimetres
1 inch = 2·540 centimetres

# COMPARISON OF CELSIUS (CENTIGRADE) AND FAHRENHEIT THERMOMETRIC SCALES

| °C | °F | °C | °F | °C | °F |
|---|---|---|---|---|---|
| 0 | 32·0 | 34 | 93·2 | 68 | 154·4 |
| 1 | 33·8 | 35 | 95·0 | 69 | 156·2 |
| 2 | 35·6 | 36 | 96·8 | 70 | 158·0 |
| 3 | 37·4 | 37 | 98·6 | 71 | 159·8 |
| 4 | 39·2 | 38 | 100·4 | 72 | 161·6 |
| 5 | 41·0 | 39 | 102·2 | 73 | 163·4 |
| 6 | 42·8 | 40 | 104·0 | 74 | 165·2 |
| 7 | 44·6 | 41 | 105·8 | 75 | 167·0 |
| 8 | 46·4 | 42 | 107·6 | 76 | 168·8 |
| 9 | 48·2 | 43 | 109·4 | 77 | 170·6 |
| 10 | 50·0 | 44 | 111·2 | 78 | 172·4 |
| 11 | 51·8 | 45 | 113·0 | 79 | 174·2 |
| 12 | 53·6 | 46 | 114·8 | 80 | 176·0 |
| 13 | 55·4 | 47 | 116·6 | 81 | 177·8 |
| 14 | 57·2 | 48 | 118·4 | 82 | 179·6 |
| 15 | 59·0 | 49 | 120·2 | 83 | 181·4 |
| 16 | 60·8 | 50 | 122·0 | 84 | 183·2 |
| 17 | 62·6 | 51 | 123·8 | 85 | 185·0 |
| 18 | 64·4 | 52 | 125·6 | 86 | 186·8 |
| 19 | 66·2 | 53 | 127·4 | 87 | 188·6 |
| 20 | 68·0 | 54 | 129·2 | 88 | 190·4 |
| 21 | 69·8 | 55 | 131·0 | 89 | 192·2 |
| 22 | 71·6 | 56 | 132·8 | 90 | 194·0 |
| 23 | 73·4 | 57 | 134·6 | 91 | 195·8 |
| 24 | 75·2 | 58 | 136·4 | 92 | 197·6 |
| 25 | 77·0 | 59 | 138·2 | 93 | 199·4 |
| 26 | 78·8 | 60 | 140·0 | 94 | 201·2 |
| 27 | 80·6 | 61 | 141·8 | 95 | 203·0 |
| 28 | 82·4 | 62 | 143·6 | 96 | 204·8 |
| 29 | 84·2 | 63 | 145·4 | 97 | 206·6 |
| 30 | 86·0 | 64 | 147·2 | 98 | 208·4 |
| 31 | 87·8 | 65 | 149·0 | 99 | 210·2 |
| 32 | 89·6 | 66 | 150·8 | 100 | 212·0 |
| 33 | 91·4 | 67 | 152·6 | | |

# A GUIDE TO PRONUNCIATION

After each entry in the dictionary the pronunciation is found in brackets. The stress mark ' shows where the emphasis should be made in a word of more than one syllable, and these are divided by hyphens.

The basic vowel and consonant sounds are listed below:

| *Vowel sound* | *Example* |
|---|---|
| a as in bat | cataract (*kat'-a-rakt*) |
| ā as in mate | flatus (*flā'-tus*) |
| ah as in father | after (*ahf'-ter*) |
| ar as in far | carbon (*kar'-bon*) |
| ā-r as in air | aerosol (*ā'-rō-sol*) |
| aw as in fall | audiometer (*aw-dē-om'-et-er*) |
| e as in get | electric (*e-lek'-trik*) |
| ē as in been | ether (*ē'-ther*) |
| ē-r as in ear | sclera (*sklē'-ra*) |
| i as in bit | nicotinic (*ni-kō-tin'-ik*) |
| ī as in bite | eye (*ī*), hydro- (*hī-drō*) |
| o as in hop | optics (*op'-tiks*) |
| ō as in hope | isotopes (*ī-zō-tōps*) |
| oo as in soon | croup (*kroop*) |
| or as in for | orbit (*or'-bit*) |
| ow as in how | sound (*sownd*) |
| oy as in boy | boil (*boyl*) |
| u as in cup | tongue (*tung*) |
| ū as in mute | cubit (*kū-bit*) |

| | *Consonant sound* | | *Example* |
|---|---|---|---|
| f | the sound of ph | as in phobia (*fō'-bi-ah*) |
| j | the sound of g | as in dermalgia (*der-mal'-jia*) |
| k | the sound of c | as in catalyst (*ka'-ta-list*) |
| ks | the sound of x | as in x-ray (*eks'-rā*) |

| *Consonant sound* | | | *Example* |
|---|---|---|---|
| kw | the sound of qu | as in quintan (*kwin'-tan*) |
| s | the sound of c | as in lucid (*loo'-sid*) |
| shon | the sound of tion | as in ablution (*ab-loo'-shon*) |
| zhon | the sound of sion | as in invasion (*in-vā'-zhon*) |

# DICTIONARY OF MEDICAL TERMS

## A

**āā.** An abbreviation used in prescriptions, when equal quantities of two or more substances are to be used.

**a-** or **an** (*ā* or *an*). Prefix indicating 'absence of' as in *amenorrhoea*, absence of menstruation, *anoxia*, absence of oxygen.

**ab** (*ab*). Prefix meaning from, away from, *e.g.* abnormal, contrary to the normal type.

**abalienation** (*ab-āl-yen-ā'-shon*). Mental derangement.

**abasia** (*ā-bā'-si-a*). Motor inco-ordination in walking.

**abdomen** (*ab-dō'-men*). The belly. The body cavity immediately below the thorax, bounded above by the diaphragm, below by the pelvis, behind by the lumbar vertebrae, and in front at the sides by muscular walls. It contains many important organs, including the stomach, intestines, liver, kidneys, spleen, pancreas, bladder, uterus and ovaries.

It is lined with a serous membrane called the peritoneum, which is reflected onto many of the organs in the abdomen.

**abdominal** (*ab-do-mi-nal*). Pertaining to the abdomen.

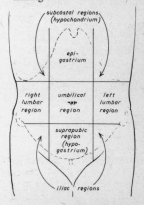

*1. Areas of the abdomen*

**abdomino-perineal** (*ab-do-mi-nō-pe-ri-nē-al*). Describes an operation with approach from both abdominal and perineal incisions.

**abducent nerves** (*ab-dū-sent nervs*). The sixth pair of cranial nerves, activating the external rectus muscle of the eyeball, which rotates the eyeball outwards.

**abduct** (*ab-dukt'*). To draw away from the mid-line.

**abduction** (*ab-duk-shon*). The act of moving a limb away from the middle line of the body.

**abductor** (*ab-duk'-ter*). A muscle which draws a limb from the median line of the body, *e.g.* deltoid.

**aberration** (*a-be-rā'-shon*). Deviation from the normal. In optics, defect in focus of a lens. *Mental a.* Mental disturbance or peculiarity.

**ablatio retinae** (*ab-lah-tē-ō re-ti-nē*). Detachment of the retina.

**ablation** (*ab-lā'-shon*). Removal or detachment of a part.

**abort** (*a-bort'*). To terminate a process before the full course is run.

**abortifacient** (*a-bor-ti-fā'-shunt*). A drug taken for the purpose of procuring abortion.

**abortion** (*a-bor'-shon*). Discharge of the gestation sac from the pregnant uterus before the fetus is viable. Abortion may be *complete* or *incomplete*; it may be *threatened* or *inevitable*, according to the cervical canal being closed or open. In *missed* abortion, the fetus is dead but not discharged immediately. In *habitual* abortion, it is thought that weakness of the muscle of the cervical canal prevents pregnancy from running to term. Also *therapeutic* abortion when there are medical or social grounds to justify it; and *criminal* and *septic* abortion.

**abortus** (*a-bor'-tus*). The aborted fetus.

**abortus fever** (*a-bor'-tus fē-ver*). *See* BRUCELLOSIS.

**abrasion** (*a-brā-zhon*). A superficial injury to the skin or mucous membrane.

**abreaction** (*ab-rē-ak'-shon*). A state of mind brought about during the process of psycho-analysis. The patient lives again through past painful experiences which may unconsciously be causing the neurosis. *See also* NARCO-ANALYSIS.

**abscess**(*ab'-ses*). A collection of pus in a cavity, the result of inflammation. *Alveolar a.* One which develops in the socket of a tooth. *Blind a.* One with no external opening. *Cold a.* One which develops slowly, without inflammation, as in tuberculosis. *Ischiorectal a*. One in the ischiorectal fossa. *Metastatic a*. Secondary to an abscess elsewhere: caused by an infected embolus. *Milk a*. One in the breast when it is secreting milk. *Pelvic a*. Arises in the pelvic peritoneum, esp. recto-uterine pouch. *Psoas a*. One due to disease of the vertebrae. The pus descends in the sheath of the psoas muscle, forming a fluctuating tumour above or below Poupart's ligament. It is sometimes tuberculous in origin. *Residual a*. One developing in old inflammatory products. *Stitch a*. One formed around a stitch or suture. *Subphrenic a*. One which develops beneath the diaphragm, esp. after peritonitis.

**absolute values** (*ab-so-lūt va'-lūs*). Actual figures, not the percentage figures, *e.g.* in blood counts, the actual numbers of cells counted.

**absorbent** (*ab-sor-bent*). Taking up by suction. Gauze and wool are absorbent dressings.

**acantholysis** (*ak-an-tho'li-sis*). Process of individual cell keratinization occurring in blistering diseases. *A. cell* is one that has undergone individual cell keratinization.

**acanthosis** (*ak-an-thō'-sis*). Thickening of the epidermis. *A. nigricans*. Pigmented warty outgrowths of epidermis.

**acapnia** (*ā-kap'-ni-a*). A lessened amount of carbon dioxide in the blood.

**acardia** (*ā-kar'-di-a*). Congenital absence of the heart.

**Acarus** (*ak'-a-rus*). The name of a group of animal parasites. *A. scabiei* is the parasite causing scabies.

**acatalasia** (*ā-ka-ta-lā'-si-a*). Genetic abnormality in which the enzyme catalase is absent from the red blood cells.

**acatalepsy** (*ā-ka-ta-lep'-si*). Uncertainty, lack of understanding.

**acataphasia** (*a-kat-a-fā'-zi-a*). Difficulty in expressing ideas in logical sequence.

**accessory nerves** (*ak-se-so-ri nervs*). The eleventh pair of cranial nerves. Developmentally a branch of the vagus.

**accidental haemorrhage** (*ak-si-den'-tal hem-o-rāj*). Bleeding from the pregnant uterus in the later months of pregnancy due to premature separation of normally situated placenta. It may be *concealed*, when the bleeding remains internal; or *external*, when the blood escapes by the vagina. *See* ANTEPARTUM HAEMORRHAGE.

**accommodation** (*a-ko-mo-dā'-shon*). The process of altering the focus of the eye by changing the curvature of the lens. When focussing on near objects, the lens becomes more convex by contraction of the ciliary muscles.

**accouchement** (*ak-koosh-mon*). Childbirth.

**accretion** (*ak-krē-shon*). Accumulation of foreign matter.

**acephalic** (*ā'-se-fa'-lik*). Headless.

**acetabuloplasty** (*a-sē-tab-ū-lō-pla'-sti*). A plastic operation performed on the hip joint for osteoarthritis.

**acetabulum** (*a-sē-ta'-bū-lum*). The cuplike socket in the hip or innominate bone into which the head of the femur fits.

**acetic acid** (*a-sē-tik*). The acid contained in vinegar. It is used in testing urine for albumin.

**aceto-acetic acid** (*as-sē-tō-a-sē-tik*). Produced at an intermediate stage of fatty acid oxidation. If metabolism is disturbed, as in diabetes mellitus, it is found in excess in the blood and the urine. *Syn.* diacetic acid.

**acetonaemia** (*as'-sē-tō-nē-mi-a*). The presence of acetone in the blood.

**acetone** (*as'-se'-tōn*). A colourless volatile solvent. This substance is formed in the body when metabolism is upset, as in starvation, excessive vomiting, diabetes mellitus. It is excreted in the urine and the breath.

**acetonuria** (*as'-sē-tō-nū-ri-a*). The presence of acetone in the urine.

**acetylcholine** (*a-sē-til-kō'-lēn*). A chemical substance causing parasympathetic effects, *e.g.* cardiac slowing, dilatation of surface blood vessels and contractions of the gut.

**achalasia** (*a-ka-lā'-zi-a*). Failure to relax. Usually *A. of the cardia* when there is a disorder of motor function of the oesophagus and a failure of the cardiac orifice of the stomach to relax.

**Achilles tendon** (*a-kil-lēz ten'-den*). The large tendon which attaches the calf muscles to the heel.

**achillorrhaphy** (*a-ki-lo-ra-fi*). Surgery to rejoin the Achilles tendon after rupture.

**achlorhydria** (*ā-klor-hī'-dri-a*). Absence of hydrochloric acid in the gastric juice; may occur in pernicious anaemia and cancer of the stomach.

**acholia** (*ā-ko'-li-a*). Absence of bile.

**acholuria** (*a-ko-lū-ri-a*). The absence of bile pigment from the urine.

**acholuric jaundice** (*a-ko-lū'-rik*). *See* JAUNDICE

**achondroplasia** (*a-kon'-drŏ-plā-zi-a*). A form of arrested development of the long bones, leading to dwarfism.

**achromasia** (*a-krŏ-mā'-zi-a*). Absence of colour. Extreme pallor associated with severe illness.

**achromatopsia** (*a-krŏ-ma-top'-si-a*). Colour blindness.

**achylia** (*a-kī-li-a*). Absence of chyle. Usually *gastric a.* when an abnormally small amount of gastric juice is secreted.

**acid** (*as'-sid*). A substance capable of combining with alkalis to form salts. Acids turn blue litmus paper red and when in liquid form have a sour taste, *e.g.* vinegar and lemon juice both contain acids. (For individual acids *see under* special name.)

**acidaemia** (*a-si-dē'-mi-a*). Abnormally acid blood, *i.e.* pH is below 7·3. Normal blood pH is 7·3 to 7·5.

**acid-base balance** (*a'-sid-bās ba'-lans*). Balance between acidic and basic components which determines the pH of the body fluids.

**acid-fast.** In bacteriology a term applied to certain bacteria which retain the red carbo-fuchsin stain after the appli-

cation of an acid solution. Other organisms are decolorized. Tubercle bacilli are 'acid-fast'.

**acidity** (*as-si'-di-tē*). The proportion of acid in a given substance. Thus gastric juice contains normally 0·2 per cent of hydrochloric acid.

**acidosis** (*a-si-dŏ'-sis*). A condition which tends to lower the pH of body fluids. Acidosis is generally classified as respiratory or metabolic. Metabolism of the central nervous system may be disturbed.

**acid phosphatase** (*a-sid fos-fa-tāz*). Phosphatases are enzymes which are able to split off phosphate groups from certain substances. The prefix 'acid' indicates that the enzyme is optimally active in acid solution, *cf.* alkaline phosphatase. Acid phosphatase is present in lysosomes in all cells. The prostate gland is the source of most of the acid phosphatase in the serum.

**acinus** (*a-sē-nus*) (pl. **acini** (*a-sē-nē*)). A minute grape-like structure whose cells secrete; as in the breast. *See also* ALVEOLUS.

**acme** (*ak'-mē*). The highest point attained; the crisis.

**acne** (*ak'-nē*). Condition, occurring particularly among adolescents, resulting from hormonally induced hyperactivity of the sebaceous glands, and characterized by blackheads and pustules. Occurs commonly on the face, neck, back and chest.

**acoustic** (*ak-koo'-stik*). Relating to sound or hearing.

**acquired** (*ak-wī-rd*). Contracted after birth, not congenital.

**acrid** (*ak'-rid*). Sharp, burning.

**acriflavine** (*ak-ri-flā'-vin*). Antiseptic yellow dye.

**acrocentric** (*ak-rō-sen'-trik*). Of chromosomes, having the centromere near to one end.

**acrocephaly** (*ak-ro-ke'-fa-li*). Congenitally malformed, cone-shaped head.

**acrocyanosis** (*ak'-rō-sī-a-nō-sis*). Cyanosis of the extremities.

**acromegaly** (*ak-rō-meg'-a-li*). A disease marked by enlargement of the face, hands and feet, due to a pathological condition of the pituitary gland.

**acromion** (*ā-krō'-mi-on*). The outward extremity of the spine of the scapula. *See* SCAPULA.

**acronyx** (*ak'-rō-niks*). An ingrowing nail.

**acroparaesthesia** (*ak-rō-pa-res-thē'-zi-a*). Numbness and tingling sensation of the extremities.

**acrophobia** (*ak-rō-fō'-bi-a*). Fear of being at a height.

**acrosclerosis** (*ak'-rō-skle-rō'-sis*). Scleroderma affecting the hands. Associated with Raynaud's phenomenon.

**acrosome** (*ak-rō-sōm*). Part of the head of sperm cells; believed to help penetration of the ovum.

**ACTH.** Adrenocorticotrophic hormone produced by the anterior lobe of the pituitary. It stimulates the release of steroid hormones from the adrenal cortex.

**actinism** (*ak'-ti'nizm*). Chemical changes produced by radiant energy, *e.g.* light rays.

**actinodermatitis** (*ak-ti-nō-der-ma-tī'-tis*). Inflammation of the skin resulting from exposure to radiant energy, esp. sunlight. The term usually implies hypersensitivity of the skin.

**Actinomyces** (*ak-tī-nō-mī'-sēz*). Group of filamentous bacteria.

**actinomycosis** (*ak-tī-nō-mī-kō'-sis*). Disease due to Actinomyces usually presenting as chronic discharging abscesses which may be localized, classically on the neck, or widespread in the body.

**action potential** (*ak-shon pō-ten'-shal*). Term applied to electrical changes which occur when a nerve conducts an impulse or when a muscle fibre contracts.

**activator** (*ak-ti-vā'-tor*). A physical or chemical agent which initiates some reaction in which the activator itself does not take part.

**active assisted movements.** Active movements aided by the physiotherapist or by mechanical devices.

**active movements.** A term used by physiotherapists to denote a movement done by the patient.

**active principle.** The substance in a drug which gives it a therapeutic effect.

**actomyosin** (*ak-tō-mī-ō'-sin*). Muscle protein complex composed of actin and myosin. The myosin component acts as an enzyme releasing energy by the breakdown to ATP.

**acuity** (*a-kū-i-ti*). Sharpness and clearness.

**acupuncture** (*a-kū-pungk-cher*). Skin puncture with fine metal needles. Used mainly by the Chinese for producing anaesthesia.

**acute** (*ak-yoot'*). Rapid; severe. *A. abdomen.* General term embracing surgical emergencies resulting from disease or damage of abdominal viscera, *e.g.* appendicitis.

**acystia** (*a-sis'-ti-a*). Congenital absence of the bladder.

**adactylia** (*ā-dak-til'-i-a*). Absence of fingers or toes.

**Adam's apple** (*a'-damz a'-pl*). Laryngeal prominence due to thyroid cartilage.

**Adams-Stokes syndrome** (*sin'-drōm*). See STOKES-ADAMS.

**adaptation** (*a-dap-tā'-shon*). (1) Adjustment by structural or functional change to new circumstances. (2) The process whereby the eye adjusts to sudden changes from light to dark and vice versa.

**addiction** (*ad-dik'-shon*). State of physical and mental dependence on one or more of many substances including alcohol, a variety of drugs, cigarettes or sweet foods.

**Addis count** (*ad-dis kownt*). Number of red blood cells in the urine. Expressed as cells found per 24 hours.

**Addison's** or **Addisonian anaemia.** See PERNICIOUS ANAEMIA.

**Addison's disease.** Syndrome, due to adrenal cortical insufficiency, characterized by wasting, hypotension, vomiting, malaise, weakness and hyperpigmentation of the skin and buccal mucosa.

**adduct** (*ad-dukt*). To draw towards the mid-line.

**adduction** (*ad-duk'-shon*). The act of moving a limb towards the mid-line of the body.

**adductor** (*ad-duk'-ter*). A muscle which draws towards the mid-line of the body, *e.g. A. muscles* of the thigh draw the legs together.

**adendritic** (*ā-den-dri'-tik*). Without dendrites.

**adenectomy** (*ad-en-ek'-to-mi*). Excision of a gland.

**adenine** (*a-de-nēn*). An amino purine base; one of two in both RNA and DNA.

**adenine flavine dinucleotide** (*a-den-ēn flā-vin dī-nū-kli-ō-tīd*). A co-factor in the electron transport system associated with the biochemical pathways of respiration.

**adenitis** (*a-de-nī'-tis*). Inflammation of a gland.

**adenocarcinoma** (*a-de-nō-kar-si-nō'-ma*). Malignant growth of glandular cells.

**adenoid** (*a'-de-noyd*). Lymphoid tissue, in the nasopharynx, which when swollen hinders breathing.

**adenoidectomy** (*a'-de-noy-dek'-to-mi*). Operation to remove adenoids.

**adenoma** (*a-de-nō'-ma*). Benign tumour of glandular cells.

**adenomyoma** (*a-de-nō-mī-ō'-ma*). Benign tumour composed of glandular and muscular elements.

**adenomyosis** (*a-de-nō-mī-ō'-sis*). Presence of adenomyomata in smooth muscle.

**adenopathy** (*a-de-no'-pa-thi*). A disease of a gland, especially a lymphatic gland.

**adenosine** (*a-de-nō-sēn*). An important member of the group of substances known as nucleosides, the phosphorylated derivatives of which are the key to energy reactions in the body.

**adenosine diphosphate** (*a-den-ō-sēn dī-fos'-fāt*). ADP. Resulting from the removal of phosphate from ATP and is re-formed into ATP by respiratory metabolism, thus making the energy available for work in the cell.

**adenosine monophosphate** (*a-den'-ō-sēn mo-nō-fos'-fāt*). AMP. Metabolically related to other adenosine phosphates. In its cyclic form (cAMP) exerts an important controlling influence on cellular physiology.

**adenosine triphosphate** (*a-den-ō-sēn trī-fos'-fāt*). ATP. A coenzyme of a large number of reactions. One of the phosphate groups is readily released by enzyme action resulting in the simultaneous liberation of utilizable energy.

**adenovirus** (*a-den-ō-vīr'-us*). A group of viruses affecting particularly the adenoids, pharynx and conjunctivae; usually associated with minor respiratory infections.

**ADH.** *See* ANTIDIURETIC HORMONE.

**adherent** (*ad-hār'-ent*). Fixed firmly to.

**adhesion** (*ad-hē'-zhon*). A sticking together of two surfaces or parts. Bands of fibrous tissue, usually the result of inflammation.

**adiaphoresis** (*a-dī-a-fo-rē-sis*). Deficiency of perspiration.

**Adie's syndrome** (*a-diz sin'-drōm*). Association of myotonic pupil with absent or diminished tendon reflexes.

**adipose** (*a'-di-pōz*). Fatty.

**aditus** (*a'-di-tus*). An entrance. A portal. *A. ad antrum* is the narrow passage between the mastoid antrum and the tympanic cavity of the ear.

**adjustment** (*ad-just-ment*). The change made by a person to adapt to circumstances.

**adjuvant** (*ad-jū'-vant*). A secondary ingredient in a preparation aiding the action of the principal drug.

**adnexa** (*ad-nek'-sa*). Appendages. Usually applied to the uterine appendages.

**adolescence** (*a-dō-les'-sens*). The period of development during which full anatomical, physiological and emotional maturity is attained.

**ADP.** *See* ADENOSINE DIPHOSPHATE.

**adrenal cortex** (*a-drē'-nal korteks*). Outer part of the adrenal gland which synthesizes and secretes the steroid hormones. Those of major importance are *glucocorticoids*, *e.g.* hydrocortisone, which tend to produce the conversion of tissue protein to glucose; *mineralocorticoids*, esp. aldosterone, regulating sodium and potassium excretion and *androgens*.

**adrenal glands** (*a-drē'-nal glans*). A pair of endocrine glands, also called suprarenal glands, situated adjacent to the upper pole of each kidney. They consist of two regions, the cortex and the medulla.

**adrenal insufficiency.** Usually adrenocortical insufficiency. *See* ADDISON'S DISEASE.

**adrenal medulla** (*a-drē'-nal me-du'-la*). Central part of adrenal gland which synthesizes and secretes adrenaline and noradrenaline.

**adrenal nerves** (*a-drē'-nal nervs*). Cholinergic, preganglionic sympathetic nerve fibres supplying the adrenal medulla. Stimulation causes the release of adrenaline into the circulation.

**adrenalectomy** (*a-drē-na-lek'-to-mi*). The removal of one or both adrenal glands.

**adrenaline** (*a-drē-na-lin*). Epinephrine. Hormone secreted by the adrenal medulla. Similar substance secreted at nerve endings of sympathetic nerves. Effects produced include increased heart rate, blood pressure and blood sugar, contraction of skin blood vessels, increase in muscle blood flow, dilatation of pupil, etc.

**adrenergic** (*a-drē-ner-jik*). Term applied to identify motor nerves by their transmitter substance, thus *cholinergic*, when the impulse is transmitted by acetylcholine and *adrenergic* when the impulse is transmitted by adrenaline, noradrenaline or a drug with comparable action.

**adrenocortical steroids** (*ā-drē-nō-kor'-ti-kal ste-royds*). See ADRENAL CORTEX.

**adrenocorticotrophic hormone** (*a-drē-nō-kor-ti-kō-trō-fik hor-mōn*). See ACTH.

**adrenogenital syndrome** (*a-drē-nō-je'-ni-tal sin'-drōm*).

Virilization occurring in women due to excessive secretion of androgens, usually as a result of hyperplasia or adenoma of the adrenal cortex. Rarely the syndrome is due to arrhenoblastoma or pituitary disorder.

**adrenolytic** (*a-drē-no-li-tik*). Substance antagonizing the action of adrenaline.

**adsorbent** (*ad-sor'-bent*). Substance causing adsorption.

**adsorption** (*ad-sorp'-shon*). The property possessed by certain porous substances, *e.g.* charcoal, of taking up other substances.

**adulteration** (*a-dul-te-rā'-shon*). Addition to any substance of a component not normally present; the original substance which may be a food or drug being made of less value.

**advancement** (*ad-vans-ment*). Operation to move a tendinous insertion forwards. Can be used in curing a squint.

**adventitia** (*ad-ven-ti-sha*). The outer coat of any organ including a blood vessel.

**Aëdes aegypti** (*a-ē-dās ā-jip'-tē*). Species of mosquito transmitting yellow fever, etc.

**aeration** (*ā-rā-shon*). Charging with air or gas.

**aerobes** (*ā-rōbs*). Term applied to bacteria requiring oxygen for respiration, *cf.* anaerobes.

**aerobic respiration** (*a-rō-bik res-pi-rā-shon*). Respiration in the presence of free oxygen.

**aerocele** (*ā-rō-sel*). A diverticulum of larynx, trachea or bronchus.

**aerodontalgia** (*ā-ō-don-tal'-ji-a*). Toothache induced by reduction of atmospheric pressure.

**aerogen** (*ā'-rō-jen*). Any gas-producing bacterium, *e.g. Clostridium welchii*, the cause of gas gangrene.

**aerophagy** (*ā-ro-fa-ji*). Excessive air swallowing.

**aerosol** (*ā'-rō-sol*). Finely atomized solution ejected under pressure.

**aesthesia** (*es-thē'-zi-a*). Feeling.

**aetiology** (*ē-tē-o'-lo-ji*). The study of the causation of disease.

**afebrile** (*ā-feb'-ril*). Without fever.

**affect** (*a-fekt*). Term used in pyschology for an emotion associated with ideas.

**affective disorders.** Group of psychiatric illnesses primarily due to reaction to internal or external stress. They include anxiety states, depression, mania and hypomania.

**afferent** (*af'-fer-ent*). Leading to the centre, applied to the lymphatic vessels and to sensory nerves.

**afferent loop syndrome** (*af'-fer-ent loop sin'-drōm*). Occasional complication of one type of partial gastrectomy.

**affiliation** (*a-fi-lē-ā'-shon*). The fixing of paternity of an illegitimate child on the putative father.

**affinity** (*af-fi'-ni-ti*). Attraction. In chemistry the property of an element which prefers to combine with some other particular element.

**afibrinogenaemia** (*ā-fī-bri-nō-je-nē-mi-a*). Also called hypofibrinogenaemia. May be found in obstetrics if thromboplastins are absorbed into the bloodstream from the damaged placenta or retained blood clot. The clotting mechanism of the blood is impaired and there may be uncontrollable haemorrhage.

**aflatoxins** (*a-fla-tok'-sinz*). Toxins present in spores of *Aspergillus flavus*, a contaminant of ground-nut meal.

**African tick fever.** Disease caused by a spirochaete, *S. duttoni*, transmitted by ticks. Occasionally also applied to typhus transmitted by these insects.

**afterbirth** (*ahf'-ter-berth*). The

placenta, cord and membranes as expelled after delivery of the infant.

**after-care** (*ahf'-ter-kār*). Care of the convalescent, including rehabilitation.

**after image** (*ahf'-ter i-māj*). A retinal impression persisting although the stimulus of light has ceased.

**after-pains** (*ahf'-ter pānz*). Pains from uterine contractions following labour.

**agammaglobulinaemia** (*ā-ga-ma-glo-bū-li-nē'-mi-a*). Absence or deficiency of gammaglobulin in plasma proteins, leading to inadequate response to infection. May be congenital or acquired.

**agar-agar** (*ā-gar-ā-gar*). Polysaccharide obtained from seaweed, used in the culture of micro-organisms.

**agenesis** (*ā-je'-ne-sis*). Failure to develop.

**agglutination** (*ag-gloo-ti-nā'-shon*). The sticking together of cells, *e.g.* red blood cells, bacteria, due to an alteration of surface charge. Usually brought about by the effect of antibodies.

**agglutinins** (*ag-gloo'-ti-nins*). Antibodies such as those found in the blood serum of persons suffering from typhoid or paratyphoid fever. They have the property of

causing bacteria to clump together or 'agglutinate'. *See* WIDAL REACTION.

**agglutinogen** (*ag-loo-ti'-nō-jen*). Factor promoting the mutual adhesion of cells.

**aggregate** (*ag-gre-gāt*). To group together.

**aggression** (*ag-gre'-shon*). A hostile attitude which may be a normal reaction to danger or a compensatory reaction to cover feelings of inferiority or frustration.

**aglutition** (*ā-glū-ti-shun*). Inability to swallow.

**agnosia** (*ag-nō-zi-a*). A disturbance in the recognition of sensory impression.

**agonist** (*a'-go-nist*). In pharmacology, substance with positive action on system.

**agoraphobia** (*a'-go-ra-fō-bi-a*). Literally a fear of the market place. In practice may mean a fear of open places.

**agranulocytosis** (*ā-gran-ū-lō-sī-tō'-sis*). Absence or marked reduction in the blood of the polymorphonuclear cells. May be caused by drugs such as the sulphonamides or irradiation of the bone marrow.

**agraphia** (*ā-gra'-fi-a*). Loss of the power to express words and ideas in writing.

**ague** (*ā-gū*). *See* MALARIA.

**AHG.** Antihaemophilic globulin. The blood-coagulating

protein factor which is deficient in haemophiliacs. *See* BLOOD COAGULATION.

**AID.** Artificial insemination by a donor.

**AIH.** Artificial insemination by a woman's legal husband.

**air** (*ār*). *See* ATMOSPHERE. *A. bed.* A mattress made of some distensible material such as rubber or plastic and filled with air. *A., tidal.* The air breathed in and out in ordinary breathing.

**air embolism.** Embolism caused by air entering the circulatory system.

**air-encephalography** (*ār-en-ke-fa-lo'-gra-fi*). Radiography of brain after introduction of air into the subarachnoid space.

**air hunger.** Respiratory distress caused by lack of oxygen.

**akathisia** (*ā-ka-thi'-si-a*). Mental state characterized by subjective feelings of unrest and outwardly by agitation and over-activity.

**akinesis** (*ā-kī-nē'-sis*). Loss or imperfection of movement.

**ala** (*ā-la*). A wing. *A. nasi.* The outer side of the external nostril.

**Albee's operation** (*al-bēz*). The hip joint is ankylosed by a plastic operation.

**Albers-Schönberg's disease** (*al-bers-shern-bārgs*). Also known as osteopetrosis or marble-bone disease because of great increase in bone density seen radiographically. There are three types, fetal, juvenile and adult.

**Albert's stain** (*al'-berts stān*). Microscopic stain showing granular structure of diphtheria.

**albinism** (*al-bin-ism*). Syndrome due to defective pigment production, resulting in deficiency of pigment in the skin, hair and eyes.

**albino** (*al-bē-nō*). A person with albinism.

**Albright's syndrome** (*al-brīts sin'-drōm*). Polyostotic fibrous dysplasia of bone. Syndrome characterized by abnormal development of bone, hyper-pigmentation of the skin and in girls, precocious sexual development.

**albumin** (*al-bū'-min*). Serum protein with relatively low molecular weight (MW = 70,000) which is of great importance in controlling the water exchanges between the blood and the tissue fluids.

**albuminuria** (*al-bū-mi-nū'-ri-a*). Albumin in the urine; occurs in diseases of the kidneys.

**alcohol** (*al-ko-hol*). Chemically the hydroxides of a great number of organic radicals are known as alcohols: the term usually refers to ethyl alcohol, the alcohol present in intoxicating drinks. *Absolute a.* May contain up to 1 per cent by weight of water. Rectified spirit is 90 per cent alcohol.

**alcoholism** (*al'-kō-hol-izm*). Physical and psychological dependence on alcohol usually preceded by a varying period of excessive drinking.

**aldolase** (*al'-dō-lāz*). Enzyme in muscle concerned in conversion of glycogen to lactic acid.

**aldosterone** (*al-dos'-ter-ōn*). One of the adrenocortical hormones which regulates metabolism of electrolytes.

**Aldrich syndrome** (*awl'-drich sin'-drōm*). Sex-linked recessive condition occurring in male infants with eczema, thrombocytopenia, recurrent infections, usually fatal.

**alexia** (*a-lek'-si-a*). Inability or difficulty in understanding the written or printed word, owing to a lesion of the brain. *See* DYSLEXIA.

**algae** (*al-jē*). Seaweeds, etc. A group of Thallophyta containing chlorophyll.

**algesia** (*al-jē-si-a*). Perception of pain.

**algogenic** (*aj-gō-jen'-ik*). Pain-inducing.

**alignment** (*a-līn'-ment*). Bringing into line.

**alimentary** (*a-limen'-ta-ri*). Pertaining to the absorption of nourishment. The *a. canal* is the whole digestive tract, extending from the mouth to the anus.

**alimentation** (*a-li-men-tā'-shon*). Nourishment.

**aliquot** (*a'-li-kwot*). A measured portion.

**alkalaemia** (*al-ka-lē'-mi-a*). Abnormally alkaline blood with a pH above 7·5.

**alkali** (*al'-ka-lī*). A substance which combines with an acid to form a salt, and with a fat to form a soap. Turns red litmus paper to blue. Ammonia, soda and potash are examples of alkalis. *A. reserve.* This term is applied to the measurement of plasma bicarbonate concentration.

**alkaline** (*al'-ka-līn*). Containing alkali. Strictly, fluid with a pH greater than 7·0.

**alkaline phosphatase** (*al-ka-lin fos-fa-tāz*). Enzyme(s), capable of splitting off phosphate groups from certain substrates, esp. active in alkaline solution, *cf.* acid phosphatase.

**alkalinity** (*al-ka-li'-ni-ti*). Proportion of alkali in a given substance.

**alkaloid** (*al'-ka-loyd*). An organic substance having some properties of an alkali, esp. that of combining with an acid to form a salt. Morphine and quinine are alkaloids. Salts of these are morphine tartrate, morphine hydrochloride, quinine sulphate, etc.

**alkalosis** (*al-ka-lō'-sis*). Circumstances tending to raise the pH of body fluids.

**alkaptonuria** (*al-kap-tō-nū'-ri-a*). Genetically determined defect of metabolism in which homogentisic acid is excreted in the urine which turns dark on standing.

**alkylating agent** (*al'-ki-lā-ting ā'-jent*). Substance causing addition of an alkyl group into an organic compound.

**all or none law.** Physiological law regarding irritable tissues, *e.g.* nerves, by which there are only two possible reactions to a stimulus, either no reaction or full response. There is no grading of response according to the strength of the stimulus.

**allantois** (*al-lan'-tō-is*). Saclike outgrowth from hindgut of embryo.

**allele** (*a-lēl*). *See* ALLELOMORPH.

**allelomorph** (*al-lē-lō-morf*). Pair of genes which occupy the same relative position on homologous chromosomes and produce different effects on the same process in development.

**allergen** (*a'-ler-jen*). Substance which causes sensitization of tissues. Usually has a protein component.

**allergy** (*a'-ler-ji*). State of abnormal tissue sensitivity to a chemical substance(s). The mechanism of sensitization is complex and involves prior contact of the allergic cells with the allergen. The release of histamine from mast cells plays a part in the reaction.

**allo-antibody** (*a-lō-an'-ti-bo-di*). Antibody which reacts with allo-antigen.

**allo-antigen** (*a-lō-an'-ti-jen*). Antigen possessed by certain members of a species.

**allograft** (*a'-lō-grahft*). Graft in which both the donor and recipient are of the same species.

**allopathy** (*a-lo'-pa-thi*). Treatment of disease by medicines that produce phenomena different from those of the disease treated. *cf.* homeopathy.

**alloplasty** (*a-lō-plas'-ti*). Surgical grafts to parts of body by foreign material.

**alloy** (*al'-loy*). A mixture of two or more metals obtained by fusing them together.

**alopecia** (*a-lō-pē'-si-a*). Absence of hair, baldness.

**alpha rays** (*al-fah rās*). Nuclear radiation consisting of two

protons and two neutrons.
Will penetrate only a few
millimetres into tissue.

**Alport's syndrome** (*awl'-pawts
sin'-drōm*). Familial deafness
associated with albuminuria
and nephritis. Fatal in early
life.

**alternating current** (*orl'-ter-nā-
ting ku-rent*). Electrical current the polarity of which is
phasically reversed.

**altitude sickness** (*al-ti-tūd sik-
nes*). Malaise due to hypoxia
resulting from decrease in
partial pressure of oxygen in
atmosphere at high altitudes.

**alveolus** (*al-vē-ō-lus*). (pl.
**alveoli**). (1) The socket of a
tooth. (2) An air cell in the
lung. (3) A secreting unit of
the breast.

**Alzheimer's disease** (*alz'-hī-
mer*). Degeneration of the
cerebral cortex. Loss of
memory, aphasia and para-
lysis occur.

**amalgam** (*a-mal-gam*). An
alloy of mercury and other
metals. *Dental a.* is of silver,
tin and mercury. Used for
filling teeth.

**amastia** (*ā-mas'-ti-a*). Absence
of breasts.

**amaurosis** (*am-aw-rō'-sis*).
Blindness from disease or
defect of the nervous system
of the eye.

**amaurotic familial idiocy** (*ā-
maw-ro'-tik*). Also known as

Tay-Sach's disease; is an
inherited inborn error of
metabolism causing degen-
eration of the nervous
system.

**ambidextrous** (*am-bi-dek'-
strus*). Equally skilful with
each hand.

**ambivalence** (*am-bi-va-lens*).
Contrary emotions, such as
love and hate, are experienced towards the same
objects or person.

**Amblyomma** (*am-blē-om'-a*). A
genus of ticks, several species
of which are carriers of
rickettsial disease.

**amblyopia** (*am-bli-ō'-pi-a*).
Indistinct vision; approach-
ing blindness.

**ambulance** (*am-bū-lanz*). A
vehicle for the conveyance of
sick and wounded.

**ambulant** (*am-bū-lant*). Able to
walk.

**ambulatory** (*am'-bū-lā-to-ri*).
Relating to walking; moving
about. *A. treatment of fractures.* Enables the patient to
remain up and at work. The
limb is immobilized in plaster
of Paris.

**amelioration** (*a-mēl-i-o-rā'-
shon*). General improvement
in the condition of the
patient.

**amenorrhoea** (*a-men-o-rē'-a*).
Absence of menstruation. In
*primary a.,* menstruation has
never been established.

*Secondary a.* occurs after menstruation has commenced. There is amenorrhoea in pregnancy, and it may occur in certain endocrine disorders, anaemia, etc.

**amentia** (*ā-men'-shi-a*). Absence of intellect; idiocy.

**ametria** (*ā-mē'-tri-a*). Congenital absence of the uterus.

**ametropia** (*a-me-trō'-pi-a*). Defective vision due to abnormal form or refractive power of the eye.

**amine oxidase.** An enzyme which oxidizes amines, *e.g.* adrenaline, with the liberation of ammonia.

**amino-acid** (*a-mī'-nō-a'-sid*). Organic compound containing both basic amino ($-NH_2$) and acidic carboxyl ($-COOH$) groups. Fundamental units in the structure of proteins. Twenty different amino-acids are commonly found in proteins; eight of these cannot be synthesized in the body and must, as with vitamins, be obtained from food. These are known as *essential* amino-acids.

**amino-aciduria** (*a-mī-nō-a-si-dū'-ri-a*). Presence of excessive amounts of amino-acids in the urine.

**amitosis** (*a-mi-tō'-sis*). Type of direct cell division without prior reduplication of

chromosomes. It is said to take place in cartilage.

**amnesia** (*am-nē'-si-a*). Loss of memory. *Anterograde a.* Inability to remember recent events. *Retrograde a.* Symptom of concussion. The patient cannot remember what happened immediately before the accident.

**amniocentesis** (*am'-nē-ō-sen-tē'-sis*). Aspiration of fluid from the amniotic cavity on which tests may be done to detect an abnormal fetus.

**amniography** (*am-nē-o'-gra-fi*). Radiographic demonstration of amniotic sac by injection of radio-opaque dye.

**amnion** (*am'-nē-on*). The sac directly encircling the fetus in utero.

**amniotic fluid** (*am-nē-o-tik floo-id*). Fluid environment for embryo which probably cushions the embryo from distortion and trauma.

**amoeba** (*a-mē'-ba*). A microscopic unicellular animal, one variety of which causes amoebic dysentery.

**amoebiasis** (*a-mē-bī'-a-sis*). Infection by pathogenic amoebae. Complications include abscesses, cysts and amoeboma.

**amoebicide** (*a-mē'-bi-sīd*). Substance lethal to amoebae.

**amoeboma** (*a-mē-bō-ma*). Amoebic granuloma which

may occur in the large intestine.

**amorphous** (*ā-mor-fus*). Formless.

**AMP.** *See* ADENOSINE MONOPHOSPHATE.

**ampère** (*ahm-pār*). Unit measure of electric current.

**amphiarthrosis** (*am-fi-ah-thrō'-sis*). A slightly movable joint, *e.g.* the articulations of the spine.

**amphoteric** (*am-fo-te'-rik*). Substance with acidic and basic groupings capable of acting both as an acid or a base.

**ampoule** (*am'-pūl*). A sealed phial containing a drug or solution sterilized ready for use.

**ampulla** (*am-pū-la*). A flask-shaped dilation esp. of a duct, *e.g. a. of Vater*, a dilation of the common bile duct just before it opens into the duodenum.

**amputation** (*am-pū-tā'-shon*). The removal of a limb or organ. It is termed primary if performed immediately after the injury; secondary if performed later.

**amylase** (*a-mi-lāz*). Group of enzymes which split complex sugars, *e.g.* starch, glycogen, to disaccharides such as maltose. Present in saliva and pancreatic juice.

**amyloidosis** (*a-mi-loy-dō'-sis*). Lardaceous disease. Characterized by deposition of globulin-like material in liver, spleen, kidneys, skin, etc. Classified as primary (cause unknown) and secondary when it follows long-standing infection.

**amylopectinosis** (*a'-mi-lō-pek-ti-nō'-sis*). Condition in which the polysaccharide amylopectin is deposited in the tissues, causing death from liver failure at an early age.

**amyoplasia congenita** (*ā-mī-ō-plā-si-a kon-je'-ni-ta*). Congenital muscular dystrophy leading to rigidity of joints.

**amyotonia** (*ā-mī-o-tō-ni-a*). A form of muscular feebleness or paralysis, often congenital.

**amyotrophic lateral sclerosis** (*a-mī-o-trō'-fik la-te-ral skle-rō'-sis*). A syndrome comprising progressive muscular atrophy with upper motor neurone involvement. The clinical picture is variable according to the stage of the disease.

**ana.** Used in prescriptions to mean so much of each. *Syn.* aa.

**anabolism** (*a-na-bo-lism*). Synthesis, by living organisms, of complex molecules from simpler ones, *cf.* catabolism.

**anacrotic** (*a-na-kro'-tik*). Refers to ascending limb

(Greek 'upstroke') of tracing of pulse wave.

**anaemia** (*a-nē'-mi-a*). Diminished oxygen-carrying capacity of the blood, due to a reduction in the numbers of red cells or in their content of haemoglobin, or both. The cause may be inadequate production of red cells or excessive loss of blood.

**anaerobe** (*an-ār-ōb*). Any micro-organism that can live and multiply in the absence of free oxygen, *e.g.* tetanus.

**anaerobic metabolism** (*a-nār-ō-bik me-ta-bo-lism*). Respiratory metabolism not involving consumption of oxygen, *cf.* aerobic respiration.

**anaesthesia** (*a-nes-thē-zi-a*). Absence of sensation; loss of feeling. *Basal a.* Partial general anaesthesia obtained by a drug such as morphine given before an inhalation anaesthetic. *Dissociated a.* Loss of sensation to pain and temperature, sense of touch being retained. *General a.* This gives loss of consciousness. *Glove a.* Loss of feeling in the area of the hand a glove covers. *Intravenous a.* A general anaesthesia produced by intravenous injection. *Local a.* Anaesthesia of a certain area only. *Nerve block a.* Local anaesthesia produced by injecting an anaesthetic near a sensory nerve. *Rectal a.* General anaesthesia by administering an anaesthetic rectally. *Refrigeration a.* Anaesthesia produced by intense cold. *Spinal a.* An anaesthetic is injected into the subarachnoid space of the spinal cord producing anaesthesia in the lower part of the body.

**anaesthetic** (*a-nes-the'-tik*). An agent which produces insensibility. As an adjective it means insensible to touch.

**anaesthetist** (*a-nēs-the-tist*). The administrator of anaesthetics.

**anal** (*ā-nal*). Of the anus.

**analbuminaemia** (*an-al-bū-mi-nē'-mi-a*). Absence of albumin from blood proteins.

**analeptic** (*a-na-lep-tik*). A restorative. A drug which restores to consciousness, *e.g.* nikethamide.

**analgesia** (*a-nal-jē'-zi-a*). Diminished sensibility to pain. A symptom in certain nervous diseases, *e.g.* syringomyelia.

**analgesic** (*a-nal-jē-zik*). Relieving pain; remedy for pain.

**analogous** (*a-na'-lō-jus*). Comparable in certain respects.

**analysis** (*a-na'-li-sis*). In chemistry, the breaking down of a substance into its constituent parts. An psychiatric medicine, psycho-analysis.

**analyst** (*a'-na-list*). The person who analyses.

**anaphase** (*an'-a-fāz*). A stage in cell division when the chromosomes move towards opposite poles of the cell. *See* MITOSIS.

**anaphoresis** (*a-na-fo-rē'-sis*). Diminished activity of the sweat glands.

**anaphylaxis** (*a-na-fi-lak'-sis*). A state of shock induced by an antigen-antibody reaction occurring in cells which causes the release of substances acting on the vascular system.

**anaplasia** (*a-na-plā-si-a*). The reversion of specialized tissue or cells to a less differentiated type.

**anastomosis** (*a'-nas-to-mō'-sis*). In anatomy the inter-communication of the terminal branches of two or more blood vessels. In surgery the establishment of some artificial connection, as, for instance, between two parts of the intestine.

**anatomy** (*a-na'-to-mē*). The science of organic structure. *A., applied.* As applied to diagnosis and treatment.

**anconeus** (*an-kō'-nē-us*). A small extensor muscle of the forearm.

**androgen** (*an'-drō-jen*). A hormone producing male sex characteristics.

**android pelvis** (*an-droyd pel-vis*). Shaped like a male pelvis. In women the narrow fore-pelvis, shallow posterior segment and straight lateral walls make child-bearing difficult.

**androsterone** (*an-dro-ste-rōn*). A breakdown product of testosterone.

**anencephaly** (*a-nen-ke'-fa-li*). Failure of development of the brain, resulting in fetal death.

**anergic** (*a-ner-jik*). Without energy. Inactive.

**aneroid** (*a'-ne-royd*). Without air.

**aneuploid** (*a-nū-ployd*). Having more or less than an integral multiple of the haploid number of chromosomes, *cf.* euploid.

**aneurysm** (*a-nū-rism*). A permanent dilatation of an artery usually with rupture of the internal and middle coats. It may be (*a*) *fusiform* or (*b*) *sacculated.* The thoracic aorta and the innominate artery are those usually affected, more rarely the abdominal aorta. *Arteriovenous a.* is a communication between an artery and a vein, usually the result of injury. *Dissecting a.* Results when blood is forced into the potential space between the layers of the arterial wall.

**angiectasis** (*an-ji-ek'-ta-sis*). Dilatation of blood vessels.

**angiitis** (*an-ji-ī-tis*). Inflammation of blood vessels.

**angina** (*an-jī-na*). Suffocating pain; thus any severe sore throat associated with swelling of the walls of the air passages may be termed angina. Ludwig's angina, Vincent's angina, are examples; but the commonest use of the term is in angina pectoris.

**angina pectoris** (*an-jī-na pek'-to-ris*). Syndrome usually characterized by pain in the chest and left arm occurring on exertion. Due to insufficiency of the blood supply to the myocardium.

**angiocardiogram** (*an-ji-ō-kar'-di-o-gram*). The x-ray film taken in angiocardiography.

**angiocardiography** (*an-ji-ō-kar-di-o'-gra-fi*). To demonstrate the activity and function of the heart and great vessels by the injection of contrast medium.

**angiogram** (*an'-ji-ō-gram*). X-ray film showing blood vessels.

**angiography** (*an-ji-o'-gra-fi*). X-ray visualization of blood vessels. *See* ANGIOCARDIO-GRAPHY.

**angioma** (*an-ji-ō'-ma*). A tumour composed of blood vessels, often called a naevus.

**angioneurotic** (*an'-ji-nū-ro'-tik*). Having to do with the nervous control of the blood vessels. Thus *a. oedema* is a persistent or intermittent swelling of parts such as the eyelid or lip. It may be an allergic symptom.

**angioparalysis** (*an-ji-ō-pa-ra'-li-sis*). Vasomotor paralysis.

**angioplasy** (*an-ji-ō-pla'-sti*). Plastic surgery of the blood vessels.

**angiosarcoma** (*an-ji-ō-sar-kō'-ma*). A sarcoma composed of vascular tissue.

**angiospasm** (*an-ji-ō-spazm*). The blood vessels contract in spasm.

**angiotensin** (*an-ji-ō-ten'-sin*). Polypeptide hormone which raises the blood pressure.

**Angström unit** (*ang-strerm ū-nit*). An obsolete unit of measurement of wavelengths of light. Replaced by nanometre (nm)—$10^{-10}$ m.

**anhidrosis** (*an-hī-drō'-sis*). Deficiency of perspiration.

**anhidrotics** (*an-hī-dro'-tiks*). Drugs which reduce sweating.

**anhydrous** (*an-hī'-drus*). Without water.

**aniline** (*a-ni-lin*). Phenylamine. Used in preparing dyestuffs.

**animalcule** (*a-ni-mal'-kūl*). Microscopic animal.

**anion** (*ā-ni'-on*). An ion bearing a negative electrical charge.

**aniseikonia** (*a'-ni-si-kō'-ni-a*). Unequal magnification between two eyes or different meridia in the same eye.

**anisochromatopsia** (*a-nī-sō-krō-ma-top'-si-a*). Partial colour blindness.

**anisocoria** (*a-ni-sō-ko'-ri-a*). Inequality of the pupils.

**anisocytosis** (*a-ni-sō-sī-tō'-sis*). Inequality of size of the red blood cells.

**anisogamy** (*a-ni-so'-ga-mi*). Condition in which gametes are unlike.

**anisomelia** (*a-ni-so-me'-li-a*). Unequal limbs which should be a pair.

**anisometropia** (*an-i'-so-met-rō'-pi-a*). Differing refraction between eyes.

**ankle** (*ang'-kl*). Joint between leg and foot. The weight is transmitted between tibia and talus.

**ankyloblepharon** (*an-ki-lō-ble'-fa-ron*). Adhesion of the edges of the eyelids.

**ankyloglossia** (*an-ki-lō-glo'-si-a*). Inability to protrude the tongue fully and tendency for it to deviate to one side, usually the result of damage to the tongue muscles.

**ankylosing spondylitis** (*an-ki-lō-sing spon-di-lī'-tis*). Disease of joints, of unknown aetiology, in which destruction of the joint space occurs and is followed by sclerosis and calcification. The sacroiliac joints are predominantly affected.

**ankylosis** (*an-ki-lō'-sis*). Immobility in a joint, following inflammation or prolonged immobilization. *False a.* Fixation or stiffness produced by conditions around the joint such as contraction of skin, *e.g.* after burns, or of tendons, by ossification of muscles, or by outgrowths of bone. *True a.* Fixation or stiffness produced by conditions in the joint such as injury or arthritis. *Fibrous a.* Fixation by fibrous tissue. *Bony a.* The articular surfaces of the bones are fused together.

**Ankylostoma duodenale** (*an-ki-lo-stō'-ma du-ō-de-nar-li*). A minute parasitic hookworm which may inhabit the duodenum in large numbers and cause profound anaemia.

**ankylostomiasis** (*an-ki-lō-stō-mī'-a-sis*). Hookworm disease. Infection with the *Ankylostoma duodenale*.

**annular** (*a'-nū-lar*). Ring-shaped. *A. ligament.* The

ligament around the wrist or ankle.

**anode** (*a-nōd*). Electrode with positive charge.

**anodyne** (*a-no-dīn*). A pain-relieving drug.

**anomalous** (*a-no'-ma-lus*). Irregular. Out of the ordinary.

**anomia** (*a-nō-mi-a*). Inability to name objects and recall names.

**anonychia** (*a-nō-ni'-ki-a*). Absence of nails.

**anoperineal** (*ā-nō-per-ri-nĕ-al*). Relating to anus and perineum.

**Anopheles** (*a-no'-fe-lēz*). A genus of mosquito. They are carriers of the malarial parasite, their bite being the means of transmitting the disease to human beings.

**anorchous** (*a-nor'-kus*). Without testes. Sometimes applied incorrectly to undescended testes.

**anorectal** (*ā-nō-rek'-tal*). Pertaining to the anus and the rectum.

**anorexia** (*a-no-rek'-si-a*). Lack of appetite, abhorrence of food. *A. nervosa.* A disease usually occurring in female adolescents. Dieting may start to lose real or imagined excess of weight and the patient becomes progressively less able to eat any food. Amenorrhoea is com-

mon. Psychiatric treatment is usually indicated.

**anosmia** (*a-nos'-mi-a*). Loss of sense of smell.

**anovulation** (*a-no-vū-lā'-shon*). Cessation of ovulation.

**anovulatory cycle** (*an-ov'-ū-lā-to-ri sī-kl*). Apparently normal menstrual cycle without ovulation.

**anoxaemia** (*a-nok-sĕ'-mi-a*). Insufficient oxygen in the blood.

**anoxia** (*a-nok'-si-a*). Absence of oxygen. Often implies insufficient oxygen available for normal respiratory metabolism, *i.e.* hypoxia.

**antacid** (*an-ta'-sid*). Any substance neutralizing an acid, *e.g.* sodium bicarbonate.

**antagonist** (*an-ta'-go-nist*). An organ such as a muscle that acts in opposition to another, or a drug neutralizing another drug.

**anteflexion** (*an-tē-flek'-shon*). Being bent forward. Term applied to uterus.

**ante mortem** (*an-tē maw-tem*). Before death.

**antenatal** (*an-tē-nā-tal*). Before birth.

**antepartum** (*an-tē-par'-tum*). Before birth. *A. haemorrhage* may be inevitable or accidental when it is due to partial separation of the placenta; incidental when it is due to diseases of the cervix.

**anterior** (*an-te'-ri-or*). In front of.

**anterior chamber of eye.** The space, between the cornea in front and the iris and lens behind, which contains the aqueous humour.

**anterior commissure** (*an-te'-ri-or kom'-mis-sūr*). A bundle of nerve fibres crossing the mid-line in front of the third ventricle and serving to connect certain parts of the two cerebral hemispheres.

**anterior fontanelle** (*an-te-ri-or fon-ta-nel*). See FONTANELLE.

**anterior poliomyelitis** (*an-te-ri-or pō-liō-mī-e-lī-tis*). See POLIOMYELITIS.

**anterior root.** Motor root, *syn.* ventral root. Nerve root emerging from the spinal cord carrying motor fibres, *cf.* dorsal or posterior root.

**anterograde** (*an-te-rō-grād*). Going forwards.

**antero-inferior** (*an-te-rō-in-fā'-ri-or*). Lying in front and below.

**antero-interior** (*an-te-rō-in-tā-ri-or*). Lying to the front and internally.

**anterolateral** (*an-te-rō-la'-te-ral*). In front and to the side.

**anteromedian** (*an-te-rō-mē'-di-an*). Lying in front and near the mid-line.

**anteroposterior** (*an-te-rō-pō-stā'ri-or*). From front to back.

**anterosuperior** (*an-te-rō-soo-pā-ri-or*). In front and above.

**anteversion** (*an'-tē-ver'-shon*). The state of being inclined forward. It is the normal position of the uterus. Also called anteflexion.

**anthelmintic** (*an-thel-min'-tik*). A remedy for intestinal worms.

**anthocyanin** (*an-thō-sī'-a-nin*). Red pigment in beetroot which may cause red colour in urine.

**anthracosis** (*an-thra-kō'-sis*). Disease caused by inhaling coal dust or soot into the lungs. Seen in miners.

**anthrax** (*an'-thrax*). An acute, infectious disease produced by the Anthrax bacillus. *Skin a.* and *Pulmonary a.* are the two main forms.

**anthropoid** (*an'thro-poyd*). Man-like. *A. apes* include animals most closely related to man. *A. pelvis.* The pelvis has a narrowed transverse inlet which is long antero-posteriorly.

**anthropology** (*an-thro-po'lo-ji'*). The natural history of mankind.

**antibiotic** (*an-ti-bī-o'-tik*). Opposed to life; drugs, derived from living cells, especially fungi, which prevent micro-organisms from multiplying, *e.g.* penicillin.

**antibody** (*an-ti-bo'-di*). Protein

substance, usually circulating in the blood, which neutralizes corresponding antigens. *Auto-a.* A. directed against a component normally present in the body. *Blocking a.* A. inhibiting effect of another A. *Forssman a.* A. specific for antigen unrelated to that providing immunizing stimulus. *Incomplete a.* A. which will not by itself form precipitate *in vitro* with corresponding antigen.

**anticholinergic** (*an-ti-kō-li-ner'-jik*). Substance antagonizing the action of acetylcholine.

**anticholinesterase** (*an-ti-kō-li-nes'-te-rāz*). Generic term for substances which prevent the action of cholinesterases and specifically acetylcholinesterase which breaks down acetylcholine.

**anticoagulant** (*an-ti-kō-a'-gū-lant*). Substance which delays the clotting of blood.

**anticodon** (*an-tē-kō-don*). Triplet of unpaired bases which are complementary to the triplet of the genetic code which specifies an amino-acid.

**anticonvulsant** (*an-ti-kon-vul'-sant*). A drug used to prevent a convulsion.

**antidepressant** (*an-ti-de-pres'-sant*). Drug used to treat depression.

**antidiuretic hormone** (*an-ti-dī-ū-re-tik hor'-mōn*). Posterior pituitary hormone regulating the amount of water re-absorbed from the uriniferous tubules into the renal substance.

**antidote** (*an'-ti-dōt*). The corrective to a poison.

**antigen** (*an'-ti-jen*). Substance capable of stimulating the formation of antibodies. *Australia a.* A. found in 25 per cent of patients with leukaemia, Down's syndrome and viral hepatitis.

**antigenic determinant** (*an-ti-je'-nik de-ter'-mi-nant*). Site on antigen molecule determining specificity of antibody evoked.

**antiglobulin test** (*an-ti-glo'-bū-lin test*). Coomb's test, used to identify abnormal antibody in the blood.

**antihaemophilic globulin** (*an-ti-hē-mō-fi'-lik glo-bū-lin*). One of the factors essential for blood coagulation. Congenital deficiency causes haemophilia.

**antihistamine** (*an-ti-his'-ta-mēn*). Drug counteracting the effects of the liberation of histamine in the tissues.

**anti-metabolite** (*an-ti-me-ta'-bo-līt*). Substitute for a metabolite which interferes with metabolism.

**antimitotic** (*an-ti-mi-to'-tik*).

Agent which inhibits cell division.

**anti-mongolism** (*an-ti-mong'-gōlizm*). Multiple congenital defects resulting from a chromosome mutation.

**antimycotic** (*an-ti-mi-ko'-tik*). Substance used to treat fungus diseases.

**antinuclear factors** (*an-tē-nū'-klēr fak'-terz*). Antibodies reacting with material in cell nuclei.

**antiperistalsis** (*an-ti-pe-ri-stal'-sis*). Reverse peristalsis, *i.e.* from below upward. *See* PERISTALSIS.

**antiphlogistic** (*an-ti-flo-jis'-tik*). Relieving inflammation.

**antipruritic** (*an-ti-proo-ri-tik*). Substance relieving itching.

**antipyretic** (*an-ti-pī-re'-tik*). A drug which reduces the high temperatures of feverish conditions.

**antirachitic factor** (*an-ti-ra-ki'-tik fak-tor*). *Syn.* vitamin D. Prevents rickets.

**antiscorbutic** (*an-ti-skor-bū'-tik*). *Syn.* vitamin C or ascorbic acid. Prevents scurvy.

**antiseptic** (*an-ti-sep'-tik*). A substance opposing sepsis by arresting the growth and multiplication of micro-organisms. Iodine, phenol, biniodide of mercury, chlorine, formalin, quaternary ammonium compounds, chloroxyl-enols, hypochlorites are common antiseptics. Many are poisonous.

**antiserum** (*an-ti-sā-rum*). Serum, usually prepared from horses, containing a high titre of antibody to a specific organism or toxin.

**antisocial** (*an-ti-sō-shal*). Disregard of the normally accepted behaviour in a particular society.

**antispasmodic** (*an-ti-spaz-mo'-dik*). An agent relieving spasm.

**antithrombin** (*an-ti-throm'-bin*). A substance in the blood having the power of retarding or preventing coagulation.

**antithyroid drugs** (*an-ti-thī'-royd*). Substances which restrict the secretion of thyroid hormones by interference in the intermediary metabolism of the gland.

**antitoxin** (*an-ti-tok'-sin*). A specific antibody produced in the blood in response to a toxin or poison. The antibody is capable of neutralizing that particular toxin.

**antitragus** (*an-ti-trā'-gus*). The prominence of the lower portion of the external ear.

**antivenin** (*an-ti-ve'-nin*). An antidote to animal or insect venom.

**Anton's syndrome** (*an'-tonz sin'-drōm*). Cortical blindness in which patient is unaware of inability to see.

**antrostomy** (*an-tro'-sto-mi*). Incision of an antrum.

**antrum** (*an'-trum*). A cave; applied to the maxillary sinus, called the antrum of Highmore, and the cavity in the mastoid bone communicating with the middle ear. *See* MAXILLARY SINUS.

**anuria** (*an-ū'-ri-a*). Cessation of the production of urine; to be distinguished from retention of urine, due to inability to empty the bladder.

**anus** (*ā'-nus*). The rectal exit. *Imperforate a.* A congenital malformation where a child is born with no anal opening, or an anus is present but does not communicate with the bowel above.

**anxiety neurosis** (*ang-zī-e-ti nū-rō'-sis*). An illness in which a patient's fears and anxieties are out of proportion to reality.

**aorta** (*ā-or'-ta*). Large artery arising from the left ventrical of the heart and from which blood is distributed to the whole body.

**aortic incompetence** (*ā-or'-tik in-kom'-pe-tens*). Blood from the aorta regurgitates back into the left ventricle, due to inefficiency of the valve.

**aortic stenosis** (*ā-or'-tik ste-*

*nō'-sis*). Narrowing of the aortic valve due to malformation and/or disease.

**aortic valves** (*ā-or'-tik valvs*). Three semilunar valves guarding the entrance from the left ventricle to the aorta and preventing the backward flow of the blood.

**aortitis** (*ā-or-tī'-tis*). Inflammation of the aorta.

**apathy** (*a'-pa-thi*). Absence of emotion or feeling.

**apepsia** (*ā-pep'-si-a*). Failure of digestion due to deficiency of gastric juice.

**aperient** (*a-pār-i-ent*). A purgative medicine, *e.g.* cascara.

**aperistalsis** (*ā-per-i-stal'-sis*). Cessation of peristalsis.

**apex** (*ā-peks*). Top, extreme point, summit. *A. of the heart.* Narrow end of heart enclosing left ventricle. *A. beat.* The heart beat as felt at its most forcible point on the chest wall. This corresponds approximately with the position of the left ventricle.

**Apgar score** (*ap'-gah skaw*). Rapid evaluation system for physical condition of newborn infants usually recorded at 1 minute and 5 minutes after birth.

**APH.** Antepartum haemorrhage.

**aphagia** (*a-fā'-ji-a*). Inability to swallow.

**aphakia** (*ā-fā'-ki-a*). Absence of lens.

**aphasia** (*a-fā'-zi-a*). Speechlessness; due to disease or injury to brain.

**aphonia** (*a-fō-ni-a*). Loss of voice.

**aphrodisiac** (*af-frō-di'-zi-ak*). An agent which increases sexual desire.

**aphthae** (*af-thē*). Small white ulcers in the mouth.

**aphthous stomatitis** (*af-thus sto-ma-tī'-tis*). Inflammation of the mucous membrane of the mouth due to herpes simplex virus, *cf. thrush*.

**apicectomy** (*ā-pi-sek-to-mi*). Excision of the root-end of a tooth.

**apicolysis** (*a-pi-ko-lī'-sis*). Stripping of the parietal pleura from the chest wall to collapse a tuberculous apex of lung.

**aplasia** (*a-plā-si-a*). Non-development of an organ or tissue.

**aplastic anaemia** (*ā-plas'-tik a-nē-mi-a*). Anaemia resulting from destruction of bone marrow cells.

**apnoea** (*ap-nē-a*). Suspended respiration.

**apocrine glands** (*a-po-krin glans*). Specialized sweat glands found in the axillae and genital regions.

**aponeurosis** (*a-po'-nū-rō'-sis*). A tendon-like fibrous tissue, which invests the muscles and transmits their movements to the structures upon which they act.

**apophysis** (*a-po'-fi-sis*). A bony protuberance or outgrowth.

**apoplexy** (*a-pō-plex'-si*). A stroke. The effects of a cerebrovascular accident.

**apothecary** (*a-po'-the-ka-ri*). A druggist or pharmacist.

**appendicectomy** (*ap-pen-di-sek'-to-mi*). Removal of the vermiform appendix. Also called appendectomy.

**appendices epiploicae** (*ap-pen-di-sēs ep-pi-plō-i-sē*). Small bags of fat projecting from the peritoneal coat of the large intestine.

**appendicitis** (*ap-pend-di-sī'-tis*). Inflammation of the appendix.

**appendix vermiformis** (*ap-pen-diks ver-mi-for'-mis*). A worm-like offshoot from the caecum, ending blindly, and 2 to 13 cm long.

**apperception** (*a-per-sep-shon*). The conscious reception of a sensory impression.

**applicator** (*ap'-li-kā-tor*). An instrument for applying local remedies, *e.g.* radium.

**apposition** (*a-po-zi'-shon*). The lying together or the fitting together of two structures.

**apraxia** (*a-prak'-si-a*). Inability to carry out purposeful voluntary movements but without loss of muscle power.

**APT.** Alum precipitated (diphtheria) toxoid.

**aptitude** (*ap'-ti-tūd*). A facility or a particular bent for certain work or actions.

**aptyalism** (*ap-tī-a-lism*). Absence of salivation.

**apyrexia** (*ā-pī-rek'-si-a*). Absence of fever.

**aqua** (*a'-kwa*). Water: abbreviation is *aq*.

**aqueduct** (*a'-kwē-dukt*). Certain canals of the body, such as the A. of Sylvius which leads from the third to the fourth ventricle of the brain.

**aqueous humour** (*ā'-kwē-us hū'-mor*). Fluid in the eye between the cornea and the iris and the lens.

**arachnodactyly** (*a-rak-no-dak'-ti-li*). With spider digits. Developmental anomaly associated with Marfan's syndrome in which the digits are excessively long.

**arachnoid** (*a-rak'-noyd*). Spider-like. *A. membrane* surrounds the brain and spinal cord. It is between the dura and pia mater.

**Aran-Duchenne's disease.** *See* DUCHENNE'S DISEASE.

**arbor vitae** (*ah-bor-vē-tī*). Tree-like appearance seen in a section of the cerebellum and also applied to a similar appearance seen in the inter-

ior folds of the cervix of the uterus.

**arborization** (*ah-bo-rī-zā'-shon*). Branching of processes of nerve cells.

**arcus** (*ar-kus*). An arch or ring. *A. senilis*. An opaque circle round the edges of the cornea, occurring in the aged.

**areola** (*a-re'-o-la*). The pigmented skin round the nipple of the breast.

**areolar tissue** (*a-rē'-ō-la ti-shoo*). Loose connective tissue.

**arginine** (*ar'-ji-nēn*). An amino-acid.

**arginino-succinuria** (*ar-ji-nē-nō-suk-sin-ū'-ri-a*). Inborn error of metabolism associated with mental retardation and sometimes abnormal hair. Inherited by a recessive gene.

**Argyll-Robertson pupil** (*ar-gīl-ro'-bert-son*). Pupil of eye which is small, reacting to accommodation but not to light. Seen in diseases of the nervous system, *e.g.* tabes dorsalis.

**argyria** (*ar-ji-ri-a*). Discoloration of the skin and sclera due to the deposition of silver. Results from prolonged ingestion of preparations containing silver.

**Arizona organisms** (*a'-ri-zō-na aw'-ga-nizmz*). Group of genus *Entorobacteriaceae* allied to *Salmonella*, producing similar infections.

**Arnold-Chiari malformation** (*ahr'-nold-ki-ahr'-i malfaw-mā-shon*). Herniation of cerebellum and elongation of medulla oblongata, associated with spina bifida.

**arrector pili** (*a-rek-tor pē-lē*). Muscle fibres around the hair follicles which on contraction produce 'goose-flesh'.

**arrhenoblastoma** (*a-rā-nō-blas-tō-ma*). A neoplasm of the ovary associated with masculinization.

**arrhythmia** (*a-rith'-mi-a*). Disturbance of rhythm, usually the heart's rhythm. *Sinus a*. Increased pulse rate during inspiration, decreased during expiration; common in the young.

**artefact** (*ar'-tē-fakt*). A lesion produced by artificial means.

**arterial** (*ar-tār-i-al*). Pertaining to an artery. Thus *arterial tension* means the pressure of the blood circulating in a given artery.

**arteriectomy** (*ar-tā-rē-ek'-to-mi*). Excision of an artery.

**arteriography** (*ar-tār-i-o'-gra-fi*). To demonstrate blood vessels following the injection of contrast medium opaque to x-rays.

**arterioles** (*ar-tā'-ri-ōls*). Small arteries with contractile muscular walls which control the supply of blood to the capillaries.

**arteriopathy** (*ah-tā-ri-o'-pa-thi*). Disease of the arteries.

**arterioplasty** (*ah-tā-ri-ō-pla'-sti*). Surgery to reform an artery, especially for aneurysm.

**arteriorrhaphy** (*ar-tā-ri-or'-ra-fi*). Suture of an artery.

**arteriosclerosis** (*ar-tā-ri-ō-skle-rō'-sis*). Degeneration of an artery with hardening of its walls, seen chiefly in old age. The condition is accompanied by high blood pressure.

**arteriotomy** (*ar-tā-ri-o'-to-mi*). Incision of an artery.

**arteriovenous aneurysm** (*ar-tā-ri-ō-vē'-nus a'-nū-rism*). *See* ANEURYSM.

**arteritis** (*ar-te-rī'-tis*). Inflammation of the arteries.

**artery** (*ar'-te-ri*). A vessel carrying blood from the heart.

**arthralgia** (*ar-thral-ji-a*). Pain in the joints.

**arthrectomy** (*ar-threk'-to-mi*). The removal by operation of the whole or part of a joint.

**arthritis** (*ar-thrī-tis*). Inflammation of a joint.

**arthroclasia** (*ar-thrō-klā-si-a*). An operation for breaking up an ankylosed joint to produce free movement.

**arthrodesis** (*ar-thrō-dē'-sis*). Fixation of a joint by means of a surgical operation.

**arthrodynia** (*ar-thrō-di'-ni-a*). Pain in the joints.

**arthrography** (*ar-thro'-gra-fi*). Radiography of joint after the injection of radio-opaque fluid to outline the joint space.

**arthropathy** (*ar-thro'-pa-thi*). Disease of the joints. Commonly used to imply secondary damage to joints as a result of other disease processes.

**arthroplasty** (*ar-thrō-plas'-ti*). The making of an artificial joint.

**arthrotomy** (*ar-thro'-to-mi*). Incision into a joint.

**Arthus phenomenon** (*ar'-thus fe-no'-mi-non*). Tissue necrosis after repeated antigen injections.

**articular** (*ar-ti'-kū-la*). Relating to the joints; the articulation of a skeleton is the manner in which the bones are joined together.

**articulation** (*ar-ti-kū-lā'-shon*). (1) A joint between two or more bones. (2) The enunciation of words.

**artificial feeding** (*ar-ti-fi-shal*). Feeding of an infant with food other than its mother's milk.

**artificial insemination** (*ar-ti-fi-shal in-se-mi-nā'-shon*). Artificial introduction of spermatozoa into the vagina.

**artificial kidney** (*ar-ti-fi-shal kid'-ni*). Dialysing apparatus through which blood from the patient is pumped so that excretory products such as urea may be extracted in the event of the patient's own kidneys not functioning.

**artificial pneumothorax.** *See* PNEUMOTHORAX.

**arytenoid** (*ar-i-tē-noyd*). The term applied to two funnel-shaped cartilages of the larynx.

**asbestos** (*as-bes'-tos*). A mineral substance which is incombustible and which does not conduct heat.

**asbestosis** (*as-bes-tō-sis*). Disease of the lung caused by inhalation of asbestos dust.

**ascariasis** (*as-ka-rī'-a-sis*). Infestation of the bowel by roundworms (ascarides).

**ascaricide** (*as-ka'-ri-sīd*). Substance lethal to intestinal worms.

**Ascaris** (*as'-ka-ris*). A genus of parasitic roundworm. *A. lumbricoides*. Long roundworm.

**Aschoff nodules** (*a-shof no'-dŭls*). The focal lesions of acute rheumatic fever consisting of perivascular necrosis of collagen. These nodules tend to occur in the heart, muscles and connective tissue.

**ascites** (*as-sī'-tēz*). Fluid collection in the abdominal cavity.

**ascitic fluid** (*a-si-tik floo-id*). Fluid of ascites which can be aspirated.

**ascorbic acid** (*a-scaw-bik a-sid*). Vitamin C. It is required for collagen formation in healing of wounds. Deficiency causes scurvy.

**asemasia** (*ā-se-mā'-si-a*). Disorder affecting non-verbal means of communication.

**asepsis** (*a-sep'-sis*). The state of being free from living pathogenic micro-organisms.

**aseptic** (*a-sep'-tik*). Free from bacteria. In aseptic surgery all instruments, dressings, etc., are sterilized before use.

**asexual** (*ā-sek-shal*). Having no sex.

**Aspergillus** (*as-per-gil-lus*). The name of a group of fungi, some species of which are pathogenic, causing aspergillosis, which may infect the ear, eye or lungs.

**aspermia** (*ā-sper'-mi-a*). Absence of live spermatozoa in semen.

**asphyxia** (*as-fik'-si-a*). Suffocation.

**aspiration** (*as-pi-rā'-shon*). The operation of drawing off fluids from the body.

**aspirator** (*as'-pi-rā-tor*). The apparatus used for aspiration.

**assimilation** (*a-si-mi-lā'-shon*). The absorption and utilization of nourishment by the living tissues. *A. pelvis*. Term indicating the incorporation of the fifth lumbar vertebra in the sacral body.

**Assmann's focus** (*as'-manz fō-kus*). Radiological opacity caused by lesion of post-primary pulmonary tuberculosis.

**association** (*as-sō-si-ā'-shon*). Co-ordination. 'Association of ideas', *i.e.* a phrase used to denote the secondary thoughts that arise on the receipt of any individual mental impression.

**asteatosis** (*ā-stē-a-tō'-sis*). Deficient action of sebaceous glands.

**astereognosis** (*a-ste-re-og-nō'-sis*). Loss of power to recognize the shape of objects by touch.

**asthenia** (*as-thē'-ni-a*). Failure of strength; debility.

**asthenopia** (*as-the-nō'-pi-a*). Weakness of sight.

**asthma** (*as'-ma*). Paroxysms of difficult breathing, with sense of suffocation. There is difficulty in expiration. The main causes are infection and allergy. Severe asthma can usually be relieved by steroids. *Cardiac a.* occurs later in life and is due to failure of left ventricle.

**astigmatism** (*as-tig'-ma-tizm*). Inequality in the curvature of the cornea or lens, with consequent blurring and distortion of the images thrown upon the retina.

**astringent** (*as-trin'-jent*). A substance applied to produce local contraction of blood vessels and inhibit secretion, *e.g.* tannin, adrenaline.

**astrocytoma** (*as-tro-sī-tō'-ma*). Tumour occurring in the central nervous system, composed of cells called astrocytes.

**astroglia** (*as-tro'-gli-a*). Star-shaped supporting cells of the central nervous system.

**asymmetry** (*ā-si'-me-tri*). Lack of symmetry.

**asynclitism** (*ā-sin'-kli-tism*). Engagement in the pelvis of a diameter of the fetal head other than the biparietal. It may occur with a contracted pelvis.

**atavism** (*a'-ta-vism*). After an interval of several generations, recurrence in descendants of a character possessed by an ancestor.

**ataxia, ataxy** (*a-tak'-sē*). Literally, disorder; applied to any defective control of muscles and consequent irregularity of movements. *See also* LOCOMOTOR ATAXIA and FRIEDREICH'S ATAXIA.

**atelectasis** (*a-te-lek'-ta-sis*). Imperfect expansion of the lungs of the newborn. Term also used for collapse of part of the lung from some other cause.

**atherogenic** (*a-the-rō-je'-nik*). Producing atheroma.

**atheroma** (*a-the-rō'-ma*). Degeneration of walls of arteries associated with the deposition of cholesterol esters in the lesions.

**atherosclerosis** (*a-the-rō-skle-rō'-sis*). Narrowing of blood vessels resulting from atheromatous deposits.

**athetosis** (*a-the-tō'-sis*). A condition marked by continuous and purposeless movements, especially of the hands and fingers.

**athlete's foot** (*ath-lēts*). Infectious disease of the skin between and under the toes due to parasitic fungi.

**atlas** (*at'-las*). First cervical vertebra.

**atmosphere** (*at'-mōs-fār*). The air surrounding the earth. The pressure, at sea level, measured by means of a barometer equivalent to approximately 15 p.s.i. or 1,055 g/cm².

**atom** (*a-tom*). The structural unit of an element.

**atomic weight** (*a-to'-mik wāt*). The weight of an atom as compared with that of an atom of hydrogen (= 1).

**atomizer** (*a'-to-mī-zer*). A spray for providing a shower of very minute droplets.

**atony** (*a'-to-ni*). Wanting in muscular tone or vigour; weakness.

**ATP.** *See* ADENOSINE TRIPHOSPHATE.

**atresia** (*a-trē'-si-a*). Absence of a natural passage. Closure of a duct.

**atria** (*ā-tri-a*). The two thin-walled chambers of the heart into which the veins drain. Formerly known as the auricles. *See Diagram of* HEART p. 173.

**atrial fibrillation** (*ā'-tri-al fī-bri-lā'-shon*). Cardiac arrhythmia caused by the independent contraction of muscle bundles in the atrial walls. There is no co-ordinated atrial contraction and the ventricular contractions are stimulated irregularly.

**atrial flutter** (*ā-tri-al flu'-ter*). Cardiac arrhythmia caused by rapid atrial contractions, 200 to 300 per minute, stimulated by an excitable focus in the atrial wall. The ventricles are unable to contract at this rate and respond only to every second or third atrial contraction. *See* HEART BLOCK.

**atrial septal defect** (*ā-tri-al septal dē-fekt*). Defect in the development of the heart leaving a hole in the wall separating the right and left atrium.

**atrio-ventricular bundle** (*ā-tri-ō-ven-tri-kū-la bun-del*). *See* AURICULO-VENTRICULAR BUNDLE.

**atrophy** (*a-tro-fi*). Wasting of a part, from disuse or lack of nutrition.

**atropine** (*a'-trō-pēn*). Active principle of belladonna. Parasympathetic antagonist.

**attenuation** (*at-ten-ū-ā-shon*). A weakening or dilution.

**atypical** (*ā-ti-pi-kal*). Not typical.

**audiogram** (*aw-di-ō-gram*). Chart showing the responsiveness of ear to sounds of differing pitch.

**audiologist** (*aw-di-o'-lo-jist*). A specialist in the diagnosis and treatment of hearing problems.

**audiometer** (*aw-di-o'-me-ter*). Instrument used for audiometry.

**audiometry** (*aw-di-o'-me-tri*). Measurement of hearing ability. The results are usually plotted as an audiogram.

**auditory** (*aw-di-to-ri*). Pertaining to the sense of hearing.

**Auer bodies** (*ow'-er bo'-dēz*). Blue-staining granules seen in myeloblasts in leukaemia.

**Auerbach's plexus** (*ow'-er-bax plek-sus*). The collection of nerve fibres (terminations of vagus and sympathetic nerves) and ganglia situated in the intestinal walls. Function: regulates peristalsis.

**aura** (*aw'-ra*). A sensation, which is usually auditory or visual, arising indigenously in the patient; it may precede an epileptic fit.

**aural** (*aw'-ral*). Pertaining to the ear.

**auricle** (*aw'-ri-kl*). (1) The external ear. (2) One of the upper cavities of the heart now usually termed atrium. *See* HEART.

**auricular** (*aw-ri'-kū-lar*). Pertaining to the ear or to the auricles of the heart. *A. fibrillation*. *See* ATRIAL FIBRILLATION. *A. flutter*. *See* ATRIAL FLUTTER.

**auriculo-temporal syndrome** (*aw-ri-kū-lō-tem'-po-ral sin'-drōm*). Frey's syndrome. Results from injury to the fibres of the auriculotemporal nerve. When the patient eats, the cheek becomes red, hot and sweats.

**auriculo-ventricular bundle** (bundle of His) (*aw-ri-kū-lō-ven-tri'-kū-lar bundl*). Also called atrio-ventricular bundle. Normally the contraction of the heart is initiated at the sinuatrial node. The impulse then passing through the atrial walls causing atrial contraction and reaching the atrio-ventricular node (A-V node) which it stimulates. The A-V node is composed of specialized tissue continuous with the A-V bundle through which the impulse is conducted to the ventricles to initiate their contraction. Defects in the A-V bundle which impair conduction of the impulse result in heart block.

**auriscope** (*aw-ri-skōp*). An instrument for examining the drum of the ear. An otoscope.

**auscultation** (*aw-skul-tā'-shon*). Listening to sounds of the body for the purposes of diagnosis. Usually a tube is employed, *e.g.* stethoscope.

**autistic** (*aw-tis-tik*). Usually describing a child who withdraws from contact with people and fails to use speech as a means of communication.

**auto** (*aw'-tō*). A prefix meaning self, of itself.

**autocatalytic** (*aw-tō-ka-ta-li'-tik*). Catalysing production of self.

**autoclave** (*aw'-tō-klāv*). An apparatus for sterilizing by steam.

**autodigestion** (*aw-tō-di-jes'-chon*). Process of self-digestion.

**auto-eroticism** (*aw-tō-e-ro'-ti-sizm*). Masturbation.

**autogenous** (*aw-to'-je-nus*). Self produced.

**autograft** (*aw-tō-grahft*). Graft taken from the patient's own body. *See* GRAFT.

**autographism** (*aw-tō-gra'-fism*). Same as dermographism.

**autohypnosis** (*aw-tō-hip-nō'-sis*). Self-induced hypnotism.

**auto-immunity** (*aw-tō-im-mū'-ni-ti*). State of sensitization to products of one's own organs, *e.g.* as in Hashimoto's disease.

**auto-infection** (*aw-tō-in-fek-shon*). Self-infection.

**auto-intoxication** (*aw-tō-in-tok-si-kā'-shon*). Poisoning by toxins generated within the body.

**autolysis** (*aw-to'-li-sis*). Process of self-digestion.

**automatism** (*aw-to'-ma-tizm*). A condition in which actions are performed without consciousness or regulated purpose; sometimes follows a major or minor epileptic fit.

**autonomic nervous system** (*aw-tō-no-mik ner-vus sis-tem*). Motor supply to smooth muscle and glands. Divided into sympathetic and parasympathetic systems and characterized by synapsing in ganglia after fibres leave the central nervous system. Generally speaking the effector fibres (postganglionic fibres) of the sympathetic system are adrenergic and the parasympathetic are cholinergic. Not directly under conscious control but there is considerable cortical representation.

**autoplasty** (*aw-tō-pla'-sti*). *See* AUTOGRAFT.

**autopsy** (*aw-top-si*). A post-mortem examination.

**autoradiography** (*aw-tō-rā-di-o'-gra-fi*). Photography showing localization of radioactive substance in a tissue section.

**autosomes** (*aw-tō-sōms*). All chromosomes excluding the sex chromosomes.

**auto-suggestion** (*aw-tō-su-jes-chon*). Self-suggestion: used in the treatment of functional nervous disorders.

**avascular** (*a-vas'-kū-la*). Bloodless.

**aversion therapy** (*a-ver'-shon the'-ra-pi*). Treatment by conditioning based on association of a disagreeable stimulus with an abnormal desire.

**avirulent** (*ā-vi-rū-lent*). Not virulent.

**avitaminosis** (*ā-vi-ta-mi-nō'-sis*). Lack of vitamins. Usually the particular vitamin deficiency is specified, *e.g.* avitaminosis A.

**avulsion** (*a-vul'-shon*). A tearing apart.

**axilla** (*ak-si-la*). The arm-pit.

**axillary artery** (*ak-si'-la-ri ar'-te-ri*). The artery of the armpit, connecting the subclavian and brachial arteries.

**axis** (*ak'-sis*). (1) The second cervical vertebra on which the atlas rotates. (2) Line passing through the centre of a body. *A. of pelvis* is a curved line which is everywhere at right angles to the planes of the pelvic cavity. *A. traction* is force so applied to the fetus by forceps that its effect is always exerted along the axis of the pelvis.

**axon** (*ak-son*). The long process of a nerve cell conducting impulses away from the cell body, *cf.* dendrite.

**axonotmesis** (*ak-so-nō-tmē-sis*). Damage causing discontinuity of axons but the supporting tissue remains intact.

**azoospermia** (*ā-zoo-sper'-mi-a*). Absence of viable sperms in the semen causing male sterility.

**azotaemia** (*ā-zo-tē-mi-a*). Excess urea in the blood.

**azoturia** (*ā-zo-tū-ri-a*). An increase of urea in the urine.

**azygos** (*ā-zī-gos*). Single, *i.e.* not paired.

**B**

**Babinski's reflex** (*ba-bin-skēz rē-fleks*). Extensor plantar response, *i.e.* the toes go up when the sole of the foot is stroked. This is normal in infants and abnormal after about two years.

**bacillary dysentery** (*ba-si-la-ri di'-sen-te-ri*). Infection of the gut with Shigella bacilli, *cf.* amoeba.

**bacilluria** (*ba-si-lū-ri-a*). Presence of bacilli in the urine.

**bacillus** (*ba-si'-lus*). See BACTERIA.

**bacteraemia** (*bak-te-rē-mi-a*). Bacteria in the blood.

**bacteria** (*bak-tā'-ri-a*). Microscopic unicellular living organisms; some cause disease and are called pathogenic. The principal forms are: (1) *Cocci*, those which are rounded in shape. When these are disposed in pairs they are called *Diplococci*. These occur in pneumonia, some forms of meningitis, and gonorrhoea. When in chains they are called *Streptococci*, when in clusters *Staphylococci*. (2) *Bacilli* are rod-shaped bacteria which include the Gram-positive organisms causing anthrax, tetanus and diphtheria; Gram-negative causing dysentery, typhoid and plague and the acid-fast organisms of tuberculosis and leprosy. (3) *Spirochaetes* are corkscrew-like germs, or spiral rods with several twists, occurring in relapsing fever and syphilis. The majority of bacteria are immobile, but some have power of movement. Bacteria have the power of multiplying by splitting across their centre; this is known as binary fission; others form spores, which are small, round, glistening bodies able to withstand great extremes of heat and cold.

**bacterial** (*bak-tā'-ri-al*). Pertaining to bacteria.

**bactericidal** (*bak-tā-ri-sī'-dal*). Capable of killing bacteria, *cf.* bacteriostatic.

**bacteriology** (*bak-tā-ri-o'-lo-ji*). The study of bacteria.

**bacteriolytic** (*bak-tā-ri-ō-li'-tik*). Capable of breaking down the cell membranes of bacteria.

**bacteriophage** (*bak-tā-ri-ō-fāj*). A virus which destroys bacteria.

**bacteriostatic** (*bak-tā-ri-ō-sta'-tik*). Preventing the growth of bacteria, *cf.* bactericidal.

**bacteriuria** (*bak'-tār-i-ū-ri-a*). The presence of bacteria in the urine.

**bagassosis** (*ba-ga-sō'-sis*). Disease of lungs caused by the inhalation of sugar cane dust.

**Bailliart dynamometer** (*bā'-yart dī-na-mo'-me-ter*). Device for measuring blood pressure in central retinal artery.

**Bainbridge reflex** (*bān-brij rē-fleks*). Inhibition of vagal impulses caused by raised right atrial pressure.

**Baker's cysts** (*bā-kers sists*). Cysts originating from synovial pouches connected with joints.

**BAL.** British Anti-Lewisite (dimercaprol), an antidote for heavy metal poisoning.

**balanitis** (*ba-la-nī'-tis*). Inflammation of the glans penis.

**Balkan beam** (*bawl'-kan bēm*). Frame erected over bed to enable limb to be suspended.

**ballooning** (*ba-loo-ning*). The distension of a cavity by air, or by its natural contents.

**ballottement** (*bal-lot'-mo*). The sensation of a return tap against the fingers when the hand is suddenly pressed on the pregnant uterus and temporarily displaces the contained fetus as it floats in the liquor amnii. Ballottement may be elicited externally, or per vaginam.

**balneotherapy** (*bal-ni-ō-the'-ra-pi*). The amelioration of disease or pain by baths.

**balneum** (*bal'-ni-um*). A bath.

**bandages** (*ban'-dā-jez*). Materials used for binding wounds, fractures, etc.

**Bandl's ring** (*ban-dels ring*). *See* RETRACTION RING.

**Bankart's operation** (*ban-kartz o-pe-rā'-shon*). Operation to repair the glenoid cavity after repeated dislocation of the shoulder joint.

**Banti's syndrome** (*ban-tiz sin'-drōm*). Characterized by anaemia with recurrent bleeding from the alimentary tract, leucopenia and splenomegaly, due to portal hypertension.

**Barany's caloric test** (*ba'-ra-nēz ka'-lo-rik test*). Test for labyrinthine function by douching ear to induce nystagmus. *B.'s chair test.* Labyrinthine function in aviators assessed by rotating chair.

**Barbados leg** (*bah'-bā-dos leg*). Elephantiasis.

**barber's rash** (*bar-berz rash*). *See* SYCOSIS BARBAE

**Barlow's sign** (*bah'-lōz sīn*). Test for congenital dislocation of the hip.

**baroreceptors** (*bā-rō-re-sep'-terz*). Aortic nerve-endings of afferent branches of vagus and glossopharyngeal nerves. Receptors of pressure stimuli in reflex control of blood pressure.

**Barr body** (*bahr bo'-di*). Sex-chromatin body. Small dark-staining mass underneath nuclear membrane in majority of female cells. Represents an inactive X chromosome.

**barrier nursing** (*ba-ri-er ner-sing*). The nursing of a patient with an infectious disease in a general ward, or a ward with patients having a variety of infectious diseases. Adequate precautions are taken so that cross-infection does not occur.

**Bartholin's glands** (*bah-tō-lins glans*). Two small glands, one each side of the vulva. An abscess may develop there or the duct may distend into a cyst.

**bartholinitis** (*bah-tō-li-nī'-tis*). Inflammation of Bartholin's glands.

**basal ganglia** (*bā-sal gang'-li-a*). Four deeply-placed masses of grey matter within the cerebral hemisphere, known as the caudate, lentiform and amygdaloid nuclei, and the claustrum. Little is known of their function but disease involving the basal ganglia gives rise to athetosis and Parkinsonism.

**basal metabolism** (*bā-sal me-ta'-bo-lism*). The rate of combustion of foodstuffs to produce energy when the body is at rest.

**basal metabolic rate** (*bā-sal me-ta-bo-lik rāt*). BMR. Also known as resting metabolic rate or RMR. The rate of consumption of oxygen by the patient after an overnight fast and at least an hour's complete rest. This figure is expressed as a percentage of the normal average. Normal range ± 15 per cent.

**basal narcosis** (*bā-sal nah-kō-sis*). Deep sleep induced by drugs.

**base** (*bās*). (1) The bottom. (2) The chief substance of a mixture. (3) In chemistry, an alkali, the substance which combines with an acid to form its salt.

**Basedow's disease** (*ba-zā-dofs di-sēz*). Exophthalmic goitre.

**basement membrane** (*bās-ment mem-brān*). Substance, probably secreted by the basal cells of an epithelium, which forms a fine membrane separating the epithelium from the underlying structures.

**basic** (*bā-sik*). (1) Basal. (2) Alkaline.

**basilic** (*ba-zi'-lik*). The name of a vein on the inner side of the arm.

**basophil adenoma** (*bā-sō-fil a-de-nō'-ma*). Tumour of basophil cells, *cf.* pituitary, anterior. The cells comprising the anterior pituitary may be classed according to their staining with acid dyes, *e.g.* eosin; or basic dyes, *e.g.* haematoxylin. The differently stained cells appear to secrete different hormones. Thus the eosinophil (acidophil) cells secrete growth hormone, *see* ACROMEGALY. The basophil cells secrete adrenocorticotrophic hormone (ACTH). Basophil adenomas usually secrete excessive amounts of ACTH and this gives rise to Cushing's syndrome.

**basophile** (*bā-sō-fil*). Readily stained with basic dyes, in which the cation is the active part. Nucleic acids are basophilic.

**basophilia** (*bā-so-fi'-li-a*). Abnormality of red blood cells found in lead poisoning in which there is punctate basophilic staining of the cytoplasm.

**Bassini's herniorrhaphy** (*ba-si'-nis her-ni-or'-ra-fi*). Method of reconstruction of the inguinal canal in repair of hernia.

**battered baby** (*ba'-terd bā'bi*). Infant physically injured by parent or guardian.

**Battle's incision** (*ba'tels in-si-zhon*). Also known as Lennander's incision. Paramedial abdominal incision allowing the rectus muscle to be retracted to one side. Sometimes used for appendicectomy.

**battledore placenta** (*ba-tel-daw pla-sen'-ta*). A placenta in which the umbilical cord is inserted into the edge instead of the centre.

**Bazin's disease** (*bā-zins di-sēz*). Purple, tender nodules which may ulcerate. Characteristically on the lower legs of young women with tuberculosis.

**BBA.** Born before arrival (of nursing or medical help).

**BCG.** Bacillus Calmette-Guérin. A vaccine used for inoculation against tuberculosis.

**bearing down** (*bār-ing down*). Popular term for the expulsive contractions during the second stage of labour when the cervix uteri is fully dilated.

**beat** (*bēt*). Applied to the beating of the heart and the pulsation of the blood.

**bed bug.** Insect, the *Cimex lectularius*, living in furniture.

**bedsores** (*bed-saws*). Ulcerated lesions occurring on pressure areas, *e.g.* buttocks, heels, ankles, elbows, in chronically debilitated patients. More commonly called pressure sores.

**behaviour** (*be-hā'-vi-a*). Conduct; or response to certain stimuli. *B. disorder*. Abnormal pattern of behaviour in child or adult. May be of physical origin but usually considered a psychological problem.

**behaviourism** (*be-hā'-vūr-ism*). Psychological analysis of behaviour patterns.

**Behcet's syndrome** (*bā-sets sin'-drōm*). Association of ulcers in the mouth and genitalia with often serious eye involvement.

**Bell's palsy** (*belz pawl-si*). Peripheral paralysis or palsy of facial nerve.

**belladonna** (*bel-a-do'-na*). Deadly nightshade, the source of atropine.

**belle indifference** (*bel in-di-fe-renz*). Abnormal lack of emotional response to distressing circumstances. The cause of this absence of integration is not known.

**Bence-Jones protein** (*bens-jōns prō'-tēn*). A protein found in the urine in myelomatosis.

**bends.** *See* CAISSON DISEASE.

**Benedict's solution** (*be-ne-diks so-lū'-shon*). Used in testing urine for sugar.

**benign** (*be-nīn*). Non-malignant.

**Bennett's fracture** (*ben-netz frak-tūr*). Fracture of the base of the first metacarpal due to a blow on the point of the thumb.

**Berger rhythm** (*ber'-ger rith'-em*). Normal wave form produced by action currents from cerebral cortex, observed by electro-encephalography.

**beriberi** (*be-ri-be-ri*).

Polyneuritis sometimes associated with oedema due to deficiency of thiamine, vitamin B₁.

**berylliosis** (*be-ri-li-ō'-sis*). Pneumoconiosis from inhalation of beryllium oxide particles.

**beryllium window** (*be-ri'-li-um win'-dō*). Apparatus designed to allow minimum penetration of the beam in x-ray therapy.

**Besnier's prurigo** (*bes-nē-ās proo-rī'-gō*). Name given to type of eczema affecting principally the flexures, *e.g.* nape of neck, behind the heels, etc. Occurs in children. Associated with asthma, hay fever and other allergic conditions.

**bestiality** (*bes-ti-a'-li-ti*). Intercourse with animals.

**beta cells** (*bē-ta sels*). Insulin-producing cells of the islets of Langerhans in the pancreas. Two types of cell are found which were originally distinguished as α and β by the differential solubilities of their cytoplasmic granules.

**beta globulin** (*bē-ta glob'-ū-lin*). One fraction of the globulin component of blood proteins.

**beta rays** (*bē-ta rās*). β-rays or β-particles are electrons emitted by radioactive substances. They will penetrate up to about one centimetre in tissue.

**Betz cells** (*bets sels*). Large motor nerve cells present in the cerebral cortex.

**bezoars** (*be'-zō-ars*). Masses of foreign material present in the gastro-intestinal tract of ruminant animals and occasionally man.

**bi** (*bī*). Prefix meaning two or twice.

**bicephalous** (*bī-kē'-fa-lus*). Having two heads.

**biceps** (*bī-seps*). The two-headed muscles in front of the humerus, *see below*, and behind the femur. The latter is known as biceps femoris.

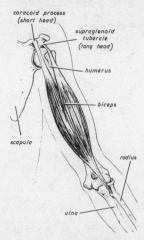

2. *The biceps muscle*

**bicornuate** (*bī-kor'-nū'-āt*). Having two horns. *B. uterus*. A congenital abnormality due to incomplete development. The uterus may be double or a single organ possessing two horns. Pregnancy may take place in one half and be normal. Very rarely twins may develop, one in each horn.

**bicuspid** (*bī-kus'-pid*). (1) Having two points or cusps. (2) The two teeth immediately behind the canines in each jaw are bicuspids. (3) Bicuspid or mitral valve, the valve between the left atrium and the left ventricle of the heart. Rarely the aortic valve is bicuspid.

**Bidwell's ghost** (*bid'-welz gōst*). Blue-violet after-image following exposure of peripheral retina to white light.

**Bielchowski's disease** (*bē-el-chow-skis di-sēz*). Also known as Batten's disease. Early juvenile cerebromacular degeneration. Characterized by mental deterioration and blindness. Inherited through an autosomal recessive gene.

**bifid** (*bī-fid*). Cleft.

**bifocal** (*bī-fō'-kal*). With a double focus. *B. spectacles* can be used for near and distant vision.

**bifurcate** (*bi-fer'-kāt*). Forked.

**Bilroth I gastrectomy.** Excision of ulcer-bearing lesser curvature of stomach, pyloric antrum and pylorus, followed by gastroduodenostomy.

**Bilroth II gastrectomy.** Excision of ulcer-bearing area of stomach or duodenum followed by gastrojejunostomy.

**bigeminal pulse** (*bī-je'-mi-nal puls*). Name applied to the pulse when a double impulse is produced by 'coupled' heart beats. An extra heart beat occurs just after the normal beat.

**bilateral** (*bī-la-te-ral*). Two-sided. Pertaining to both sides.

**bile** (*bīl*). Gall. The secretion of the liver; greenish, bitter and viscid. Alkaline. Specific gravity 1010 to 1040. It consists of water, inorganic salts, bile salts, bile pigments. About 570–850 ml secreted daily.

**bile duct** (*bīl dukt*). Duct transporting the bile from the liver to the duodenum.

**bile pigments** (*bīl pig'-ments*). Breakdown products of haemoglobin. When red blood cells are broken down their content of haemoglobin is split into two fractions: an iron-containing part which is retained by the body, an iron-free part, porphyrin, from which bilirubin is derived. Bilirubin is converted to a water-soluble glucuronide (conjugated) by the liver and this conjugated bilirubin passes in the bile into the duodenum where it is converted to stercobilinogen which gives the faeces their normal colour. Some of this is reabsorbed and small quantities occur in the urine, urobilinogen.

**Bilharzia** (*bil-har'-zi-a*). The same as Schistosoma. A parasitic worm infesting the portal vein and lymph spaces. The worm's eggs are the main cause of the symptoms in those affected; they are spiny, and therefore cause bleeding wherever they lodge. They are found in enormous numbers in the bladder and rectum.

**biliary cirrhosis** (*bil-yu-rē si-rō'-sis*). Liver disease which is considered to affect first the cells adjacent to the bile canaliculi. Two forms are recognized, *primary biliary cirrhosis* of unknown cause and *obstructive biliary cirrhosis*.

**bilious** (*bi-li-us*). Connected with bile. Term often used to denote nausea.

**bilirubin** (*bi-li-rū'-bin*). *See* BILE PIGMENTS.

**biluria** (*bi-li-ū-ri-a*). Presence of bile in the urine. Choluria.

**biliverdin** (*bi-li-ver'-din*). Bile pigment related to bilirubin.

**bimanual** (*bī-ma'-nū-al*). With two hands. By the use of both hands.

**binary fission** (*bi-na-ri fish-on*). Division of a cell into two equal parts.

**binaural** (*bi-naw'-ral*). Pertaining to both ears.

**binocular** (*bi-no'-kū-lar*). Relating to both eyes.

**binovular** (*bi-no'-vū-la*). Produced by two ova. Binovular twins develop from two separate ova fertilized at the same time.

**bio-assay** (*bī-ō-a-say*). Quantitative estimation of biologically active substances, *e.g.* hormones, by comparing, with a standard preparation, their action on living organisms.

**biochemistry** (*bī-o-ke-mi-stri*). The chemistry of life-processes.

**biogenesis** (*bī-ō-je'-ne-sis*). The birth of living matter from living matter.

**biology** (*bī-ol-o-ji*). The science of life and living organisms.

**biometry** (*bī-o-me-tri*). Application of mathematics to biological problems.

**biophysics** (*bī-ō-fi-siks*). Application of physics to biology.

**biopsy** (*bī-op'-si*). Removal of

living tissue from the body for examination.

**bios** (*bī-os*). The Greek word for life; hence the derivation of such words as 'biology', 'biogenesis'.

**biosynthesis** (*bī-ō-sin-the-sis*). Synthesis by living things.

**biotin** (*bī-o-tin*). Part of vitamin B complex. Formerly called vitamin H.

**Biot's respiration** (*bē-os res-pi-rā-shon*). Completely irregular respiration seen in meningitis.

**biparous** (*bī-pa-rus*). Having borne two children.

**bipolar version** (*bī-pō-la ver-shon*). *See* VERSION.

**birth** (*berth*). Being born. *B. injury*. Injury to the newborn sustained at birth. These may be relatively slight, *e.g.* bruising of the scalp, or may be severe, *e.g.* fracture of skull or long bones, various nerve injuries causing paralysis. *B. mark*. Congenital skin defect. Usually denotes abnormal development of dermal blood vessels which give rise to florid areas of skin. *B. paralysis*. Birth injury. *B., premature*. An infant is said to have been born prematurely if its birth weight is 5½ lb (2½ kg) or less. The premature baby tends to be

drowsy, to suck feebly, and does not cry.

**bisalbuminaemia** (*bis-al'-bū-min-ē'-mi-a*). The presence in the blood of two types of albumin with different electrophoretic mobilities.

**bisexual** (*bī-sek-shal*). Being of both sexes. Hermaphrodite.

**bistoury** (*bis'-too-ri*). A surgical knife.

**bitemporal hemianopia** (*bī-tem-po-ral he-mi-a-nō'-pi-a*). Loss of vision in the outer part of the visual field of each eye.

**Bitot's spots** (*bē'-tōz spots*). Conjunctival lesions found in vitamin A deficiency.

**blackhead.** *See* COMEDONES.

**black stools** (*blak stools*). Sign of bleeding from the intestine. May also occur in patients taking large quantities of iron tablets.

**blackwater fever** (*blak-waw-ter fē'-ver*). Acute haemolysis occurring in malaria and leading to excretion of altered haemoglobin in the urine.

**bladder.** A hollow organ for the reception of fluid. *Urinary b.*, receives the urine from the kidneys. *See* GALL BLADDER.

**Blalock's operation** (*blā-lok*). The subclavian artery is anastomosed to the pulmonary artery. Performed in cases of congenital pulmonary stenosis. *See* FALLOT'S TETRALOGY.

**bland.** Mild, non-irritating.

**blast cell** (*blahst sel*). Primitive cell which can usually divide to yield more mature forms.

**blast injury** (*blahst in-jū-ri*). Injury sustained as a result of blast wave from explosion.

**blastoderm** (*blas-tō-derm*). Germinal membrane of ovum.

**blastomycosis** (*blas-tō-mī-kō'-sis*). A skin disease caused by the invasion of a yeast-like organism.

**blastula** (*blas'-tū-la*). Early stage in development of fertilized ovum.

**BLB mask.** Designed by Boothby, Lovelace and Bulbulian of the Mayo Clinic for oxygen administration.

**bleb** (*bleb*). *See* BLISTER.

**bleeder.** *See* HAEMOPHILIA.

**bleeding time.** The duration of bleeding following puncture of the skin.

**blennophthalmia** (*blen'-of-thal'-mi-a*). Mucoid discharge from the eye.

**blennorrhoea** (*blen-ō-rē'-a*). Mucous discharge from urethra.

**blepharadenitis** (*ble-far-a-de-nī-tis*). Inflammation of the Meibomian glands. Terms commencing 'blephar' refer to the eyelids.

**blepharitis** (*ble-fa-rī-tis*). Inflammation of the eyelids.

**blepharoptosis** (*ble-fa-rop-tō'-sis*). *See* PTOSIS.

**blepharospasm** (*ble-fa-rō-spazm*). *See* BLINKING.

**blind-loop syndrome** (*blīnd loop sin'-drōm*). Disconnection of a loop of small intestine from alimentary tract mainstream which causes a decrease in fat absorption from intestine.

**blindness** (*blind-nes*). Lack of sight. *Colour b.*, an inability to distinguish certain colours. *Cortical b.*, blindness due to a lesion of the visual centre in the brain. *Night b.*, or nyctalopia, vision subnormal at night, thought to be due to a deficiency of vitamin A in the diet. *Snow b.*, dimness of vision with pain and lacrimation due to the glare of sunlight upon the snow. *Word b.*, inability to recognize familiar written words owing to a lesion of the brain.

**blind spot** (*blīnd*). Point where the optic nerve enters the retina.

**blinking** (*blin-king*). Normal spasmodic closure of eyelids. Increased frequency commonly due to a foreign body in the eye.

**blister** (*bli-ster*). Usually refers to collection of fluid in or under the epidermis. Blisters greater than 5 mm in diameter are termed bullae; those smaller are termed vesicles.

**blood** (*blud*). Fluid circulating through blood vessels which serves as a transport system for oxygen, food materials, waste products, etc. It may be divided into cellular and non-cellular components. The cellular component consists of the red blood cells (RBCs or erythrocytes) and a smaller number of white cells (leucocytes). The non-cellular component (plasma) is a complex solution containing many proteins. One of these, fibrinogen, is important in the blood-clotting mechanism and can be removed by allowing the plasma to clot. This leaves the *serum* which contains albumin and globulins.

**blood-brain barrier** (*blud-brān ba-ri-er*). Term used to denote the fact that a number of substances which are found in the blood do not appear in the cerebrospinal fluid. Apart from academic interest, it is important as some antibiotic drugs are unable to cross the blood-brain barrier.

**blood casts** (*blud kahsts*). Small shreds of coagulated blood present in the urine in renal injury.

**blood cells** (*blud sells*). Usually divided into red blood cells (RBCs or erythrocytes) and white blood cells (WBCs or leucocytes). The RBCs are biconcave in shape and measure about 7 microns in diameter. They have no nuclei and contain haemoglobin. The WBCs are divided into three groups: (1) Cells which contain granules in the cytoplasm; these are classed as basophil, neutrophil or eosinophil (acidophil) granulocytes according to the staining of the granules. (2) Lymphocytes, which have an even nucleus and relatively little clear cytoplasm. (3) Monocytes, relatively large cells with kidney-shaped nuclei. The function of the RBCs is to transport oxygen. The function of the various WBCs is in the defence of the body against infection by phagocytosis and the production of antibodies.

**blood coagulation** (*blud kō-a-gū-lā-shon*). Clotting of blood is essential to prevent the loss of this vital fluid when blood vessels are injured. About twelve factors are known to influence clotting. When one or more of these factors are missing, the clotting mechanism fails as, for instance, in haemophilia, Christmas disease, afibrinogenaemia.

**blood colour index** (*blud ku-la in-deks*). This is a measure of the mean haemoglobin content of a single RBC. It is obtained by dividing the haemoglobin percentage by the number of RBCs per mm³ expressed as a percentage of the normal figure of five million.

**blood count** (*blud kownt*). By the use of special dilution techniques and a counting chamber the number of cells in a sample of blood may be estimated by microscopic examination. The figure is expressed as the number of cells per mm³. The normal range is approximately 5 million RBCs, and 5 to 10 thousand WBCs. In a *differential* count, the numbers of different types of WBC *see above*, are expressed as a percentage of the total WBC count.

**blood destruction.** The normal processes of destruction of old blood cells occur in the spleen. Abnormal destruction of RBCs may take place in the blood vessels and this is known as haemolysis. *See* HAEMOLYTIC.

**blood dyscrasias** (*blud dis-kra'-zi-ahs*). Any abnormal features of the blood cells.

**blood formation** (*blud for-mā'-shon*). Except in infants and in certain disease states the blood cells are manufactured in the bone marrow. Some lymphocytes are produced by lymphoid tissue (lymph glands).

**blood grouping** (*blud groo-ping*). For a blood transfusion it is essential that the blood of the donor be compatible with that of the patient. Blood grouping is decided according to the presence or absence of certain agglutinogens in the corpuscles, two in number, A and B. The international nomenclature of the different groups is as follows: AB, A, B, O. In Group AB are those who may receive blood from any other group and are called universal recipients. Group A may receive blood from Groups A and O. Group B may receive blood from Groups B and O. Group O may receive only from Group O. From the above it will be seen that Group O can give blood to all other groups, and therefore is a universal donor. Before transfusion a direct match is always made between the red cells of the donor and the serum of the recipient. Any clumping together or agglutination of the corpuscles which can be seen even with the naked eye means incompatibility. *The Rhesus (Rh) Factor.* In human beings of most races 85 per cent possess this agglutinogen in their red cells, and are termed 'Rh positive'. The remaining 15 per cent, 'Rh negative', are liable to form an antibody (agglutinin) against the agglutinogen, if it is introduced into their circulation. It may occur in an 'Rh negative' woman if she becomes pregnant with a fetus whose blood cells are 'Rh positive' or if an 'Rh negative' person is transfused with 'Rh positive' blood. *Other blood groups* include M, N, P, Lewis, Duffy, Kell, Lutheran, etc.

**bloodless operation** (*blud'-les o-pe-rā'-shon*). An operation unaccompanied by loss of blood. In the case of operation on a limb the blood is expelled from the part operated upon by raising the limb and applying a tourniquet or by applying an elastic bandage.

**blood-letting** (*blud le-ting*). Bleeding, phlebotomy, venesection. The withdrawal of blood for therapeutic purposes from a vein.

**blood plasma.** *See* PLASMA.

**blood platelets** (*blud plāt-lets*). These are small fragmentary bodies produced by the breakdown of special cells, megakaryocytes, in the bone marrow. Platelets are important in initiation of clotting in blood vessels.

**blood pressure** (*blud pre-sher*). The pressure exerted by the blood in the vessels in which it is contained. It is taken in the brachial artery and estimated in terms of the number of millimetres pressure of mercury required, on the upper arm, just to obliterate the pulse at the wrist. This figure is the *systolic b. pressure.* The average systolic pressure in a young adult is 100–120. The *diastolic b. pressure* is the pressure in the artery during the resting phase of the cardiac cycle, *i.e.* the lowest pressure. The average diastolic pressure is 70 to 90 in a young adult. It rises with age. High blood pressure is present in arteriosclerosis, and some kinds of kidney and heart disease.

**blood sedimentation rate** (*blud se-di-men-tā-shon rāt*). Also called erythrocyte sedimentation rate (ESR). It is a measure of the rate at which red cells clump together. Clumping of RBCs, and therefore a raised sedimentation rate, is increased by the presence of certain proteins in the blood. The test is a non-specific index of disease.

**blood serum** (*blud sā-rum*). See SERUM.

**blood sugar** (*blud shoo-ger*). The amount of sugar normally in the blood is about 0·08 to 0·12 per cent or 4·6 to 7·0 mmol/l of blood. This figure rises slightly after a meal, but not to more than about 10 mmol/l and returns to a normal level within 2 hours. Above this figure, sugar leaks through into the urine. The amount in the blood can be raised artificially by a meal of glucose; and the blood sugar is raised in diabetes mellitus.

**blood transfusion** (*blud tranz-fū'-zhon*). The transference of blood from a healthy individual to one suffering from a grave degree of anaemia due to either haemorrhage or disease. The donor must be free from syphilis, and his blood must belong to the same or to a compatible group. *See* BLOOD GROUPING. Clotting is prevented by the addition of 3·8 per cent sodium citrate solution. The blood is taken from a suitable vein of the arm; the quantity is usually 1 pint. This is allowed to flow from the needle in the arm, along a piece of short tubing into a vacuum bottle containing citrate solution; all needles and tubing have previously been run through with citrate solution. The blood is injected into the patient by (1) the closed method, through a thick hollow needle into the vein, (2) the vein of the patient is cut down upon, isolated and lifted; an incision is made into it, a small cannula slipped into the opening and tied there. The blood is then slowly run in from a giving set through a drip cannula. After the cannula in the arm is withdrawn, the vein is tied above and below and the skin incision closed.

**blood urea** (*blud ū-rē-ah*). Normally between 2·5 to 6·6 mmol/l of blood, rising to a higher figure with increasing age. An abnormal amount of urea present usually shows deficient kidney function.

**blood volume** (*blud vo-lŭm*). The calculated amount of blood in the whole body.

About 8 pints or 4½ litres in the normal adult.

**blue baby.** Cyanosed infant due to circulatory defects which prevent adequate oxygenation of the blood, or which mix venous and arterial blood.

**blue-dome cyst** (*bloo-dōm sist*). A bluish-coloured benign cyst which appears in the female breast at age 40–50, associated with fibrous overgrowth of surrounding stroma.

**blue line.** Present on gums in lead poisoning.

**blue sclerotics** (*skle-ro'-tiks*). Blue colour of sclerotics, characteristic of imperfect osteogenesis (fragilitas ossium), a disease of bone found in children.

**BMR.** Abbreviation for basal metabolic rate. *See* BASAL METABOLISM.

**BNA.** Abbreviation for *Basle Nomina Anatomica*. Naming of anatomical terms agreed in Switzerland in 1895.

**Bodecker index** (*bō'-de-ker in-deks*). The ratio between the number of tooth surfaces (five to a tooth) which are carious and the total number of surfaces of the teeth which could be affected.

**body rocking.** One of a variety of rhythmic movements seen in infancy and childhood. Occurs most commonly in children deprived of an adequate feeling of security.

**Boeck's disease** (*berks di-sēz*). *See* SARCOIDOSIS.

**Böhler's iron** (*ber'-lerz īr-en*). Metal heel incorporated into leg plaster.

**boil** (*boyl*). Furuncle. A staphylococcal infection of the skin, causing inflammation round a hair follicle.

**bolus** (*bō-lus*). A large round mass such as that of food before it is swallowed.

**bomb.** Container for radioactive material, *e.g.* cobalt bomb, used to enable the beams of radiation to be directed accurately.

**bone** (*bōn*). Hard material forming the skeleton. It is made up of organized connective tissue in which calcium salts are deposited.

**bone graft** (*bōn grahft*). A portion of bone is transplanted to remedy a defect.

**bone marrow** (*bōn ma-rō*). Fatty substance contained within the marrow cavity of bones. In the flat bones, and with children in the long bones as well, the fat is replaced by active blood-forming tissue, which is responsible for production of the granular leucocytes, the red cells and platelets. *B.m.*

*puncture.* Method by which specimen of blood-forming marrow tissue is obtained. The bone is punctured and a specimen of marrow cells withdrawn through a needle.

**Bonnevie-Ullrich syndrome** (*bo'-ne-vi' ool'-rik sin'-drōm*). Congenital short stature with multiple ectodermal defects, pterygium colli, lymphoedema of hands and feet, and bone and muscle hypoplasia.

**borborygmus** (*bor-bo-rig'-mus*). Rumbling of intestinal flatus.

**Bordet Genjou bacillus** (*bor-dā gen-jew ba-si-lus*). The haemophilus pertussis causing whooping cough.

**Bornholm disease** (*bawn-hōm di-sēz*). Epidemic diaphragmatic pleurodynia.

**boss** (*bos*). A projection.

**Botallo's foramen** (*bot-al-ōs faw-rā-men*). The foramen ovale in the interatrial septum of the fetal heart.

**botulism** (*bo-tū-lism*). Food poisoning by *Bacillus botulinus.* Usually fatal.

**bougie** (*boo'-je*). Instrument used to dilate passages.

**bougienage** (*boo'-ji-nahj*). Dilation of a structure by bougie.

**bouillon** (*boo-i-yo*). (1) A broth or soup. (2) A liquid nutritive medium for culture purposes.

**bowel** (*bow'-el*). The intestine.

The gut. It consists of the small and large intestine. The small intestine is about 6·1 m long and divided into: (*a*) *Duodenum,* 30 cm long; (*b*) *Jejunum*, about 2·4 m long; (*c*) *Ileum*, about 3·65 m long. The large intestine is about 152 cm long and consists of: (1) the *Caecum* (*sē-kum*) with the *Vermiform appendix;* (2) *Ascending colon*, running up the right side; (3) *Transverse colon*, running from right to left; (4) *Descending colon*, running down left side; (5) *Sigmoid* or *Pelvic colon*, passing to (6) *Rectum* which opens externally via (7) the *Anal canal.*

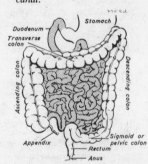

*3. The bowel*

**Bowen's disease** (*bo-wens di-sēz*). A type of intra-epidermal carcinoma.

**bow-leg** (*bō-leg*). Genu varum.

**Bowman's capsules** (*bō-mans kap-sūls*). Malpighian capsules which surround glomeruli in the kidney. *See* MALPIGHIAN CORPUSCLE.

**BP.** 1. Blood pressure. 2. British Pharmacopoeia. *See* FORMULARY.

**B.P.C.** British Pharmaceutical Codex.

**brachial** (*brā-ki-al*). Pertaining to the arm. *B. artery*, the main artery of the arm; it is a continuation of the axillary artery. *B. plexus*, the plexus of nerves supplying the arm, forearm, and hand. *B. neuralgia. Syn.* brachial neuritis. Pain in arm due to pressure on the roots of the brachial plexus. Comparable with sciatica in the leg.

**brachium** (*brā'-ki-um*). The arm.

**brachycephaly** (*bra-ki-ke-fa-li*). Descriptive of shape of head in which the anteroposterior diameter is relatively short. Principally of anthropological interest but may be of some importance in obstetrics.

**bradycardia** (*bra-di-kar'-di-a*). Slow heart beat.

**bradykinin** (*bra'-di-kī-nin*). Peptide formed by enzymatic degradation of protein.

**brain** (*brān*). The main integrating mass of nervous tissue situated in the skull. It may be divided into cerebral hemispheres, cerebellum and brain stem.

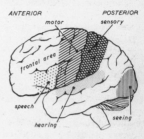

*4. The brain*

**branchial** (*bran'-ki-al*). Pertaining to the gills. Thus *B. cysts* are sometimes found in certain regions of the neck as vestiges of the gill stage of fetal development.

**Braun's splint** (*brawnz splint*). Type of lower limb splint with extension frame.

**breast** (*brest*). (1) The milk-secreting gland. (2) The anterior surface of the thorax. *See* MAMMAE.

**breath** (*breth*). Air taken into and expelled from the lungs. *B. of life*. Kiss of life. Mouth-to-mouth respiration used as a resuscitatory measure. *B. sounds*, the sounds heard by auscultation of the chest during respiration.

**breath holding.** A behaviour

disorder of infants and children.

**breathing exercises** (*brē-thing ek-ser-sī-zes*). Physiotherapy to improve ventilation of lungs.

**breech** (*brēch*). The buttocks. *B. presentation*, presentation of buttocks of fetus.

**bregma.** *See* FONTANELLE.

**Brenner tumour** (*bren'-er tū-mer*). Fibromatous ovarian tumour with epithelial cells generally benign.

**Bright's disease** (*brītz di-sēz*). Kidney disease, now classified as Type II nephritis characterized by albumin in the urine and oedema.

**Brill's disease** (*brilz di-sēz*). Typhus fever, appearing after long latent period following infection.

**brittle bones** (*bri-tel bōns*). Osteogenesis imperfecta (fragilitas ossium). A bone disease characterized by bones which break easily. It is often associated with blue sclerotics.

**Broadbent's sign** (*brawd-bents sīn*). Retraction of the lower left part of the chest wall when the pericardium is adherent.

**broad ligaments** (*brawd li-ga-ments*). The folds of peritoneum with the contained ligaments, blood vessels, Fallopian tubes, etc., which pass outwards on each side of the uterus.

**Broca's area** (*brō-kers ār-i-a*). On left side of brain exercising control of movement of lips, tongue and vocal cords, and therefore the motor speech area. *See* APHASIA.

**Broder's classification** (*brō-derz klas'-i-fi-kā-shun*). Classification for malignant tumours, where the degree of malignancy is shown by the degree to which cells are differentiated.

**Brodie's abscess** (*brō-dis ab-ses*). Chronic abscess of bone. The tibia is most commonly affected.

**bromidrosis** (*bro-mi-drō-sis*). Offensive sweating, most common in the feet.

**bromism** (*brō'-mizm*). Poisoning by bromides.

**bronchi** (*bron-kī*) (sing. **bronchus**). Tubes into which the trachea divides.

**bronchial breathing** (*bron-ki-al brē-thing*). Abnormal breath sounds heard on auscultation over diseased lung.

**bronchial carcinoma** (*bron-ki-al kar-si-nō'-mer*). Cancer arising from the lining of a bronchus.

**bronchial tubes** (*bron-ki-al tūbs*). *See* BRONCHI.

**bronchiectasis** (*bron'-ki-ek'-ta-sis*). Pathological dilatation of bronchi.

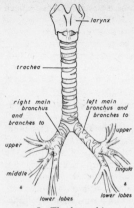

larynx

trachea

right main bronchus and branches to

left main bronchus and branches to

upper

upper

middle

lingula

&

&

lower lobes

lower lobes

5. *The bronchi*

**bronchiocele** (*bron'-ki-ō-sēl*). A local dilatation of a bronchiole.

**bronchiole** (*bron'-ki-ōl*). A small bronchus.

**bronchiolitis** (*bron-kē-o-lī-tis*). Inflammation of the bronchioles.

**bronchitis** (*bron-kī'-tis*). Inflammation of the bronchial tubes.

**bronchocele** (*bron'-ko-sēl*). A diverticulum of a bronchus.

**bronchogenic** (*bron-kō-je'-nik*). Originating from a bronchus.

**bronchography** (*bron-ko-gra-fē*). Instillation of radio-opaque dye in the bronchi, so that they are apparent on x-ray.

**broncholith** (*bron-kō-lith*). A bronchial calculus.

**bronchophony** (*brong-ko'-fo-ni*). Voice resonance heard over bronchi.

**broncho-pneumonia** (*bron-kō-nū-mō'-ni-a*). Pneumonia, beginning in the bronchioles, affecting scattered lobules of the lung and also the finest or capillary bronchioles.

**bronchoscope** (*bron'-kō-skōp*). An instrument for seeing into the main bronchi.

**bronchoscopy** (*bron-kos'-kō-pi*). Examination of the bronchi with a bronchoscope.

**bronchospasm** (*bron-kō-spasm*). Spasm of the muscles in the bronchial walls, usually associated with copious secretion of mucus into the bronchi, results of respiratory difficulty.

**bronchospirometry** (*bron-kō-spi-ro'-me-tri*). Method of assessing the function of each lung separately by passing a catheter down the trachea into the right or left main bronchus.

**brow presentation.** Presentation of brow of fetus.

**Brown's splints** (*brownz splints*). Metal splints for correction of talipes equinovarus.

**Brownian movement** (*brow-ni-an moov-ment*). Oscillatory movement seen under the microscope in fine particles suspended in a liquid.

**Brown-Séquard syndrome.** Complex neurological syndrome resulting from damage to one half of the spinal cord.

**Brucella abortus** (*broo-se-ler a-bor'-tus*). Organism causing brucellosis. It causes abortion in cows and is present in the milk of infected cows. Similar organisms are present in infected goat's milk.

**brucellosis** (*broo-se-lō-sis*). Undulant fever. It is an infection with an organism of the Brucella group.

**Brudzinski's sign** (*broo-dzin-skis sīn*). Passive flexion of the thigh causes spontaneous flexion of the opposite thigh. Sign of meningeal irritation.

**bruise** (*brooz*). A contusion. The skin is not broken but is discoloured due to bleeding in the underlying tissues.

**bruit** (*broo-ē'*). The French for 'sound', used with regard to the sounds heard in auscultation.

**Brunhilde virus** (*broon-hil-de vī'-rus*). A strain of poliomyelitis virus. Others are Lansing and Leon strains.

**Brunner's glands** (*broo-ners glans*). Glands of the duodenum.

**bubo** (*bū'-bō*). Inflammatory swelling of lymph glands, particularly of groin.

**bubonic plague** (*bū-bo-nik plāg*). Oriental plague, which in some forms is characterized by the development of buboes.

**buccal** (*buk-kal*). Pertaining to the mouth.

**buccinator** (*buk'-sin-ā-tor*). The muscle of the cheek; one of the muscles of mastication.

**Budd-Chiari syndrome** (*bud ki-ah'-ri sin'-drōm*). Syndrome consisting of vomiting, jaundice and enlargement of the liver and ascites due to thrombosis of the hepatic vein.

**Buerger's disease** (*ber-gerz dis-ēz*). Thrombo-angiitis obliterans. Rare disease of blood vessels resulting in reduction of blood supply to extremities.

**buffer.** A substance stabilizing changes in the pH of a solution.

**Buffy coat** (*bu-fi kōt*). Name given to a layer of blood cells obtained by a standard centrifuging technique. Most of the cells are white blood cells and these are used in tissue culture techniques.

**bulb.** A rounded expansion of an organ.

**bulbar palsy** (*bul'-ba pawl'-zē*).

Paralysis due to disease of medulla oblongata.

**bulimia** (*bū-li'-mi-a*). Abnormal hunger.

**bullae** (*boo-lē*). Large blisters, *cf.* vesicles.

**bundle branch block** (*bun-del brahnch blok*). Term applied to ECG evidence of delay in conduction in either the left or right branch of the auriculo-ventricular bundle.

**bundle of His.** *See* AURICULO-VENTRICULAR BUNDLE.

**bunion** (*bun'-yon*). Inflammation of a bursa situated over the metatarsophalangeal joint of the great toe.

**burette** (*būr-et*). Graduated tube with a tap which allows measured volumes of a reagent to be dispensed.

**Burkitt's tumour** (*ber'-kits tūmer*). Lymphoma, especially of jaws, retroperitoneal area and larger glands. Occurs in high altitude, high temperature and high humidity areas of Central Africa, New Guinea and Columbia. First human malignancy for which there is evidence of a viral origin.

**burns** (*berns*). Burns may be produced by various physical and chemical agents. They may be local or widespread and are classified according to the depth of tissue destruction. (1) First degree burns involve only the epidermis. (2) Second degree burns involve dermis and epidermis. (3) Third degree burns extend into deep structures. *cf.* scald.

**Burns-Marshall technique** (*berns-mah-shal tek-nēk*). Method of delivering a breech presentation.

**burr hole** (*ber hōl*). Circular hole cut in cranium to allow access to the brain.

**bursa** (*ber'-ser*). A small sac interposed between movable parts.

**bursitis** (*ber-sī'-tis*). Inflammation of a bursa.

**buttock** (*bu-tok*). Breech. Nates.

**byssinosis** (*bi-si-nō'-sis*). A type of pneumoconiosis caused by inhalation of cotton dust.

## C

**cachet** (*ka'-shā*). Capsule in which powders of disagreeable taste are enclosed.

**cachexia** (*kā-kek'-si-a*). A chronic state of malnutrition and debility produced by absorption of toxins.

**cadaver** (*ka-da-ver*). A corpse.

**caeco-sigmoidostomy** (*sē'-kō-sig-mōy-dos'-to-mi*). Operation for establishing direct communication between the caecum and sigmoid colon.

**caecostomy** (*sē-kos'-to-mi*).

Operation to provide an opening into the caecum through the abdominal wall.

**caecum** (*sē'-kum*). The blind intestine, a cul-de-sac at the commencement of the large intestine. *See* BOWEL and APPENDIX VERMIFORMIS.

**caesarean section** (*se-za'-rē-an sek'-shon*). Delivery of the fetus through an incision in the abdominal and uterine walls.

**café-au-lait pallor** (*ka-fā-oh-lā pa-lor*). Curious pallor resembling milky coffee, characteristic of subacute bacterial endocarditis.

**caffeine** (*kaf'-fēn*). The alkaloid of coffee and tea; a cerebral stimulant and diuretic.

**Caisson disease** (*kā-son di-sēz*). Also known as 'the bends'. Is the effect on those working under a greater atmospheric pressure than normal, *e.g.* in deep mines or under water. Return to normal pressure should be effected gradually or nitrogen bubbles form in the blood and tissues.

**calcaneal spur** (*kal-kā-nē-al sper*). A bony outgrowth from the calcaneum leading to persistent local tenderness on the sole of the foot.

**calcaneus** (*kal-kā'-nē-us*). The os calcis or heel bone.

**calcareous** (*kal-kār-i-us*). Containing calcium phosphate.

**calciferol** (*kal-si-fe-rol*). Vitamin D. Its function is to regulate calcium metabolism.

**calcification** (*kal-si-fi-kā-shon*). Deposition of insoluble calcium salts, *e.g.* calcium phosphate, in tissue. This is normal in bone but may occur in other sites.

**calcitonin** (*kal-si-tō-nin*). Hormone which regulates blood calcium levels.

**calculus** (*kal'-kū-lus*). A stone. The term generally refers to a concretion in the urinary tract.

**Caldwell-Luc operation** (*kawl-dwel-lūk o-pe-rā-shon*). Operation to drain the maxillary antrum.

**calibrate** (*ka-li-brāt*). To graduate an instrument for measuring according to a given standard.

**calipers** or **callipers.** (*ka-li-pers*). (1) Surgical instruments for measuring the chest, the pelvis, etc. (2) *Icetong caliper*, a two-pointed instrument used for fixing a bone by actual penetration of some of it, as in the treatment of fractures. (3) *Walking caliper*, an instrument fixed at the lower end to a boot. At the upper end is a padded ring which fits round the groin and under the ischial tuberosity. This takes the weight off an injured leg when walking.

**callosity** (*ka-lo-si-ti*). Thickened horny layer of epidermis formed on palmar and plantar surfaces which are subject to much friction.

**callous** (*kal'-lus*). Hard, insensible, thickened.

**callus** (*kal-lus*). (1) Material which first joins broken bone. It consists predominantly of connective tissue and cartilage, which later calcifies. (2) Callosity.

**calor.** Heat.

**calorie** (*ka-lo-ri*). Scientific term for the standard unit of heat. One kilocalorie (C) is the amount of heat required to raise 1 litre of water by 1 degree Celsius. The amount of heat produced in the body by the combustion of food can be estimated. A diet should yield an adequate number of calories per day. One calorie (c) is the amount of heat necessary to raise 1 gram of water by 1 degree Celsius. The unit is now the joule. 1 kcal = 4·2 kJ.

**calorific** (*ka-lo-ri-fik*). Producing heat.

**calorimeter** (*ka-lo-ri-mē-ter*). An apparatus for determining the amount of heat yielded by combustion of a substance.

**calvarium** (*kal-vā-ri-um*). The upper half of the skull. The cranial vault.

**calyx** (*kā-liks*). A cup-shaped organ or cavity such as those of the recesses of the pelvis of the kidney.

**canal of Nuck.** A narrow passage along which the round ligament passes to the region of the pubes; it is sometimes the seat of inguinal hernia and occasionally of cysts.

**canaliculus** (*ka-na-li'-kū-lus*). A small canal.

**cancelli** (*kan'-se-lē*). The uncalcified spaces of bone.

**cancer** (*kan'-ser*). A malignant growth.

**cancerophobia** (*kan-ser-o-fō'-bē-a*). Excessive fear of cancer.

**cancroid** (*kan'-kroyd*). Cancer-like.

**cancrum oris** (*kan'-krum o'-ris*). Ulceration of the mouth. Has nothing to do with cancer.

**Candida** (*kan'-di-da*). A genus of fungi which may cause thrush.

**canicola fever** (*ka-ni-kō-ler fē-ver*). Disease produced by *Leptospira canicola*. Characterized by malaise, fever, muscle pains, and occasionally jaundice.

**canine teeth** (*kā-nīn tēth*). The four eye teeth, next to the incisors. *See* TEETH.

**canker** (*kang'-ker*). Ulceration.

**cannabis** (*ka'-na-bis*). Hemp, hashish.

**cannula** (*kan'-nū-la*). Surgical name for a tube used to withdraw fluid from a cavity. *See* TROCAR.

**canthus** (*kan'-thus*). The angle of the eyelids, outer or inner.

**capelline** (*kap'-e-lin*). Bandage for the head.

**Capgras' syndrome** (*cap'-grahs sin'-drōm*). Psychotic state in which patient recognizes but denies identity of person confronting him. Insists he is 'double' of that person.

**capillaries** (*ka-pi-la-rēz*). The network of microscopic vessels which communicate with the arterioles and the venules. The walls are formed of a single layer of endothelium.

**capillarity** (*ka-pi-la-ri-ti*). Effect of surface tension in causing liquid to rise up inside a small tube.

**capillary fragility test** (*ka-pi-la-ri fra-ji-li-ti test*). Fragility of capillary vessels is measured by applying suction to a small area of skin and recording the negative pressure required to produce haemorrhage. *See also* HESS'S TEST.

**capillary naevus** (*ka-pi-la-ri nē-vus*). Also known as a congenital abnormal dilatation of capillary blood vessels.

**capitate** (*ka'-pi-tāt*). (1) Like a head. (2) One of the carpal bones.

**capsular ligament** (*kap'-sū-lar lig'-a-ment*). A ligament surrounding a movable joint.

**capsule** (*kap'-sūl*). Connective tissue sheath investing an organ.

**capsulotomy** (*cap-sū-lo'-to-mi*). An incision of the capsule of the lens of the eye.

**caput succedaneum** (*suk-sē-dā-ni-um*). Swelling on infant's scalp, due to pressure during labour.

**carbohydrate** (*kar-bō-hī'-drāt*). Compound of the general formula $C_x (H_2O)_y$ such as sugar and starch. Carbohydrates are of central importance in cell metabolism.

**carbon dioxide** (*dī-ok'-sīd*). $CO_2$. A gas which is a product of combustion. It is formed in the system by the metabolic process of the body, and excreted through the lungs. It is a respiratory stimulant and is administered diluted with oxygen when respiration is depressed. At extremely low temperatures this gas forms a liquid, and lower still a substance resembling snow. The latter is often used for destroying naevi and similar superficial growths on the skin.

**carbon monoxide poisoning.** Poisoning by inhalation of carbon monoxide, CO, *e.g.* from coal gas or motor vehicle exhaust. *Symptoms* begin as giddiness and singing of ears, then lividity of face and body; later, owing to combination of the gas with the blood, the patient may have a rosy tinge; loss of muscular power; violent action of heart and lungs; fixed dilated pupils, convulsions, coma or asphyxia. *Treatment*: fresh air, oxygen and artificial respiration if necessary.

**carboxyhaemoglobin** (*kar-bok-si-hē-mō-glō'-bin*). A compound of carbon monoxide and haemoglobin formed in coal-gas poisoning.

**carbuncle** (*kar'-bunk-l*). Severe staphylococcal inflammation of an area of skin and subcutaneous tissue. There is necrosis and liquefaction of the subcutaneous tissue and several points of discharge.

**carcinogenic** (*kar-si-nō'-je'-nik*). Term applied to substances producing or predisposing to cancer.

**carcinoid tumour** (*kar-si-noyd*

*tū-mer*). *See* ARGENTAFFI-NOMA.

**carcinoma** (*kar-si-nō'-mer*). Cancer of epithelial tissue.

**carcinoma-in-situ** (*kar-si-nō-mer-in-sē-too*). Early stage of carcinoma in which the growing cells have not invaded surrounding tissues.

**carcinomatosis** (*kar-sin-ō-ma-tō-sis*). The spread of carcinomatous metastases.

**cardia** (*kar'-dē-a*). (1) The heart. (2) The aperture between the oesophagus and the stomach.

**cardiac** (*kar-di-ak*). Relating to the heart. *C. arrest.* Stopping of the heart. *C. catheterization.* Investigation carried out to diagnose certain heart conditions. A catheter is introduced through a vein in the arm into the chambers of the heart from which pressure recordings can be obtained. *C. cycle.* The recurrent train of events which produce a heart beat. *C. failure.* When the contraction of the heart is insufficient to expel a volume of blood equal to that which fills it there is a damming back of blood on the venous side of the circulation with the consequent production of the clinical signs of congestive cardiac failure (CCF). *C. massage.* Direct cardiac massage consists of squeezing the heart rhythmically to stimulate the normal heart beat in an attempt to restart the circulation, having first gained access to the heart through an incision in the chest. More recently external cardiac massage has been widely used to restart the heart. This consists of pressing on the chest with patient lying flat on his back so that the heart is rhythmically compressed between the front and back of the thoracic cage. *C. tamponade.* The action of the heart is impeded by the accumulation of fluid in the pericardium.

**cardinal** (*kar-di-nal*). Chief.

**cardinal ligaments** (*kar-di-nal li-ga-ments*). Fan-shaped fibro-muscular expansions passing from the cervix and vault of the vagina to the pelvic wall which forms part of the support of the uterus and vagina.

**cardiogram** (*kar'-di-ō-gram*). The tracing obtained by the use of the cardiograph.

**cardiograph** (*kar-di-ō-graf*). Also known as electrocardiograph (ECG or EKG). Instrument which records the electrical potentials which reflect the conduction of impulses and other electrical events in the heart.

**cardiology** (*kar-di-o'-lo-ji*). Study of the heart and circulatory diseases.

**cardiomyopathy** (*kar-di-ō-mī-o'-pa-thi*). Disease of heart muscle not caused by specific infection.

**cardiomyotomy** (*kar-di-ō-mī-o'-to-mi*). Operation to relieve muscular spasm at the lower end of the oesophagus.

**cardio-omentopexy** (*kar-di-ō-o-men-tō-pek'-si*). An operation consisting of grafting part of the omentum on to the surface of the heart. The omentum is taken through the diaphragm. The object is to provide a better blood supply in cases where the coronary circulation is deficient.

**cardiopathy** (*kar-di-o'-pa-thi*). Disease of the heart.

**cardiospasm** (*kar-di-ō-spasm*). Achalasia of cardia.

**cardiovascular** (*kar-di-ō-va'-skū-ler*). Pertaining to the heart and circulatory system.

**carditis** (*kar-dī'-tis*). Inflammation of the heart muscle.

**caries** (*kā-rēz*). Decay of teeth.

**carina** (*ka-rē-na*). Literally a 'keel'. Term sometimes applied to ridges.

**carminative** (*kar'-min-a-tiv*). A remedy for flatulence, *e.g.* oil of peppermint.

**carneous** (*kar'-nē-us*). Flesh-like.

**carneous mole** (*kar-nē-us mōl*).

Term sometimes used to describe retained products of conception.

**carotene** (*kar-o-tēn'*). A yellow pigment occurring in some plants. It is a precursor of vitamin A.

**carotid** (*ka-rot'-id*). Name given to the two great arteries of the neck, and to structures connected with them. *C. body*. Specialized tissue found at the bifurcation of the carotid artery (into internal and external carotoids) which is sensitive to chemical changes in the blood. *C. sinus*. Region of the carotid artery just below its bifurcation which is sensitive to pressure and acts as one of the blood pressure regulating mechanisms. *Carotid sinus syncope* may occur in individuals who have hypersensitive carotid sinuses; loss of consciousness may follow pressure on the sinus by an abrupt movement of the neck, etc.

**carpal tunnel syndrome** (*karpal tu-nel sin'-drōm*). Numbness and tingling in the fingers and hand as a result of compression of the median nerve at the wrist.

**carpometacarpal** (*kar-pō-meta-kar-pal*). Relating to a carpus and metacarpus.

**carpopedal spasm** (*kar-pō-pe-dal spasm*). Cramp in hands and feet which occurs typically in conditions in which there is a deficiency of ionized calcium in the blood.

**carpus** (*kar'-pus*). The wrist.

**carrier** (*ka'-ri-er*). An individual who transmits disease without showing symptoms of it. (1) Genetic defects may be masked by other genes in a carrier. (2) Micro-organisms may be harboured in the body, *e.g.* typhoid bacilli. In families with inherited diseases an unaffected female may carry the defect in her genes and if sex-linked her sons may inherit the disease and her daughters become carriers.

**cartilage** (*kar'-ti-lāj*). Gristle; a transparent substance of the body, very elastic and softer than bone.

**caruncle** (*ka-run-kl*). Small pedunculated granulomatous mass. *Lacrimal c*. The small red globe at the inner corner of the eye. *Urethral c*. Pea-sized vascular growth in the urethra which may give rise to urinary symptoms in elderly women.

**caseation** (*kā-sē-ā'-shon*). Conversion into cheesy material, as in breaking down of tuberculous glands.

**casein** (*kā-sēn*). An albuminous component of milk.

**Casoni test** (*ka-so-ni test*). Intradermal test used for the diagnosis of hydatid disease.

**Castle's factors** (*kar-sels fak'-tors*). Two factors leading to megaloblastic anaemia were described by Castle. *Intrinsic factor* is a constituent of normal gastric juice necessary for the absorption of *extrinsic factor* (vitamin $B_{12}$).

**castration** (*kas-trā-shon*). Removal of the testes, *cf.* sterilization.

**casts** (*karsts*). Pieces of material taking shape of cavity from which they have been expelled, *e.g.* blood or epithelial debris found in the urine in kidney disease, membranous casts from large bowel in mucous colitis.

**CAT scan.** *See* COMPUTERIZED AXIAL TOMOGRAPHY.

**cat scratch fever.** Fever transmitted by the scratch of apparently healthy cats. The causative organism has not been isolated.

**catabolism** (*ka-ta-bo-lism*). Biochemical reactions taking place in living tissues (metabolism) are divided into those involved in building up or synthesis of material (anabolism) and those involved in breaking down or lysis of material (catabolism).

**cataclysm** (*kat'-a-klizm*). Sudden shock; a deluge.

**catacrotic** (*ka-ta-kro-tik*). Waverings in the downward mark of the sphygmograph.

**catalepsy** (*ka-ta-lep'-si*). A period of trance, during which the limbs remain in any position in which they are placed.

**catalyst** (*ka-ta-list*). A substance which takes part in a reaction, not itself being changed. Enzymes are catalysts.

**cataphoresis** (*ka-ta-fo-rē'-sīs*). Iontophoresis consists of the introduction through the unbroken skin of ionized substances by the means of an electric current. Cataphoresis is the introduction of positively charged ions (cations) by this means.

**cataplasm** (*ka-ta-plasm*). A poultice.

**cataplexy** (*ka-ta-plek'-si*). A rigid muscular condition produced by fear or shock.

**cataract** (*ka-ta-rakt*). Opacity of the lens of the eye, causing blindness.

**catarrh** (*ka-tar'*). Inflammation of the mucous membrane, generally applied to the nose and throat, and also to internal organs, *e.g.* the bile ducts.

**catatonia** (*ka-ta-tō-ni-a*). State of generalized muscular inhibition in schizophrenia.

**catgut.** Material prepared from

sheep's intestine and used for absorbable ligatures.

**catharsis** (*ka-thar-sis*). Emotional relief brought about by the conscious realization of suppressed desire.

**cathartic** (*ka-thar'-tik*). Literally can be a drastic purge. Can also be used in sense of release of pent-up emotions.

**catheter** (*ka-the-ter*). Instrument used for the passage of fluids; usually from the bladder where there is urethral obstruction. *Nasal c.* (Ryle's tube). Used for the administration of fluid feeds. The tube passes through the nose down the throat into the stomach. *Eustachian c.* A special tube used to inflate the pharyngotympanic tube (Eustachian tube).

**cathode** (*ka-thōd*). The negative pole of an electric battery.

**cation** (*kat'-i-on*). A positive ion which in electrolysis passes to the negative electrode or cathode.

**cation exchange resin.** Resins which have a differential preference for certain cations. They are used in medical practice for purposes such as a stringent sodium-free diet. The resins are taken with the food and exchange hydrogen ions for cations in the food. These cations are then excreted with the resins in the faeces.

**cauda equina** (*kaw'-da ek-wī'-na*). The bundle of sacral and lumbar nerves at the base of the spine.

**caudal analgesia** (*kaw-dal a-nal-jē-si-a*). Regional anaesthesia of the rectum and perineum produced by injecting local anaesthetics into the sacral canal through the sacral hiatus.

**caul** (*kawl*). Fetal membranes about the face and head of some infants at birth.

**causalgia** (*kaw-sal-ji-a*). Pain referred to the distribution of a cutaneous nerve which persists long after an injury to that nerve. Causalgia often follows herpes zoster (shingles). The cause is not known.

**caustic** (*kaw-stik*). Substance, usually a strong alkali or acid, which destroys cells and causes chemical 'burns'.

**cautery** (*kaw'-ter-i*). Application of heated metal to living tissue in order to destroy it or to arrest haemorrhage.

**cavernous naevus** (*ka-vern-us nē-vus*). Abnormal development of blood vessels which are greatly enlarged and dilated.

**cavernous respiration** (*ka'-vern-us res-pī-rā'-shon*). A hollow sound, heard on auscultation, when there is a cavity in the lung.

**cavernous sinus** (*sī'-nus*). A blood sinus on the body of the sphenoid bone.

**cavernous tumour** (*ka'-ver-nus tū-mer*). Angioma.

**cavitation** (*ka-vi-tā-shon*). Process whereby cavities are formed.

**cavity of pelvis.** The space between the pelvic inlet and outlet.

**CCC.** Cathodal closing contraction.

**cell** (*sel*). Discrete mass of protoplasm bounded by a membrane which forms the basic reproducible structural unit of living organisms. There are about $10^{12}$ cells in a man. Generally speaking cells contain a *nucleus* which harbours the genetic material—the DNA blueprints—which provide the instructions for the synthesis of materials by the *cytoplasmic* component. The advent of electron microscopy has revealed the cytoplasm to be exceedingly complex. The nuclear material (which contains one or more nucleoli, the function of which is unclear) is discontinuously bounded by a double membrane which projects and branches into the cytoplasm forming a complex network of inter-

connecting canals. In places this network opens exteriorly to the cell, becoming continuous with the cell wall. The canalicular system in the cell is called the *endoplasmic reticulum* (ER) and it is thought that it is made by the *Golgi apparatus*. In some places the endoplasmic reticulum is closely associated with *ribosomes*, tiny granular structures which are the sites of protein synthesis. The cytoplasmic material between the canals of the endoplasmic reticulum contains *mitochondria* which are the centres housing the respiratory enzymes, and *lysosomes* which are specialized organelles containing catabolic enzymes.

**cellulitis** (*se-lū-lī-tis*). Inflammation of cellular tissue. Pelvic c., *see* PARAMETRITIS.

**cellulose** (*se-lū-lōs*). The woody, fibrous part of plants. It has no food value but forms bulk in the colon and so stimulates peristalsis. In the form of wood wool, cellulose is used as an absorbent dressing.

**Celsius** (*sel-si-us*). In SI units the equivalent of the centigrade scale which is now obsolete. *See* CENTIGRADE.

**censorship** (*sen-so-ship*). Freudian term for the barrier

83 **CEP**

preventing repressed memories, ideas and impulses from easily coming into consciousness.

**Centigrade** (*sen'-ti-grād*). The scale of thermometers for scientific purposes, now known as the Celsius scale; the freezing-point is 0 deg., normal body temp. 37 deg., boiling-point 100 deg. *See* p. 13 for conversion of Celsius into Fahrenheit, etc.

**centimetre** (*sen-ti-mē-ter*). Metric unit of length. One hundredth of a metre. Approximately 2½ cm equal 1 inch.

**Central Midwives Board.** The statutory authority which formerly controlled the practice of obstetrics by those who are not qualified medical practitioners.

**central nervous system** (*sen-tral ner'vus sis-tem*). Abbreviation CNS. General term incorporating the brain and spinal cord, as opposed to the *peripheral nervous system*, which includes the nerves and sensory receptors outside the brain and spinal cord.

**centrifugal nerve fibres** (*sen-tri-fūgal nerv fī-bers*). Usually called *efferent* nerves; those which conduct impulses leaving the central system.

**centrifuge** (*sen-tri-fūj*). An instrument for separating liquids of different specific gravity by rotation.

**centriole** (*sen-tri-ōl*). Small granule situated just outside the nuclear membrane and found in many resting cells. Just before mitosis this granule divides and at mitosis the two resulting centrioles move apart and form the poles of the spindle.

**centripetal nerve fibres** (*sen-tri-pē-tal nerv fibers*). Usually called *afferent* nerves; those which conduct impulses entering the central nervous system.

**centromere** (*sen-tro-mār*). Spindle-attachment. The region of the chromosome which attaches it to the spindle which is composed of long protein molecules passing between chromosomes and the centriole when the cell is dividing.

**centrosome** (*sen-trō-sōm*). Region of differentiated cytoplasm in which the centriole is situated.

**cephalhaematoma** (*kef-al-hē-ma-tō'-ma*). A subperiosteal haemorrhage on the head of an infant, usually due to pressure during a long labour. It is gradually absorbed.

**cephalic version** (*kef-al'-ik ver'-shon*). The production artificially of a cephalic presentation, from a breech presentation or transverse lie. *See also* VERSION.

**cephalocele** (*ke-fa-lō-sēl*). Hernia of the brain.

**cephalometry** (*ke-fa-lo-me-tri*). Estimation of the size of the head of a fetus, usually by radiographic means.

**cephalotribe** (*ke-fa-lō-trib*). An instrument consisting of two blades and a screw, used to crush the fetal head when intact delivery is impossible.

**cerebellum** (*se-re-be-lum*). Outgrowth from the hindbrain overlying the medulla oblongata. Concerned with the co-ordination of movement.

**cerebral cortex** (*se-re-bral kor'-teks*). Outer rim of grey matter of the brain.

**cerebral embolism** (*se-re-bral em-bo-lism*). Embolism of vessels supplying the cerebral cortex and its major connections.

**cerebral haemorrhage** (*se-re-bral he-mo-rāj*). Rupture of an artery of the brain, due to either high blood pressure or disease of artery. Escape of blood causes destruction of brain tissue, and paralysis occurs of that side of the body which is opposite to the injured side of the brain. If the haemorrhage has occurred on the left side of the brain, then speech is affected in right-handed subjects.

**cerebral palsy** (*pawl'-zē*). A condition in which the control of the motor system is affected due to a lesion in the brain resulting from a birth injury or prenatal defect. The popular term is 'spastic'.

**cerebral thrombosis** (*se-re-bral throm-bōsis*). Thrombus formation in vessels supplying the cerebral cortex or its major connections.

**cerebration** (*se-re-brā'-shon*). Thinking: activity of the brain related to conscious thought processes.

**cerebrospinal fever** (*se-re-brō-spī-nal fē-ver*). Epidemic meningitis of the brain and spinal chord, caused by the meningococcus. The fever is often accompanied by a rash; hence the popular name 'spotted fever'.

**cerebrospinal fluid** (*se-re-brō-spīnal floo'-id*). CSF. The clear watery fluid which lies in the subarachnoid space, surrounding the brain and spinal chord. It also fills the cavities or ventricle of the brain.

**cerebrovascular accident** (*se-re-brō-vas'-kū-ler ak'-si-*

*dent*). General term referring to cerebral embolism, thrombosis or haemorrhage.

**cerebrum** (*se-re-brum*). The larger part of the brain occupying the cranium. *See* BRAIN.

**cerumen** (*se-rū-men*). Secretion of the ceruminous glands situated in the external auditory meatus. The secretion is a wax-like substance closely related to sebum, the oily secretion of the sebaceous glands.

**cervical** (*ser-vī'-kal*). Pertaining to the neck or cervix of the uterus.

**cervical dystocia** (*ser-vī-kal dis-tō-si-a*). Failure of relaxation of the external os of the cervix. A rare cause of mechanical obstruction to the delivery of a child.

**cervical rib** (*ser-vī'-kal rib*). Outgrowth from the seventh cervical vertebra, passing out and down to join the rib below. It may press on nerve trunks to the arm giving rise to pins and needles in hands and fingers.

**cervical smear** (*ser-vī-kal smē-a*). Sample of mucus taken from the cervix uteri, smeared on to a glass slide and examined for the appearance of the cells it contains. *See* PAPANICOLAU STAIN.

**cervical spondylosis** (*ser-vī-kal spond-di-lō-sis*). Degenerative changes in the intervertebral discs of the cervical spine with associated secondary osteoarthritic changes in the intervertebral joints of the neck.

**cervicectomy** (*ser-vi-sek'-to-mi*). Excision of the cervix uteri.

**cervicitis** (*ser'-vi-sī-tis*). Inflammation of the cervix of the uterus.

**cervix uteri** (*ser-viks ū'-te-rī*). The neck of the uterus. The lowest third of the uterus, about 2½ cm in length. It is traversed by a canal which opens into the vagina.

**Cestoda** (*ses-tō-der*). Class of Platyhelminths: tapeworms.

**CFT.** Complement fixation test.

**chalazion** (*ka-lā-zi-on*). Meibomian cyst. A small retention cyst in the eyelid, due to blocking of a meibomian follicle.

**chancre** (*shang'-ker*). Syphilitic ulcer of the first stage; occurs at the site of infection. Contagious.

**chancroid** (*shang-kroyd*). A venereal ulcer due to infection by *Haemophilus ducreyi*.

**change of life.** Popular term for the menopause.

**character** (*ka-rak-ter*). Applied to a person's mental features and according to which his actions are unique and individual to that person.

**Charcot's joint** (*shar-kōs joynt*). Painless destructive changes in a joint due to loss of sensation.

**Charcot-Marie-Tooth disease** (*shar-kō-ma-rē-tooth di-sēz*). Peroneal muscular atrophy. A familial condition of unknown cause in which there is atrophy of the spinal nerves and neuritis affecting the peroneal nerves with resultant wasting of the muscles of the feet and lower legs. The hands may also be affected.

**Chediak-Higashi syndrome** (*che'-di-ak hi-gash-i sin'-drōm*). Anomalies of leucocytes with azurophil granules in cytoplasm. Associated with fatal form of granulocytopenia. Autosomal recessive inheritance. Death is usually in childhood.

**cheilitis** (*kī-lī-tis*). Inflammation of the lip.

**cheiloplasty** (*kī-lo-plas-ti*). Plastic operation on the lips.

**cheilosis** (*kī-lō-sis*). Condition affecting the lips and angles of the mouth which can be caused by riboflavin deficiency.

**cheiropompholyx** (*kī-rō-pom'-fo-liks*). An eczematous eruption on the hands characterized by the appearance of tense vesicles.

**chelating agent** (*kē-lā-ting ā-jent*). Substance which forms a complex with metals, thus rendering them chemically inactive.

**chemoreceptor** (*ke-mō-rē-sep-tor*). Nerve-ending capable of detecting and differentiating substances according to their chemical structure by contact with the molecules of the substances, *e.g.* taste, smell.

**chemosis** (*kē-mō'-sis*). Oedema of the conjunctiva.

**chemotaxis** (*ke-mo-tak'-sis*). Tendency for cells to move through a chemical gradient.

**chemotherapy** (*ke-mō-the-ra-pi*). Healing by chemical means, administration of drugs.

**chemotropism** (*ke-mō-trō-pism*). Syn. chemotaxis.

**cherubism** (*che'-roo-bizm*). Genetically determined condition in which cysts, arising in infancy in maxilla and mandible, regress in later life.

**Cheyne-Stokes breathing** (*chān-stokes brē'-thing*). Irregular respiration, at first shallow, then increasing in depth till a maximum is reached, when it decreases again until imperceptible and a pause ensues, during which breathing is absent. Usually a bad sign, and due to a poor supply of oxygen to that part of the brain containing the respiratory centre.

**chiasm** (*kī-asm*). A crossing.

**chiasma opticum** (*kī-as-ma op'-ti-kum*). Also called optic chiasm. Site at which there is a partial exchange of fibres between the optic nerves. It is situated close to the pituitary and is often affected by tumours of the pituitary gland.

**chicken-pox** (*chi'-ken poks*). A virus disease. Varicella. Rash appears on the chest on the first day; the disease runs its course in a fortnight. Incubation period 10 to 16 days. Quarantine period for contacts, 20 days.

**chilblain** (*chil-blān*). Pernio. Inflammation of the skin due to cellular damage as a result of local deficiency in the circulation.

**chimera** (*kī-mā-ra*). Organism whose tissues are composed of cells of two or more genetically different sorts.

**chiropodist** (*kī-ro'-pō-dist*). One qualified in the treatment of the feet and hands.

**chirurgical** (*ki-rur'-ji-kal*). Surgical.

**chloasma** (*klō-az'-ma*). Usually *chloasma gravidarum*. A patchy hyperpigmentation of face associated with pregnancy.

**chloroform** (*klo-rō-form*). Anaesthetic agent. In disrepute since it may cause sudden cardiac arrest and liver damage.

**chloroma** (*klo-rō-ma*). A green-coloured sarcoma especially affecting the bones of the skull.

**choana** (*ko-ā-na*). An opening like a funnel such as one of the posterior nasal openings.

**cholaemia** (*ko-lē-mi-a*). Lit. bile in the blood.

**cholagogue** (*ko-la-gog*). Preparation reputed to increase flow of bile.

**cholangiogram** (*kō-lan-jē-o-gram*). X-ray showing the biliary system.

**cholangitis** (*kō-lan-jī'-tis*). Inflammation of the biliary system.

**cholecystectomy** (*ko'-lē-sis-tek'-to-mi*). Removal of the gall bladder.

**cholecystenterostomy** (*ko'-lē-sis-ten-ter-os'-to-mi*). Operation for forming an artificial communication between the gall bladder and the intestine.

**cholecystitis** (*ko'-lē-sis-tī'-tis*). Inflammation of the gall bladder.

**cholecystography** (*ko-lē-sis-tog'-ra-fi*). Radiographic examination of the gall bladder and bile duct by the introduction of a radio-opaque substance which is usually ingested some time before the procedure is undertaken.

**cholecystolithiasis** (kō-lē-sis-toŏ-li-thī'-a-sis). Removal of a stone from the gall bladder.

**cholecystostomy** (ko'-lē-sis-tos'-to-mi). Operation for making the gall bladder open to the exterior.

**choledocholithotomy** (ko-lē-dok-ō-li-tho-to-mē). Incision of the common bile duct for the removal of gallstone.

**choledochotomy** (ko-lē-do-ko-to-mi). Incision of the common bile duct.

**cholelithiasis** (ko-lē-li-thī'-a-sis). Formation of gallstones.

**cholemesis** (kō-le-me-sis). Vomiting of bile.

**cholera** (ko'-le-rer). Epidemic tropical disease due to infection by the cholera vibrio.

**cholesteatoma** (ko-lē-stē-a-tō'-mer). Small tumour containing fat-like material which occasionally is found in the external auditory meatus.

**cholesterol** (ko-les'-te-rol). A sterol widespread in animal tissues, first isolated from bile. One of the substances which on precipitation gives rise to gallstones.

**choline** (kō-lēn). An organic base which is a constituent of some important substances, e.g. phospholipids, acetylcholine.

**cholinergic** (kō-li-ner-jik). Nerves which release acetylcholine as a transmitter substance.

**cholinesterase** (kō-li-nes-te-rāz). Specific or acetylcholinesterase: an enzyme found at motor end-plates and other sites, which breaks down and inactivates acetylcholine. Non-specific or pseudocholinesterases are found in the blood.

**choluria** (ko-lū-ri-a). Bile in the urine.

**chondralgia** (kon-dral-ji-a). Pain in cartilage.

**chondrin** (kon'-drin). Cartilaginous tissue.

**chondritis** (kon-drī-tis). Inflammation of cartilage.

**chondroma** (kon-drō'-mer). Benign tumour of cartilage cells.

**chordae tendineae** (kor-dē ten-di-ni-ē). Thin musculotendinous bands extending between the walls of the ventricles of the heart and the tricuspid and mitral valves.

**chordee** (kor-dē'). Painful erection of penis, common in gonorrhoea.

**chorditis** (kor-dī-tis). Inflammation of the vocal cords.

**chordotomy** (kor-do-to-mi). Division of an anterolateral column of the spinal cord.

**chorea** (ko-rē-a). Huntington's

*c.* Dominantly inherited disease with an incidence of about 6 per 100,000 of the population. The disorder does not manifest itself till the age of about 40 and begins with choreiform movements with progressive dementia. *Sydenham's c.,* also known as St. Vitus' dance. It is a disease of children associated with rheumatic fever which is characterized by involuntary movements.

**chorion** (*ko'-ri-on*). Layer enclosing embryonic structures and forming the placenta. *C. epithelioma.* Malignant tumour arising from chorion.

**chorionic villi** (*ko'-ri-o-nik vi-lī*). Vascular processes developing on the external surfaces of the chorion.

**choroid** (*ko'-royd*). The posterior five-sixths of the middle coat of the eye, containing blood-vessels and pigment. It lies between the retina and the sclerotic.

**choroid plexus** (*ko-royd plek-sus*). Specialized vascular epithelium which produces the cerebrospinal fluid. One choroid plexus is situated in each of the four ventricles of the brain.

**choroiditis** (*ko-roy-dī-tis*). Inflammation of the choroid.

**choroidocyclitis** (*ko-roy-dō-sī-klī-tis*). Inflammation of the choroid and ciliary body.

**Christmas disease** (*kris'mas di-sēz*). Rare defect of blood coagulation.

**chromatography** (*krō-ma-tog'-ra-fi*). Separation of components of a mixture by their physical properties.

**chromatosis** (*krō-ma-tō-sis*). Abnormal pigmentation.

**chromophil adenoma** (*krō'-mō-fil a-de-nō-ma*). Anterior pituitary tumour.

**chromophobe adenoma** (*krō'-mō-fōb a-de-nō-ma*). Posterior pituitary tumour.

**chromosomes** (*krō-mō-sōmz*). When a cell divides, the genetic material present in the nucleus becomes segregated into thread-shaped bodies which are visible under the microscope. These are known as chromosomes and consist of connected strands of DNA molecules known as genes. In man there are forty-six chromosomes per cell: twenty-two pairs of *autosomes* and two *sex chromosomes*; females have two X chromosomes, males one X and one Y. The Y chromosome is shorter than the X chromosome.

**chronic** (*kro-nik*). A lengthy disease, reverse of acute.

**Chvostek's sign** (*shfos-teks sīn*).

A spasm of the facial muscles produced by tapping the facial nerve. This sign is present in tetany.

**chyle** (*kīl*). Lymph draining from the villi of the small intestine.

**chylomicron** (*kī-lō-mī'-kron*). Tiny emulsified droplets of neutral fat which are absorbed into the lymphatics of the small intestine.

**cicatrical** (*si-ku-tri-shal*). Pertaining to a scar, or cicatrix.

**cicatrix** (*si-ku-triks*). The scar of a healed wound or ulcer.

**cilia** (*si-li-er*). Fine protoplasmic threads projecting from the surface of a cell which beat in a constant direction moving material surrounding it.

**ciliary body** (*si'-li-a-ri bo'-di*). Consists of the ciliary muscle and processes, forming part of the middle coat of the eye.

**ciliated epithelium** (*si-li-ā-ted e-pi-thē'-li-um*). Epithelial cells with cilia forming the lining of certain tubes, *e.g.* respiratory passages.

**cimex lectularius** (*sē-meks lek-tū-lā-rē-us*). The common bed-bug.

**cinchonism** (*sin'-ko-nizm*). Intolerance to quinine, indicated by buzzing in the ears, nausea, vomiting.

**circa** (*ser-ker*). About.

**circadian** (*ser-kā-di-an*). Relating to 24-hour cycle of physiological events.

**circinate** (*ser-ki-nāt*). Ring-shaped.

**circle of Willis** (*ser-kel of wi-lis*). Circular intercommunication of arteries supplying the brain.

**circulation** (*ser-kū-lā'-shon*). *See* HEART. *Systemic or General circulation.* Arterial blood received into the left atrium passes through the mitral valve to the left ventricle. It then passes into the aorta and through its smaller branches to the capillaries, into small veins, then larger, until on reaching the superior and inferior venae cavae it passes into the right atrium. *Pulmonary circulation.* The venous blood which is received into the right atrium passes through the tricuspid valve into the right ventricle. From there into the pulmonary artery, which divides into two branches, one going to each lung. The artery divides in the lung into capillaries, and here the blood by means of the haemoglobin in the red cells takes up oxygen from the inspired air. Oxygenated blood returns to the heart by the four pulmonary veins, two from each lung, entering the left atrium. *Portal circulation.* Veins

91 **CLA**

from the pancreas, spleen, stomach, intestines, unite behind the pancreas and form the portal tube or vein. This takes blood, rich in the products of digestion, to the liver where it divides into smaller vessels and capillaries. Blood leaves the liver by the hepatic veins which enter the inferior vena cava.

**circumcision** (*ser-kum-si'-zhon*). Surgical removal of the foreskin.

**circumduction** (*ser-kum-duk'-shon*). Circular movement of limb.

**circumflex nerve** (*ser-kum-fleks nerv*). This arises from the brachial plexus to supply the deltoid and teres minor muscles.

**circumoral** (*sir-kum-or'-al*). Around the mouth. *C. pallor*, especially seen in scarlet fever, when the white area around the mouth is in great contrast to the colour of the rest of the face.

**circumvallate** (*ser-kum-val-lāt*). Surrounded by a wall.

**cirrhosis** (*sir-rō'-sis*). Usually referring to the liver: generic term applied to chronic diffuse liver damage of multiple aetiology. Characterized by destruction of the normal liver architecture and fibrosis.

**cirsoid** (*sir'-soyd*). Resembling a varix.

**cisterna magna** (*sis-ter-ner mag'-ner*). A subarachnoid space at the back of the hind-brain between cerebellum and medulla oblongata.

**cisternal puncture** (*sis-ter-nal pungk-cher*). A puncture made with a hollow needle at the nape of the neck into a space called the cisterna magna which contains cerebrospinal fluid. Used when the fluid cannot be obtained by lumbar puncture.

**cistron** (*sis'-tron*). Smallest unit of genetic material coding for a functional protein.

**citric acid cycle** (*si-trik a-sid sīkl*). Krebs cycle or tricarboxylic acid cycle (TCA): cycle of enzyme initiated reactions whereby pyruvic acid is broken down yielding water, carbon dioxide and energy. It is the final oxidative step in the breakdown of carbohydrates and occurs in the mitochondria.

**clamps** (*klamps*). Instruments used to compress vessels or to secure a grip on a structure.

**claudication** (*klaw-di-kā'-shon*). Limping. *Intermittent c.* Limping with severe pain on walking which disappears with rest; due to insufficient blood supply.

**claustrophobia** (*klaw-stro-fō'-*

*bi-a*). Fear of confined spaces.

**clavicle** (*kla-vikl*). Collar bone.

**clavus** (*klā-vus*). A corn.

**claw foot** (*klor*). The foot is shaped like a claw and has a very pronounced arch.

**claw hand.** Claw-shaped hand due to flexor spasm followed by contracture of the muscles flexing the fingers. Often caused by ulnar nerve damage.

**cleft palate** (*kleft pa-lāt*). Failure of fusion of the lip and palate during development. The cleft is variable in extent. The deformity can be remedied by plastic surgery.

**cleidocranial dysostosis** (*klī-dō-krā-ni-al di-so-stō'-sis*). Rare hereditary condition in which there is a failure of development of membranous bone, consequently there may be partial or total absence of the clavicles and imperfect ossification of the skull in the region of the fontanelle. The striking feature is the ability to approximate the shoulders in front of the chest.

**cleidotomy** (*klī-do-to-mi*). Cutting the collar bone.

**climacteric** (*klī-mak-ter-ik*). Time in a woman's life involving hormonal, physical and emotional changes and preceding end of menstruation. The menopause.

**climatology** (*klī-ma-to-lo-ji*). The study of climates as affecting the treatment of disease.

**clinic** (*kli-nik*). An institution to treat patients.

**clinical** (*kli-ni-kal*). Relating to disease.

**Clinitest** (*kli-ni-test*). Proprietary tablets containing reagent for testing urine for sugar.

**clitoris** (*kli-to-ris*). A small organ of erectile tissue, found in the female in front of the urethra.

**clone** (*klōn*). Descendants by division of a single cell and therefore of the same genetic constitution.

**clonic** (*klo-nik*). Spasmodic contractions, short and irregular. They occur in the second stage of an epileptic convulsion and in certain other fits.

**clonus** (*klō-nus*). Reflex irregular contractions of muscles.

**Clostridium** (*klos-tri-di-um*). Large spore-bearing anaerobic bacilli. The genus includes *Cl. botulinum*, *Cl. tetani* and the gas gangrene group.

**clotting time** (*klo'-ting tīm*). Time taken for blood to clot when bleeding has occurred. Normal time is 4 to 13 minutes at 37°C.

**clubbing** (*klu-bing*). The appearance of fingers and sometimes toes when the normal angle at the base of the nail is lost. It results from hyperplasia of connective tissue. Clubbing is associated with long-standing respiratory or cardiovascular disease.

**club foot** (*klub-foot*). *See* TALIPES.

**clumping** (*klum-ping*). Packing together of cells, usually red blood cells, due to loss of membrane charge resulting from reaction with antibody.

**Clutton's joints** (*klu'-tonz joynts*). Swelling of the knee joints found in congenital syphilis.

**CNS.** *See* CENTRAL NERVOUS SYSTEM.

**coagulase test** (*kō-a-gū-lās test*). Test used for identification of pathogenic staphylococci which depends on the demonstration of the enzyme coagulase which breaks down fibrinogen and clots plasma.

**coagulation** (*kō-a-gū-lā'-shon*). Thickening of a fluid into curds or clots. Almost always applied to blood. *See* BLOOD and BLOOD TRANSFUSION.

**coarctation** (*kō-ark-tā'-shon*). The compression of the walls of a vessel. When this occurs in the aorta it is narrowed where it is joined by the ductus arteriosus.

**cobalt** (*ko-bolt'*). Trace element. Its absence from the diet of young animals may lead to anaemia. *C. bomb*. Source of irradiation in deep x-ray therapy.

**cocaine** (*ko-kān'*). A powerful local anaesthetic, much used by oculists. It enlarges the pupil of the eye. Included in the Misuse of Drugs Act because it is a drug of addiction.

**coccobacillus** (*ko'-kō-ba-sil'-us*). Micro-organism intermediate in shape between coccus and bacillus.

**coccus** (*kok'-us*). (plu. **cocci**). Any spheroidal-shaped micro-organism. *See* BACTERIA.

**coccydynia** (*kok-si-di-ni-er*). Pain in the coccygeal region.

**coccyx** (*kok'-siks*). The tail-like termination of the spine.

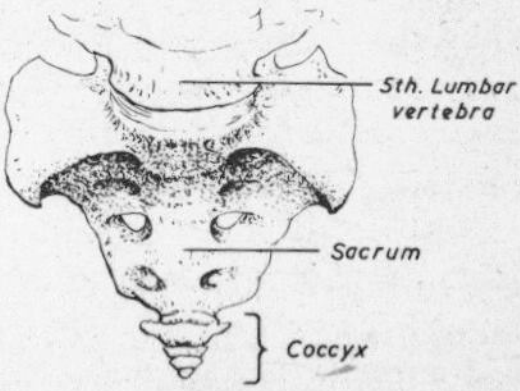


*6. The coccyx*

**cochlea** (*ko-kli-a*). The spiral cavity of the internal ear, containing the nerve endings of the eighth cranial or auditory nerve (*See illustration of* EAR, p. 125).

**cock-up splints** (*kok'-up*). For hand and wrist. Usually made of metal or polythene.

**codeine** (*kō-dēn*). One of the alkaloids of opium. It allays cough, and is used in diarrhoea for its constipating effect.

**co-dominance** (*kō-do'-mi-nans*). Of genetically transmitted conditions in which two traits are expressed in heterozygote.

**codon** (*kō-don*). Triplet of consecutive bases in unit of messenger RNA.

**coeliac** (*sē-li-ak*). Related to the abdominal cavity.

**coeliac disease** (*sē-li-ak di-sēz*). A condition caused by the inability of the intestine to absorb gluten. It is usually diagnosed in infancy. Marked by failure to thrive, diarrhoea and marked wasting of the buttocks and thighs.

**coelioscopy** (*sē-li-os'-ko-pi*). *See* LAPAROSCOPY.

**coenzyme** (*kō-en'-sīm*). Compound which plays an essential role in a reaction or reactions catalysed by an enzyme, usually acting as a carrier of an intermediate product of the reaction.

**coffee ground vomit** (*ko-fē ground vo-mit*). Appearance of vomit when it contains partly digested blood.

**cognition** (*cog-ni-shon*). Awareness. Part of a mental process. There is cognition when there is perception or memory of a material thing or idea.

**coitus** (*kō-i-tus*). Sexual intercourse.

**colectomy** (*ko-lek'-to-mi*). The operation of removing the colon.

**colic** (*ko'-lik*). Severe abdominal pain due to muscular spasm of a hollow viscus. Frequently caused by obstruction.

**coliform** (*ko-li-form*). Bacteria resembling *Esch. coli*.

**colitis** (*ko-lī-tis*). Inflammation of the colon. *Acute, ulcerative c.*, due to an infection, *e.g.* dysentery. *Chronic ulcerative c.*, cause unknown. *Mucous c.*, thought to be of nervous origin and associated with constipation.

**collagen** (*ko-la-jen*). Fibrous protein forming a major part of the intercellular connective tissue.

**collagen diseases.** A group of diseases in which one of the principal pathological features is the presence of fibrinoid necrosis usually in relation to blood vessels. To what extent the collagen is affected has not been determined but it seems that basically there is a deposition of abnormal material, possibly globulins, in the connective tissue rather than an alteration in the material normally present. Diseases such as systemic lupus erythematosus, scleroderma and periarteritis nodosa are examples of 'collagen' diseases.

**collapse** (*ko-laps*). Severe sudden prostration. *Symptoms*: see SHOCK.

**collar bone** (*ko'-la-bōn*). Clavicle.

**collar-stud abscess** (*ko'-la-stud ab'ses*). Abscess having two cavities joined by a narrow channel.

**collateral** (*ko-la'-te-ral*). Accompanying or accessory.

**Colles' fracture** (*ko-les frak'-tūr*). Transverse fracture of the radius just above the wrist with displacement of the hand backwards and outwards.

**collodion** (*ko-lō-di-on*). Pyroxylin dissolved in alcohol and ether; used in surgery to form a false skin. When painted over an incipient pressure sore it forms a protection over the skin. Highly inflammable.

**colloid** (*ko-loyd*). Physicochemical state of certain non-electrolytes in solution. Colloids are unable to pass through semi-permeable membranes and thus exert an osmotic pressure (colloid osmotic pressure).

**collutorium** (*ko-lū-to-ri-um*). A mouthwash; a gargle.

**collyrium** (*ko-lir'-i-um*). An eyewash.

**coloboma** (*ko-lo-bō'-ma*). A fissure or gap in the eyeball or in one of its component parts, *e.g.* coloboma iridis.

**colon** (*kō-lon*). The part of the large intestine between the caecum and the rectum. See BOWEL.

**colony** (*ko'-lo-ni*). A group of cells. Usually refers to circular collections of bacteria growing on culture medium.

**colorimeter** (*ko-lo-ri'-me-ter*). An instrument for estimating the depth of colour of a liquid.

**colostomy** (*ko-lo'-sto-mi*). Operation to make an artificial opening so that the colon opens on to the anterior abdominal wall.

**colostrum** (*ko-los'-trum*). A milky fluid flowing from the breasts the first 2 or 3 days after confinement, before the true milk comes.

**colotomy** (*ko-lo-to-mi*). An incision into the colon.

**colour blindness** (*ku'-ler blīnd-nes*). Inability to

distinguish certain colours, known sometimes as Daltonism.

**colour index** (*in'-deks*). Is a measure of the amount of haemoglobin contained in each red cell, compared to the normal amount. It is calculated thus:

Haemoglobin percentage

Red cell percentage

Normal

$$\frac{100}{100} = 1$$

**colpitis** (*kol-pī'-tis*). Inflammation of the vagina.

**colpocele** (*kol'-po-sēl*). A tumour or hernia in the vagina.

**colpocystopexy** (*kol-pō-sis-tō-pek'-si*). Operation for stress incontinence of urine involving the suture of the bladder neck and vaginal wall to the periosteum of the pubic symphysis.

**colpohysterectomy** (*kol-pō-hister-ek'-to-mi*). Removal of the uterus through the vagina. Usually called vaginal hysterectomy.

**colpomicroscope** (*kol'-pō-mī'-kro-skōp*). Apparatus for microscopic examination of cervix uteri.

**colpoperineorrhaphy** (*kol'-po-per-i-nē-ōr'-af-i*). Operation for repairing a torn vagina and perineum.

**colporrhaphy** (*kol-por'-af-i*). Operation for repairing a torn vagina or for preventing prolapse of the vaginal walls. *Anterior c.* Repairing the anterior vaginal wall and preventing recurrence of a cystocele. *Posterior c.* Repairing the posterior vaginal wall and preventing the recurrence of a rectocele.

**colpotomy** (*kol-po-to-mi*). Incision of the vagina.

**coma** (*kō-ma*). Insensibility, stupor, sleep.

**comatose** (*kō'-ma-tōs*). In a state of coma.

**comedones** (*ko-me-dōns*). Accumulations of sebaceous secretion in the hair follicles, commonly called blackheads. *See* ACNE.

**commensal** (*ko-men-sal*). Refers to members of different species living in close association but without influencing each other, *cf.* symbiosis.

**comminuted fracture** (*ko-mi-nū-ted frak'-tūr*). Fracture in which the bone is broken into more than two pieces.

**commissure** (*ko-mi-sūr*). Bundle of nerve fibres connecting the right and left sides of the brain and spinal cord.

**communicable disease** (*ko-mū-ni-kabl di-sēz*). Disease caused by micro-organisms which can be transmitted directly or indirectly between hosts.

**compact tissue** (*kom-pakt ti-sū*). Term infrequently used referring to the cortex of bone.

**compatability** (*kom-pa'-ti-bi-li-ti*). Able to be mixed together without ill result: thus *compatible blood* is used for transfusion since it can be mixed with that of the recipient. *Compatible drugs* are those which can be mixed without producing undesirable chemical interactions.

**compensation** (*kom-pen-sā'-shon*). A psychological way of making up for real or imagined deficiencies in personality.

**compensatory hypertrophy** (*kom-pen-sā'-to-ri hī-per-tro-fi*). Increase in size of residual organ or part of tissue in response to the removal of part, *e.g.* if one kidney is removed then the other enlarges.

**competence** (*kom'-pe-tens*). Ability of a cell of the immunological system to react to specific antigenic stimuli.

**complement** (*kom-ple-ment*). A protein present in the blood which forms an essential component of certain antibody–antigen reactions.

**complement fixation test.** The disappearance of complement from the serum is used to detect antigen–antibody reactions. This complement 'fixation' forms the basis of certain serological tests such as the Wassermann reaction.

**complex** (*kom'-pleks*). A group of ideas with an emotional background. Partially or entirely repressed in the unconscious mind, it may be the underlying cause of a neurotic illness.

**complicated fracture** (*kom-pli-kā-ted frak-tūr*). Fracture combined with injury to other important structures.

**complication** (*kom-pli-kā'-shon*). In illness, a disorder arising from the circumstances produced by the primary disease.

**compos mentis** (*kom-pos men'-tis*). Of sound mind.

**compound** (*kom-pownd*). Consisting of more than one element.

**compound fracture.** Fracture communicating with the surface.

**comprehension** (*kom-prē-hen-shon*). The understanding of ideas and the relationship between them.

**compress** (*kom'-pres*). (1) A tightly folded pad of lint, gauze, or other material used to secure local pressure. (2)

A sterile dressing applied over an area which has been prepared for a surgical operation.

**compression** (*kom-pre'-shon*). The state of being compressed. *Cerebral c.*, increased intracranial pressure from a tumour, etc.

**computerised axial tomography.** Abbrev. to CAT scan or CT scanning. The technique of examining body sections in the axial plane using very sophisticated equipment.

**concave** (*kon-kāv*). With outline curved like interior of a circle.

**concavity** (*kon-ka'-vi-ti*). A depression.

**concentration** (*kon-sen-trā-shon*). The amount of dissolved substance in a solution and therefore its strength.

**concentric** (*kon-sen-trik*). With a common centre.

**conception** (*kon-sep'-shon*). (1) The impregnation of the ovum. (2) An idea.

**concha auris** (*kon'-ka aw'-ris*). Deepest hollow of pinna of the outer ear.

**concordance** (*kon-kor'-dens*). Of twins, when both have same physical trait.

**concretion** (*kon-krē-'shon*). A calculus. An abnormal deposit in the body such as stone in the gall bladder.

**concussion** (*kon-ku'-shon*). Interruption of function of the brain as the result of compression wave set up by a blow to the head. The wave of compression transmitted through the cerebrospinal fluid and the brain substance obliterates momentarily the blood capillaries supplying the brain. Recovery may take many hours.

**condensation** (*kon-den-sā'-shon*). Transformation of gas into liquid.

**condenser** (*kon-den'-ser*). Apparatus to cool and thus cause condensation of gas.

**conditioned reflex** (*kon-di'-shond rē-flexs*). A reflex which is modified by experience in such a way that the original afferent (sensory) stimulus is replaced by a different 'learned' stimulus. Pavlov's dog salivated at the sound of a bell, associating this with the introduction of food into its mouth.

**condom** (*kon-dom*). Rubber sheath for the penis preventing conception.

**conduction** (*kon-duk-shon*). Passage of a physical disturbance through matter. Biologically, the passage of a nerve impulse.

**conductor** (*kon-duk-tor*). An instrument used to direct surgical knives, called also a director. In electricity, a substance which allows the passage of electric currents.

**condyle** (*kon'-dīl*). A round projection at the ends of some bones. *See* HUMERUS.

**condyloma** (*kon-dē-lō'-ma*). Wartlike growth about the anus or pudendum.

**cone biopsy** (*kōn bī-op-si*). Excision of cone of tissue from cervix uteri to confirm suspected carcinoma.

**confabulation** (*kon-fa-bū-lā'-shon*). The narration of fictitious occurrences.

**confection** (*kon-fek-shon*). Medication with sweet covering.

**confinement** (*kon-fīn'-ment*). Childbirth.

**conflict** (*kon-flikt*). Psychological term to denote antagonism between conflicting desires.

**confluent smallpox** (*kon-flū-ent'*). A severe form of smallpox in which the individual papules coalesce.

**confusion** (*kon-fū-zhon*). Inability to think clearly.

**congenital** (*kon-je-ni-tal*). Existing at birth.

**congenital heart disease.** Heart disease present from birth. Due to developmental abnormalities of the cardiovascular system.

**congestion** (*kon-jes-chon*). Hyperaemia. Accumulation of blood in a part of the body, as in the lungs or brain. *C. of the lungs,* pneumonia.

**conisation** (*ko-nī-zā-shon*). Part of the cervix is removed by excision or diathermy.

**conjugate diameter** (*kon'-jū-gāt dī-a'-me-ter*). An important diameter of the pelvis, measured from the most prominent part of the upper half of the sacrum to the nearest point on the back of the symphysis pubis. This is the *true* conjugate, which should measure not less than 10 cm (4¼ in), and is sometimes as large as 12 cm (4½ or 4¾ in). If less than 10 cm (4¼ in), the pelvis is a deformed one. The *diagonal* conjugate is measured from the lower edge of the symphysis to the sacrum, and can be determined clinically, whereas the true conjugate cannot. The diagonal conjugate is about 1 to 2 cm (½ to ¾ in) longer than the true conjugate. The *external* conjugate is measured from the spine of the last lumbar vertebra to the front of the symphysis pubis (this can only be done with calipers), and is normally about 20 cm (8 in).

**conjunctiva** (*kon-junk-tī'-va*). The mucous membrane which covers the sclerotic and lines the eyelids.

CON 100

**conjunctivitis** (*kon-junk-ti-vī'-tis*). Inflammation of the conjunctiva.

**connective tissue** (*kon-nek-tiv ti-shū*). Supporting or packing material consisting of a fibrous gel made up of collagen and elastin fibres in a mucopolysaccharide ground substance, bathed in extracellular fluid with scattered cells, blood vessels, lymphatics and nerve fibres traversing it.

**Conn's disease** (*kons di-sēz*). Also called *primary aldosteronism*. Rare disease characterized by periodic attacks of severe muscular weakness, tetany, paraesthesiae, hypertension and impaired renal function. The cause is usually an adenoma of the adrenal cortex with over-production of aldosterone, which results in reduced levels of potassium and raised sodium in the blood.

**consanguinity** (*kon-san-gwi-ni-ti*). Blood relationship.

**conservative** (*kon-ser'-va-tiv*). Aiming at preservation or repair, *e.g.* conservative treatment of a tooth.

**consolidation** (*kon-so-li-dā'-shon*). Becoming solid, as with a lung in pneumonia.

**constipation** (*kon-sti-pā'-shon*). Undue delay in the passage of the residue of a meal.

**constitutional** (*kon-sti-tū'-shon-al*). Affecting the whole body, not local.

**constrict** (*kon-strikt*). Contract or draw together.

**consumption** (*kon-sum-shon*). Popular term for tuberculosis.

**contact** (*kon-takt*). One who has been exposed to an infectious disease. *C. lens,* plastic or glass lens worn directly on the cornea.

**contagious** (*kon-tā-jus*). Communicable disease which is transmitted by contact, *i.e.* not communicable through atmosphere.

**contraception** (*kon-tra-sep'-shon*). Preventing conception.

**contraceptives, oral.** Drugs, usually a combination of synthetic oestrogens and progestogens, which inhibit ovulation and thus depress fertility. They prevent blastocyst implantation and make cervical mucus unfavourable to sperm migration.

**contracted pelvis** (*kon-trak'-ted pel-vis*). Pelvis in which any of the diameters are less than normal. A contracted pelvis may lead to difficulty during delivery.

**contraction** (*kon-trak'-shon*). Shortening. A drawing together.

**contraction ring.** See RETRACTION RING.

**contracture** (*kon-trak-tūr*). Permanent contraction of structure due to the formation of fibrous tissue which is inelastic. *Dupuytren's c.* Localized thickening of palmar fascia which involves the overlying skin of the palm. There is a strong tendency for this to contract, drawing the affected fingers into rigid flexion.

**contra-indication** (*kon-tra-in-di-kā-shon*). Reason for considering a particular treatment to be unsuitable.

**contralateral** (*kon-tra-la'-te-ral*). On the opposite side.

**contre-coup** (*kon-tre-koo*). Injury due to the transmission of the force of a blow. Contre-coup injuries often affect the brain which is damaged by striking the skull at a point diametrically opposite the site of the blow.

**contusion** (*kon-tū-zhon*). A bruise.

**convalescence** (*kon-va-le'-senz*). Period of regaining full health after an illness.

**convection** (*kon-vek'-shon*). The heat of liquids and gases transmitted by a circulation of heated particles.

**convergence** (*kon-ver'-jens*). A coming together.

**conversion** (*kon-ver'-shon*). C.

*symptom.* Term used in psychiatry for a symptom representing an emotional rather than a physical cause. Commonly occurs in a hysterical personality.

**convex** (*kon-veks*). With outline curved like exterior of circle.

**convolutions** (*kon-vo-lū-shons*). The folds and twists of the brain or the intestines. See BOWEL and BRAIN.

**convulsions** (*kon-vul'-shons*). Violent spasms of alternate muscular contraction and relaxation, due to disturbance of cerebral function. A fit.

**convulsive therapy** (*kon-vul-siv the-ra-pi*). See ELECTRO-CONVULSIVE THERAPY.

**Cooley's anaemia** (*koo-lis-a-nē-mi-a*). Also called thalassaemia major. It is a dominantly inherited haemolytic anaemia found in Mediterranean peoples. It is due to a metabolic fault leading to the continued production of fetal haemoglobin.

**Coomb's test** (*kooms test*). Test for the presence of globulin on the surface of red cells such as may occur in certain haemolytic anaemias in which anti-red cell antibody is produced. *Direct C.t.* Cells on which the antibody has combined with the antigen and thus coated the surface with globulin, are suspended in a medium containing anti-human globulin which reacts with the coating globulin causing agglutination of the coated red cells. *Indirect C.t.* Normal (compatible) red cells are incubated with the serum thought to contain antibody and subsequently tested for adsorbed antibody.

**copulation** (*ko-pū-lā'-shon*). Sexual intercourse.

**cor pulmonale** (*kor pul-mo-nah-lē*). Heart disease resulting from affection of the lung.

**coracoid** (*kor'-a-koyd*). A process of bone on the scapula which resembles a crow's beak. *See* SCAPULA.

**cord** (*kawd*). Any string-like body such as the spinal cord or umbilical cord.

**corium** (*ko-ri-um*). *See* DERMIS.

**corn** (*kawn*). Local hyperkeratosis due to pressure on the skin. Frequently occurs on the foot, *cf.* callus.

**cornea** (*kor'-ne-a*). Transparent epidermis and connective tissue which forms the front surface of the eye.

**corneal graft** (*kor-nē-al grahft*). Healthy cornea is given by grafting to replace a diseased cornea.

**corneal reflex** (*kor-nē-al rē-fleks*). Important superficial reflex whereby a light touch on the cornea provokes a blink in both eyelids.

**corona dentis** (*ko-rō'-na dentis*). Crown of a tooth.

**coronal suture** (*ko-rō'-nal sū'-tūr*). The suture which joins the parietal and frontal bones of the skull.

**coronary vessels** (*ko'-ro-na-ri ve-sels*). Arteries and veins carrying the blood supply of the heart muscle.

**coronoid** (*ko-ro-noyd*). Like a crow's beak as with certain bony processes.

**corpora quadrigemina** (*kor'-por-ah kwod-ri-jem'-in-ah*). Four rounded bodies consisting chiefly of grey matter in the midbrain.

**corpulence, corpulency** (*kaw'-pū-len-si*). Undue fatness. Obesity.

**corpus callosum** (*ka-lō-sum*). The band of nervous tissue which connects the two hemispheres of the cerebrum.

**corpus luteum** (*kor-pus loo-tē-um*). A temporary organ secreting the hormone progesterone which favours the establishment and continuity of a pregnancy. It is formed, under the influence of luteinizing hormone of the pituitary, by growth of the wall of a Graafian follicle after ovulation. If ovulation does not result in fertilization, the corpus luteum degenerates, but if fertilization occurs, the corpus luteum persists.

**corpus striatum** (*kor-pus strē-ā-tum*). *See* BASAL GANGLIA.

**corpuscle** (*kor'-pusl*). Usually refers to a cell, esp. red blood cell.

**corrective** (*kor-rek'-tiv*). A drug which modifies the action of another drug.

**Corrigan's pulse** (*ko-ri-ganz puls*). Known also as waterhammer pulse, occurs in aortic regurgitation. The artery distends forcibly and then appears to empty suddenly and completely.

**corrosive** (*kor-rō'-siv*). Eating into, consuming.

**cortex** (*kaw'-teks*). The outer layer of an organ.

**Corti's organ** (*kaw-tēz aw'-gan*). The collection of nerve endings of the auditory nerve in the cochlea.

**corticosteroids** (*kor-ti-kō-ste-royds*). Generic term used to refer to steroid hormones from the adrenal cortex and also synthetic steroids with similar metabolic actions.

**corticotrophin** (*kor-ti-kō-trō-fin*). Hormone from the anterior pituitary gland stimulating the adrenal cortex.

**Corynebacterium diphtheriae**

(*ko-rin-e-bak-tār-i-um dif-thā'-ri-ē*). The bacillus causing diphtheria.

**coryza** (*ko-rī'-za*). The common cold.

**costal** (*ko'-stal*). Relating to the ribs.

**costive** (*ko'-stiv*). Constipated.

**costochondritis** (*kos-tō-kon-drī'-tis*). Inflammation of the costal cartilage. The cause is unknown.

**costoclavicular syndrome** (*ko-stō-kla-vi-kū-la sin'-drōm*). Also called *thoracic outlet compression syndrome.* Characterized by pain in the arm, wasting of the muscles of the hand, paraesthesiae, sensory loss and sometimes transient obliteration of the blood supply to the hand. It is due to compression of vessels and nerves between the clavicle and the top rib.

**cotyledon** (*ko-ti-lē-don*). Portion of the placenta.

**coudé** (*koo'-dā*). Having a bend near the tip (of catheters and sounds).

**counter-extension** (*kown'-ter-ek-sten-shon*). Technique of traction used in the treatment of certain orthopaedic conditions in which the upper part of a limb is held back while the lower part is pulled.

**counter-irritation** (*kown'-ter i-ri-tā-shon*). The application of an irritant stimulus to the skin in order to divert attention from sensory information coming from another site, *e.g.* application of hot water bottle to relieve abdominal pain.

**coupling** (*ku'pling*). Abnormal heart beat which occurs in overdose of digitalis. The normal heart beat is followed by an extra ventricular contraction (ventricular extrasystole). The latter may be too weak to transmit a pulse.

**Courvoisier's law** (*koor-vuw-sē-ās law*). An adage to the effect that in jaundice the palpation of an enlarged tender gall bladder favours the diagnosis of obstructive jaundice, since a gall bladder which is the seat of chronic inflammation is usually incapable of distension.

**Cowper's glands** (*koo-perz glands*). Two small glandular structures associated with the male urethra. Their function is unknown.

**cowpox.** *See* VACCINIA.

**coxa** (*kok'-sa*). The hip joint.

**coxalgia** (*kok-sal-ji-a*). Pain in the hip joint.

**coxa valga** (*kok-sa val-ga*). Deformity of the hip joint in which the angle made by the neck and shaft of the femur is greater than normal. *C. vara.* In this case the angle is less than normal. (*See illustration of* FEMUR, p. 146.)

**Coxsackie virus** (*kok-sa-ki vī'-rus*). Group of viruses which may cause epidemic myalgia, Bornholm disease, and benign lymphocytic meningitis, and possibly other relatively mild diseases.

**crab louse** (*krab' lows*). The phthirus pubis which infests the pubic region.

**cramp** (*kramp*). Sudden painful tonic contraction of the muscles.

**cranial nerves** (*krā-ni-al nervs*). Peripheral nerves emerging from the brain, as distinct from those emerging from the spinal cord. There are twelve pairs of cranial nerves: (1) *Olfactory*—the sensory nerves of the nose; (2) *Optic*—the sensory nerves from the eyes; (3) *Oculomotor*—motor nerves supplying the eye muscles; (4) *Trochlear*—supplying eye muscles; (5) *Trigeminal*—sensory from parts of face and tongue and motor to jaw muscles; (6) *Abducens*—supplying eye muscles; (7) *Facial*—sensory from face and motor to muscles of expression; (8) *Auditory*—sensory nerves from the ear and vestibular apparatus; (9) *Glossopharyngeal*—concerned with sensory and motor aspects of swallowing; (10) *Vagus*—a para-sympathetic nerve, with motor and sensory fibres distributed to oesophagus, stomach, heart and lungs; (11) *Accessory*—nerve to trapezius and ster .omastoid muscles; (12) *Hypoglossal*—motor nerve to muscles below the pharynx.

**cranioclast** (*krā'-ni-ō-klast*). An instrument for breaking up the fetal skull when it is impossible to deliver the fetus intact.

**craniometry** (*krā-ni-o-me-tri*). Measurement of skulls.

**craniopharyngioma** (*krā-ni-ō-fa-rin-ji-ō'-ma*). Syn. Rathke pouch tumour. Cystic tumour arising from remnants of a developmental pouch in the pituitary region of the skull.

**craniostenosis** (*krā-ni-o-ste-nō'-sis*). Abnormally early fusion of bones of the vault of the skull with the effect that further growth of the skull in the direction at right angles to the line of the obliterated suture is prevented. Compensatory growth elsewhere in the skull produces a distorted head.

**craniotabes** (*krā-niō-tā'-bēz*). Thinning of the bones of the vault of thé skull; occurs in rickets.

**craniotomy** (*krā-ni-o'-to-mi*).

Operation in which openings are made in the skull.

**cranium** (*krā-nē-um*). The skull.

**creatine** (*krē-a-tin*). A constituent of muscle. Creatine phosphate acts as an energy storage substance.

**creatinine** (*krē-a-ti-nin*). A substance formed from creatine and excreted in the urine.

**Credé's method** (*krā-dāz method*). Expelling the placenta by means of compression of the fundus of the uterus.

**crepitation, crepitus** (*kre-pi-tā'-shon, kre-pi-tus*). (1) The grating of ends of a fractured bone. (2) Type of 'clicking' sound heard on auscultation of the chest when the alveoli contain fluid.

**cretinism** (*kre-ti-nism*). Congenital deficient thyroid secretion, causing impaired mentality, small stature, coarseness of skin and hair and deposition of fat on the body. Treated early with thyroid extract, great improvement may result.

**Creutzfeld-Jacob disease** (*kroyts'-felt jā-kob di-sēz*). Fatal presenile cerebral degeneration.

**cribriform** (*kri'-briform*). Perforated like a sieve.

**cricoid cartilage** (*kri'-koyd kar'-ti-lāj*). A ring-shaped cartilage below the thyroid.

**'cri du chat' syndrome**
(*krē-doo-shu sin'-drōm*).
Congenital abnormalities
causing mental retardation
and characteristic mewing
sound.

**Crigler-Najjar syndrome**
(*krig'-ler na'-jah sin'-drōm*).
Inherited defect of bilirubin
metabolism which causes
non-haemolytic neonatal
jaundice.

**crisis** (*krī'-sis*). The deciding
point of a disease, from which
the patient either begins to
recover or sinks rapidly;
often marked by a long sleep,
profuse perspiration, or
other phenomena.

**Crohn's disease** (*krōns*).
Chronic form of enteritis
affecting the terminal part of
the ileum.

**crossed laterality** (*krost la-te-
ra'-li-ti*). Combination of
either right-handedness with
left-eyedness or of left-
handedness with right-
eyedness.

**cross-infection.** Hazard in hos-
pitals where, owing to
proximity of patients to each
other, infection is easily
transferred. Particularly
dangerous in surgical and
obstetric wards where
wound infection is a problem
despite stringent efforts
to minimize the spread of
bacteria.

**cross-resistance.** Micro-
organisms which are resistant
to one antibiotic tend to have
resistance to other antibiotics
of the same type.

**croup** (*kroop*). Dyspnoea and
stridor due to obstruction of
the larynx. It may be due to
inflammation, or spasm of
the muscles.

**crucial** (*kroo-shal*). Critical or
decisive.

**cruciate** (*kròo-shē-āt*). Cross-
shaped.

**crural** (*krū'-ral*). Relating to
the thigh.

**crus** (*kroos*). Latin for leg. A
limb-like structure.

**crush syndrome** (*krush sin-
drōm*). As the result of extensive crushing of muscles,
toxic substances pass into the
circulation which cause the
medullary circulation of the
kidney to be opened up so
that blood is diverted from
the glomeruli in the renal
cortex. This results in
oliguria.

**crutch paralysis** (*kru'-ch pa-ra-
li-sis*). Caused by pressure on
the axillary nerves and
vessels by a crutch.

**cryosurgery** (*krī'-o-ser'-je-ri*).
Method of surgical removal
of tissue by local freezing.

**cryotherapy** (*krī'-ō-the-ra-pi*).
Application of cold as means
of treatment.

**cryptomenorrhoea** (*krip-tō-*

*me-no-rē-a*). Apparent
amenorrhoea due to obstruction to the flow of menstrual
blood.

**cryptorchism** (*krip-tor-kism*).
Failure of one or both testes
to descend into the scrotum.

**crypts of Lieberkühn** (*kripts of lē-ber-koon*). Glands found
in the mucous membrane of
the small intestine. They secrete a mixture of digestive
enzymes collectively termed
intestinal juice.

**crystalloids** (*kris'-ta-loyds*).
Substances which will pass
through a semi-permeable
membrane. They easily crystallize and are readily
soluble, *e.g.* salt, sugar. *Cf.*
colloids.

**crystalluria** (*kris-ta-lū-ri-a*).
The presence of crystals in
the urine.

**CSF.** *See* CEREBROSPINAL
FLUID.

**cubit** (*kū-'bit*), **cubitus** (1) The
forearm. (2) The elbow.

**culdoscopy** (*kul-do'-sko-pi*).
Inspection of internal pelvic
organs by passing illuminated
instrument through posterior
vaginal fornix.

**culture** (*kul-cher*). Artificial
cultivation of tissues, cells or
viruses. *C. media*. Substances
used as food source for cultures.

**cumulative action** (*kū'-mū-la-tiv*). A term applied to certain
drugs which are excreted
slowly. After several doses
have been given, symptoms
of poisoning may arise, *e.g.*
mercury, digitalis.

**cuneiform** (*kū-ne-form*).
Wedge-shaped.

**curare** (*kū'-rah'-rē*). A poison
derived from a South American plant. It paralyses motor
nerves.

**curettage** (*kū-re-tahj*). Operation of scraping away tissue
with a curette.

**curette** (*kū-ret*). A spoon-shaped instrument.

**curie** (*kū-rē*). Unit of radioactivity (Ci).

**Curling's ulcer** (*ker-lings ul'-ser*). An acute ulcer occurring
in the second part of the
duodenum following severe
burns.

**Cushing's suture** (*ku'-shingz soo'-tūr*). Continuous invaginating suture for internal
anastomosis. *C.'s syndrome.*
Syndrome due to oversecretion of adreno-cortical hormones and characterized by
moonface, redistribution of
body fat, polycythaemia, hirsutism, acne, amenorrhoea,
osteoporosis, glycosuria,
hypertension, purpura,
muscular weakness and
occasionally mental
derangement.

**cutaneous** (*kū-tā'-ne-us*). Pertaining to the skin.

**cuticle** (*kū-tikl*). The layer of flattened cells forming the outer coat of hair.

**cutis** (*kū'-tis*). Dermis.

**cyanocobalamin** (*sī-a-nō-kō-ba'-la-min*). Vitamin B$_{12}$. A cobalt-containing substance the lack of which interferes with cell division. How it acts is not known. It is the extrinsic antipernicious anaemia factor of Castle.

**cyanosis** (*sī-a-nō'-sis*). Blue appearance; due to deficient oxygenation of the blood. It occurs in heart failure, diseases of the respiratory tract, and congenital heart disease. *See* BLUE BABY.

**cyclamate** (*sik'-la-māt*). Salt of cyclohexylsulphamic acid. A sweetening agent.

**cycle** (*sī-kl*). Repeated series of events.

**cyclical vomiting** (*si'-kli-kal*). Recurrent attacks of vomiting occurring in childhood with headache, and signs of acidosis.

**cyclitis** (*sī-klī'-tis*). Inflammation of ciliary body of eye.

**cyclodialysis** (*sī-klō-dī-a'-li-sis*). Drainage of anterior chamber of eye.

**cycloplegia** (*sī-klō-plē'-ji-a*). Paralysis of the ciliary muscle of the eye.

**cyclothymia** (*sī-klō-thī-mi-a*). A type of personality in which there are marked swings of mood from happiness to depression.

**cyclotomy** (*si-clo-to-mi*). Incision through the ciliary body.

**cyesis** (*sī-ē-sis*). Pregnancy.

**cyst** (*sist*). A tumour containing fluid in membranous sac. *Daughter c.* One developed from the walls of a large cyst.

**cystadenoma** (*sis-ta-de-nō'-ma*). Benign growth containing cysts.

**cystectomy** (*sis-tek-to-mi*). Removal of urinary bladder.

**cystic duct** (*sis'-tik*). The duct leading from the gall bladder to the common bile duct.

**cysticercosis** (*sis-ti-ser-kō-sis*). Infection by larval stage of a tapeworm, usually from pork. The parasites may become widespread in the body, invading muscle and nervous tissue and cause serious symptoms, *e.g.* epilepsy.

**cystine** (*sis-tin*). A sulphur-containing amino-acid.

**cystinosis** (*sis-ti-nō'-sis*). A rare inborn error of metabolism of cystine and other amino-acids described by Lignac and Fanconi. It is characterized by dwarfism, vitamin D-resistant rickets, anorexia, polyuria, thirst, vomiting and cystine deposits in the tissues.

**cystinuria** (*sis-ti-nū-ri-a*). Presence of abnormal amounts of cystine in the urine as occurs, for example, in cystinosis.

**cystitis** (*sis-tī'-tis*). Inflammation of the urinary bladder.

**cystocele** (*sis'-tō-sēl*). Hernia of the bladder into the vagina.

**cystogram** (*sis-tō-gram*). X-ray of urinary bladder.

**cystolithiasis** (*sis-to-li-thī'-a-sis*). Stone in the bladder.

**cystometry** (*sis-to-me-tri*). Measurement of tone of the bladder.

**cystoscope** (*sis-to-skōp*). An instrument for examining the bladder.

**cystostomy** (*sis-tos'-to-mi*). Operation of producing an opening from the bladder to the exterior.

**cystotomy** (*sis-to-to-mi*). Incision of the bladder or division of the anterior capsule of the lens of the eye.

**cytochromes** (*sī-tō-krōms*). A number of iron-containing proteins found in cells which form the intermediary link between the electron transport chain, which accumulates hydrogen from oxidation actions taking place in cellular metabolism, and molecular oxygen.

**cytogenetics** (*sī-tō-je-ne'-tiks*). Study of genetics in relation to cytology.

**cytology** (*sī-to-lo-ji*). The study of cells.

**cytolysis** (*sī-tol'-is-is*). Cell disintegration.

**cytomegalovirus** (*sī-tō-me-ga-lō-vī'-rus*). Herpes virus causing cytomegalic inclusion-body disease.

**cytometer** (*sī-to'-me-ter*). An instrument for counting cells.

**cytoplasm** (*sī-tō-plasm*). *See* CELL.

**cytotoxic** (*sī-tō-tok'-sik*). Substance which is damaging to cells.

**cytotoxin** (*sī-tō-tok'-sin*). Cytotoxic antibody.

**cytotrophoblast** (*sī-tō-trō-phō-blast*). Inner portion of trophoblast differentiation.

# D

**dacryadenitis** (*dak-ri-a de-nī'-tis*). Inflammation of the lacrimal gland.

**dacryocystitis** (*dak'-ri-ō-sis-tī'-tis*). Inflammation of the tear sac.

**dacryocystorhinostomy** (*dak-ri-ō-sis-tō-rī-nos'-to-mi*). Operation to establish a communication between the tear (lacrimal) sac and the nose. It is performed when the tear duct, through which the lacrimal secretion normally drains, is obstructed, thus causing epiphora.

**dacryolith** (*dak'-ri-ō-lith*). Stone in the lacrimal duct.

**dacryoma** (*dak-ri-ō-mah*). Benign tumour arising from lacrimal epithelium.

**dactyl** (*dak-til'*). A digit of the hand or foot.

**dactylitis** (*dak-ti-lī'-tis*). Nonspecific term, usually applied to periostitis of the bones of the digits.

**dactylology** (*dak-ti-lol'-o-jē*). Talking by the fingers; deaf and dumb language.

**Daltonism** (*dal-tō-nism*). Red–green colour blindness inherited as a sex-linked recessive trait and therefore much more common in males than females who act as carriers for the gene, *cf.* haemophilia. There are other forms of colour blindness but they are rare.

**dandruff** (*dan'-druf*). Accumulation of desquamated keratinized cells usually in the scalp.

**Danysz phenomenon** (*dā-nis fe-no'-me-non*). When toxin is added to antitoxin, the toxicity of the product is increased the more slowly the addition is made.

**dark adaptation.** Time required for the physiological readjustment of the eye necessary to permit vision in the dark. This is critically affected by the amount of carotene available to retinal cells, *cf.* light adaptation.

**Darwinism** (*da-wi-nism*). Theory of evolution by natural selection as propounded by Darwin.

**db.** Decibel.

**d.d.** *de die*, daily.

**DDA.** Dangerous Drugs Act. Act designed to control the manufacture, distribution and sale of certain addiction-producing drugs. Now superseded by the Misuse of Drugs Act (1971).

**deaf mute** (*def mūt*). A person who is both deaf and dumb.

**deamination** (*dē-a-mi-nā'-shon*). The removal of amino ($NH_2$) group. Occurs in the liver and kidneys by the action of deaminating enzymes which remove the amino groups from aminoacids. The reaction produces ammonia which is converted to urea by enzymes in the liver.

**debility** (*de-bi'-li-ti*). Weakness, loss of power.

**debridement** (*dā-brēd'-mo*). Thorough cleansing of a wound and excision of the edges.

**decalcification** (*dē-kal-si-fi-kā'-shon*). Loss or removal of calcium salts from bone.

**decapitation** (*dē-ka-pi-tā'-shon*). The operation of severing the fetal head from the body, very rarely necessary in cases of obstructed labour.

**decapsulation** (*dē-kap-sū-lā'-shon*). Removal of the capsule of an organ, *e.g.* of the kidney.

**decerebrate** (*dē-se-ri-brāt*). Without brain. Usually applied to experimental situation in which the brain stem of an animal is sectioned, leaving the brain intact but severing the connections with the spinal cord. This results in *d. rigidity* when the limbs are rigidly extended. A similar spasticity may occur clinically as the result of severe brain damage.

**decidua** (*de-si-dū-a*). Mucous membrane lining the uterus (endometrium) in the thickened and modified form it acquires during pregnancy. Some or all of the decidua is shed with the placenta at birth.

**deciduous teeth** (*de-si-dū-us tēth*). First dentition or milk teeth.

**decompensation** (*dē-kom-pen-sā'-shon*). Failure of physiological compensation to some stimulus; for example, failure of hypertrophy of a chamber of the heart to overcome obstruction due to a defective valve.

**decomposition** (*dē-kom-pō-si-shon*). Putrefaction. Breakdown of substances by hydrolytic enzymes.

**decompression** (*dē-kom-pre'-shon*). An operation performed to relieve internal pressure, *e.g.* trephining of the skull. *D. sickness*. Otherwise known as 'the bends' or Caisson disease. Occurs in deep-sea divers and is due to nitrogen in compressed air which at the pressure under which it is breathed goes into solution in the blood but which, at ordinary atmospheric pressure, comes out of solution and forms small bubbles in the tissues.

**decortication** (*dē-kor-ti-kā'-shon*). Surgical removal of the outer layer of an organ.

**decubitus** (*de-kū'-bi-tus*). The recumbent or horizontal position.

**decussation** (*dē-ku-sā'-shon*). (1) An interlacing or crossing of fellow parts. (2) The point at which the crossing occurs. *D. of the Pyramids*. The crossing of the motor fibres from one side of the medulla to the other.

**deep x-ray therapy.** Treatment of disease, esp. malignant disease, by x-rays. They penetrate the tissue and destroy cells which are rapidly multiplying.

**defaecation** (*dē-fē-kā'-shon*). The act of evacuating the bowels.

**defemination** (*dē-fe-mi-nā-shon*). **defeminization**. Loss of female characteristics.

**defibrillator** (*dē-fĭ-bri-lā'-tor*). Apparatus which applies electrical impulses to the heart. Designed to stop fibrillation and restore the normal cardiac cycle.

**deficiency diseases** (*de-fi-shen-si di-sē-sez*). Due to an inadequate supply of vitamins in the diet, *e.g.* rickets, scurvy, beriberi.

**degeneration** (*dē-je-ne-rā'-shon*). Deterioration in structure or function of tissue. When the structural changes are marked, descriptive terms are sometimes used, *e.g.* colloid, fatty, hyaline, etc.

**deglutition** (*dē-glū-ti-shon*). Act of swallowing.

**dehydration** (*dē-hī-drā'-shon*). Loss of water.

**dehydrogenase** (*dē-hī-drō-je-nās*). Enzyme which oxidizes a substrate by removing hydrogen from it.

**déjà vu phenomenon** (*dā-ja vū fe-no-me-non*). Illusion of familiarity when experiencing something new.

**deletion** (*dē-lē'-shon*). Loss of genetic material.

**Delhi boil** (*de-li boyl*). Also known as 'oriental sore'. Cutaneous leishmaniasis.

**delirium** (*de-li-ri-um*). Extra-vagant talking, raving, generally due to high fever.

**delirium tremens** (*de-li-ri-um tre-menz*). An acute psychosis usually associated with chronic alcoholism. The patient is disorientated, has hallucinations and is excited. There is a coarse tremor of the fingers, tongue and facial muscles.

**delivery** (*de-li-ve-ri*). Parturition. Childbirth.

**deltoid** (*del'-toyd*). The muscle which covers the prominence of the shoulder and abducts the arm.

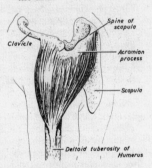

7. *The deltoid muscle*

**delusion** (*de-lū'-zhon*). A false idea, entirely without foundation in the facts of the environment.

**demarcation** (*de-mar-kā'-shon*). The marking of a boundary. *Line of d.*, red line which forms between dead and living tissue in gangrene.

**dementia** (*de-men-shi-a*). Feebleness of the mental faculties, inconsequent ideas. A form of insanity. May occur in children as a result of inborn error of metabolism. *Senile d.* occurs in older people.

**demulcents** (*de-mul'-sents*). Agents which protect sensitive surfaces from irritation.

**demyelinating diseases** (*dē-mī-e-li-nā-ting di-sē-sez*). A group of diseases, of which multiple sclerosis is the most common example, where the major visible pathological lesion is the destruction and loss of myelin sheaths round nerve fibres.

**denaturation** (*dē-na-tū-rā'-shon*). Alteration in the tertiary structure of a polymer (e.g. protein) as the result of the action of heat or chemicals rendering the molecule less soluble.

**dendrites** (*den-drīts*). Branching cytoplasmic projections of a cell.

**denervated** (*de-ner-vā-ted*). Deprived of nerve supply.

**dengue** (*deng'-ge*). A virus disease of the tropics, transmitted by mosquitoes and characterized by fever, headache, limb pains and rash.

**Denis Browne splints.** A number of splints designed to correct congenital deformity, as that of the hip, bear this surgeon's name. His padded metal splints to correct congenital talipes equinovarus are widely used.

**density** (*den-si-ti*). Compactness. Defined as mass per unit volume.

**dental** (*den'-tal*). Pertaining to the teeth.

**dental caries** (*den-tal kā-rēz*). Destruction of teeth by the action of micro-organisms. Holes in the teeth.

**dental cyst** (*den-tal sist*). Cyst, occurring at the root of a tooth, usually sterile and containing cholesterol.

**dental formula** (*den-tal for-mū-la*). Formula indicating the number of each type of teeth, *viz*. incisors, canines, premolars and molars. The numbers are written for the upper and lower jaws on one side thus: $i\frac{2}{2}; c\frac{1}{1}; p\frac{2}{2}; m\frac{3}{3}$

**dentine** (*den'-tēn*). The substance which forms the body of a tooth. *See* TEETH.

**dentition** (*den-ti-shon*). Teething. *See* TEETH.

**denture** (*den'-tūr*). A set of artificial teeth.

**deodorant** (*dē-ō-do-rant*). Substance which prevents or masks unpleasant smells.

**deoxidation** (*dē-ok-si-dā-shon*).
Removal of oxygen from a
chemical compound.

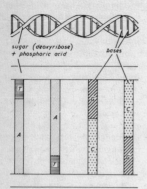

sugar (deoxyribose)
+ phosphoric acid          bases

8. *Deoxyribonucleic acid*
   *T = Thymine*
   *A = Adenine*
   *G = Guanine*
   *C = Cytosine*

**deoxyribonucleic acid** (*dē-ok-
si-rī-bō-nū-klā-ik      a-sid*).
Formed from nucleotides
containing the sugar deoxyribose and one of four bases,
adenine, cytosine, guanine
and thymine, which are
arranged in chains to give a
series. The genetic information of the cell is stored in the
DNA molecule in the form of
a three base code which has
been deciphered by molecular biologists. A gene is
envisaged as a chain of base
triplets. DNA is capable of
self-replication. In the model
proposed by Crick and Wat-
son a helix of one strand of
DNA is complementary to a
second helix to which the
bases are paired adenine–
thymine, cytosine–guanine,
*see* Fig., thus when the DNA
is duplicated the two helices
separate and each becomes a
template for the complementary pair.

**depersonalization** (*dē-per-so-
na-lī-zā'-shon*). A neurotic
state when the person feels
that he has in reality no existence but is only an onlooker
at his own behaviour and
actions.

**depilatory** (*de-pi-la-to-ri*). An
agent for removing super-
fluous hairs from the body.

**depletion** (*de-plē-shon*). Act of
emptying; bleeding; purging.

**deposit** (*de-po'-zit*). A sediment.

**depot injection** (*de'-pō*). Quantity of a drug, several times a
single dose, injected in slowly
absorbable form.

**depressant** (*de-pre'-sant*). An
agent reducing functional
activity.

**depression** (*de-pre'-shon*). A
feeling of gloom due to disappointment, loss or failure.
In *reactive d.*, due to stress,
the patient does not lose

touch with reality. *Severe d.* is a psychotic state and there is usually a predisposition to it in the person's make-up. He then loses all touch with reality and needs expert help. *Involutional d.* occasionally occurs at the menopause. In all types of depression there is a risk of suicide.

**de Quervain's disease** (*de kār-vāns di-sēz*). Stenosing tenosynovitis; a fibrous thickening of the tendon sheath usually of the abductor pollicis longus.

**Derbyshire neck** (*dah-bi-shu nek*). Term used to describe a swollen neck due to goitre. Once common in parts of Derbyshire because of local iodine deficiency in the soil and water.

**Dercum's disease** (*der-kums di-sēz*). Multiple painful lipomata.

**derma** (*der'-ma*). Dermis.

**dermatitis** (*der-ma-tī'-tis*). Inflammation of the skin. The numerous causes may be of external or internal origin.

**dermatitis herpetiformis** (*der-ma-tī-tis her-pe-ti-faw'-mis*). Blistering disease associated with intense pruritus characterized by subepidermal bullae and an eosinophil polymorphonuclear leucocyte infiltrate.

**dermatoglyphics** (*der'-ma-tō-gli'-fiks*). Study of skin ridge patterns.

**dermatology** (*der-ma-to-lo-ji*). The science of the skin and its diseases.

**dermatome** (*der-ma-tōm*). Instrument for cutting a skin graft.

**dermatomycosis** (*der-ma-to-mī-kō'-sis*). A skin disease caused by a fungus.

**dermatomyositis** (*der-ma-tō-mī-ō-sī'-tis*). A rare disease classified as a 'collagen disease' characterized by weakness and muscle tenderness and frequently associated with an erythematous rash. Occasionally the myocardium is affected. The cause is unknown.

**dermatophytes** (*der-ma-tō-fīts*). Fungi which grow on the skin.

**dermatosis** (*der-ma-tō'-sis*). Any skin disease.

**dermis** (*der-mis*). Specialized connective tissue supporting the epidermis and the epidermal appendages (hair follicles, sweat glands).

**dermographism** (*der-mō-gra-fizm*). The production of weals on the skin, resembling urticaria, on gently stroking the skin.

**dermoid cyst** (*der-moyd sist'*). A cyst containing epithelial substances, especially hair, teeth, and sebaceous material.

**Descemet's membrane** (*des-mās mem-brān*). Lining membrane behind the cornea of the eye.

**desensitization** (*dē-sen-sit-tī-zā-shon*). To remove sensitivity to a substance. A method of treatment used for the allergic state.

**desiccation** (*de-si-kā'-shon*). The act of drying.

**desmoid** (*des'-moyd*). Like a bundle. Fibrous tissue.

**desquamation** (*de-skwa-mā'-shon*). Loss of squamous cells from the surface of an epithelium.

**detergent** (*de-ter-jent*). Substance which effectively lowers the surface tension of a fluid.

**deterioration** (*de-tār-i-o-rā-shon*). A worsening condition.

**detoxicated** (*dē-tok-si-kā-ted*). With toxic properties removed.

**detritus** (*de-trī'-tus*). Debris. Accumulation of disintegrated material.

**detrusor** (*dē-trū-sor*). An expelling muscle.

**deuteranomaly** (*dū'-te-ra-no'-ma-li*). Anomalous trichromatic colour vision where red, blue and green are seen, the green imperfectly due to

inadequate discrimination in yellow part of spectrum.

**dexter** (*dek'-ster*). Right. Upon the right side.

**dextran** (*dek-stran*). A blood-plasma substitute.

**dextrin** (*dek-strin*). An intermediate product in the conversion of starch into sugar.

**dextrocardia** (*dek-stro-kar'-dia*). Congenital transposition of the heart from the left to the right side of chest.

**dextrose** (*dek-strōs*). Grape sugar. Glucose.

**dhobie itch** (*dō'-bē*). Ringworm, mainly in the inguinocrural region. Also called tinea cruris.

**diabetes insipidus** (*dī-a-bē-tēz in-si-pi-dus*). Syndrome caused by deficient secretion of antidiuretic hormone (ADH) by the pituitary gland, and characterized by polyuria, the urine being of low specific gravity.

**diabetes mellitus** (*dī-a-bē-tēz me-li-tus*). Usually diabetes. Syndrome caused by a relative deficiency of insulin. Insulin is secreted by the $\beta$ cells of the islets of Langerhans in the pancreas and in some manner facilitates the uptake of glucose by cells. In the absence of insulin there is a failure to utilize glucose which leads to biochemical disturbances resulting in ketosis, electrolyte disturbances, etc. The glucose meanwhile is secreted in the urine together with its water of solution and this results in polyuria; the urine, being loaded with sugar, is of high specific gravity. Rarely the findings in the urine of diabetes mellitus are mimicked by a low renal threshold for glucose or some other sugar (galactose, pentose).

**diabetic coma** (*dī-a-be-tik kō-ma*). Unconsciousness resulting from extreme ketosis.

**diabetic neuropathy** (*dī-a-be-tik nū-ro-pa-thi*). Asymmetrical affection of peripheral nerves which is a complication of unregulated diabetes.

**diabetic retinopathy** (*dī-a-be-tik ṛe-ti-no'-pa-thi*). Complication of unregulated diabetes; the retina shows micro-aneurysms of the blood vessels and circular haemorrhages and exudates.

**diacetic acid** (*dī-a-sē-tik a-sid*). Aceto-acetic acid. This is a substance occasionally present in the urine: especially in serious cases of diabetes.

**diagnosis** (*di-ag-nō'-sis*). The decision as to the nature of an illness, arrived at by clinical assessment of the patient and results of investigations.

**dialysis** (*dī-a'-li-sis*). Method of separating small molecules (crystalloids) from colloids by placing the mixture in a container made of a membrane which is permeable only to small molecules (semi-permeable membrane). The container is placed in water into which the small molecules diffuse leaving the colloids in the container.

**diameters of pelvis** (*dī-a-me-terz*). Besides the three conjugate diameters (described under CONJUGATE), the most important pelvic measurements are as follows: *The right and left oblique*, from the right and left sacro-iliac joints to the left and right pectineal eminences respectively; these should measure 12 to 13 cm (4¾ to 5 in). The *transverse*, which at the brim measure 12 cm (4¾ in) and at the outlet about 10 cm (4 in). *The distance between the anterior superior spines* of the ilia should not be less than 26 cm (10 in), and *between the iliac crests* at least an inch more than this.

**diameters of skull** (*dī-a-me-terz*). The important diameters of the fetal skull at term are as follows: Suboccipito-bregmatic, 9 cm (3¾ in); cervico-bregmatic, 9 cm (3¾ in); fronto-mental, 9 cm (3½ in); occipito-mental, 13 cm (5 in); supra-occipito-mental, 15 cm (5½ in); occipito-frontal, 12 cm (4½ in); suboccipito-frontal, 10 cm (4 in); biparietal, 9 cm (3¾ in); bitemporal, 9 cm (3½ in) (Jellett).

**diapedesis** (*dī-a-pe-dē-sis*). The passage of leucocytes through the walls of blood vessels. It occurs in inflammation.

**diaphoresis** (*dī-a-fo-rē'-sis*). Perspiration.

**diaphoretics** (*dī-a-fo-re-tiks*). Agents which increase perspiration, *e.g.* pilocarpine.

**diaphragm** (*dī-a-fram*). The muscular septum separating the chest from the abdomen.

**diaphragmatic hernia** (*dī-a-fra-ma-tik her-ni-a*). Herniation of abdominal viscera through the diaphragm into the chest. Usually congenital as a result of defective development of the diaphragm.

**diaphyseal aclasis** (*dī-a-fi-sē-al a-klā-sis*). A hereditary defect in the action of osteoclasts in the reshaping of the shaft of the long bones during growth which results in multiple osteomas or exostoses.

**diaphysis** (*dī-a-fi-sis*). The middle part of long bones; the shaft. *See* BONE.

**diarrhoea** (*dī-a-rē-a*). Frequent loose evacuations of the bowels.

**diarthrosis** (*dī-ar-thrō'-sis*). A freely movable joint permitting movement in any direction.

**diastase** (*dī-a-stāz*). An enzyme which converts starch into sugar with intermediate dextrins.

**diastasis** (*dī-a-atā'-sis*). Dislocation.

**diastole** (*dī-a-sto-lē*). That part of cardiac cycle when the ventricles fill with blood, *cf.* systole.

**diastolic** (*dī-a-sto'-lik*). Relating to diastole.

**diathermy** (*dī-a-ther-mi*). The passage of high-frequency electric current through a tissue. Because of the electrical resistance of the tissue, heat is generated. This is diffuse when large electrodes are used, and as such constitutes a physiotherapeutic aid. Tissues may be cauterized by using a small electrode.

**diathesis** (*dī-a'-the-sis*). Constitutional disposition to a particular disease.

**dichotomy** (*dī-ko-to-mi*). Division into two parts.

**dicrotic** (*dī-kro'-tik*). Having two beats. Usually applies to secondary pulse wave due to the closure of the semi-lunar valves since, when this is marked as in conditions associated with vasodilatation, *e.g.* high fever, it gives the impression of a double pulse.

**didactyle** (*dī-dak'-til*). Having only two fingers, or two toes.

**didymitis** (*di-di-mī'-tis*). Orchitis.

**dielectric** (*dī-e-lek-trik*). The non-conducting material separating the conducting surface in an electrical condenser.

**diet** (*dī-et*). System of food. Food intake.

**dietetics** (*dī-e-te-tiks*). The study of food values.

**Dietl's crises** (*dē-tels krī-sēs*). Severe attacks of renal pain accompanied by scanty, blood-stained urine. Occurs in some cases of movable kidney probably due to kinking of the ureter.

**differential blood count** (*di-fe-ren-shal blud kownt*). The determination of the proportion of each type of white cell in the blood, carried out by microscopical examination. Useful in diagnosis.

**differential diagnosis.** Discrimination between diseases with similar symptoms.

**diffraction** (*di-frak-shon*). Dispersion of light by the edge of the iris and colloidal particles in the cornea and lens of the eye.

**diffusion** (*di-fū-zhon*). The gradual assumption of an even distribution of molecules of gases or fluids within a given volume brought about by their random movement.

**digestion** (*di-jes-chon*). Process by which food is rendered absorbable.

**digit** (*di-jit*). A finger or toe.

**digitalis** (*di-ji-tā'-lis*). An extract of foxglove leaves containing a number of alkaloids which affect the heart muscle. The most widely used of these 'cardiac' glycosides is digoxin. The effect on the heart is to slow down the rate of conduction of the cardiac impulse.

**dilatation** (*dī-la-tā'-shon*). Increase in size, enlargement. The operation of stretching.

**dilator** (*dī-lā'-tor*). An instrument for dilating any narrow passage, as the rectum, uterus, urethra.

**dilution** (*dī-lū-shon*). Solution in which the ratio between solute and solvent has been reduced usually by the addition of solvent.

**dioptre** (*dī-op'-ter*). The unit of refractive power of lens. A lens of one dioptre has a focal length of 1 metre.

**dioxide** (*dī-ōk'-sīd*). A compound containing two atoms of oxygen, *e.g.* carbon dioxide ($CO_2$).

**diphallus** (*di-fa-lus*). A rare developmental abnormality in which there is duplication of the penis together with associated urological deformities such as double bladder.

**diphtheria** (*dif-thār-i-a*). Infectious disease caused by *Corynebacterium diphtheriae* and characterized by the formation of a membranous slough on mucous membranes, usually of the throat. A soluble exotoxin is produced by the virulent strains of *C. diphtheriae* and may cause damage to the heart muscle and nervous system.

**diphyllobothrium latum** (*dī-fi-lō-both-ri-um lah-tūm*). Fish tapeworm which may infest humans. The tapeworm absorbs vitamin $B_{12}$ and may cause megaloblastic anaemia.

**diplegia** (*dī-plē-ji-a*). Paralysis of both sides of the body.

**diplococci** (*di-plō-ko-kī*). Cocci arranged in pairs.

**diploe** (*di-plō-ē*). A cellular osseous tissue separating the two cranial tables.

**diploid** (*di-ployd*). Having chromosomes in pairs. The paired members are homologous.

**diplopagus** (*di-plō'-pa-gus*). Conjoined twins, sharing one or more vital organs.

**diplopia** (*dī-plō-pi-a*). Double vision.

**dipsomania** (*dip-sō-mā'-ni-a*). Pathological craving for alcohol.

**director.** Grooved instrument used to guide other instruments.

**disaccharide** (*dī-sa-ka-rīd*). A sugar consisting of two monosaccharides.

**disarticulation** (*di-sar-ti-kū-lā-shon*). Amputation at a joint.

**disc** (*disk*). Circular plate. *Intervertebral d.* is a fibrocartilaginous articulating layer between vertebrae. *Optic d.* is the area on the retina where the fibres of the optic nerve collect (blind spot).

**discharge** (*dis-charj*). Emission of material, *e.g.* fluid, pus, light, electricity, etc.

**discission** (*dis-si'-shon*). Also called needling. Surgical rupture of the lens capsule of the eye.

**discrete** (*dis-krēt*). Separate, distinct; opposed to confluent.

**disease** (*di-sēz*). A process

which disturbs the structure or functions of the body.

**disinfectants** (*di-sin-fek'-tants*). Substances which destroy micro-organisms. Usually for external use and affecting fungi and bacteria. Many are poisonous.

**disjunction** (*dis-junk'-shon*). Separation of halves of chromosome in cell division.

**dislocation** (*dis-lo-kā'-shon*). Displacement of articular surfaces of bone.

**disorientation** (*di-so-ri-en-tā'-shon*). Loss of the ability to locate one's position in the environment, or the mental confusion seen in psychiatric disorders.

**dispensing** (*dis-pen'-sing*). The preparing of medicines.

**disproportion** (*dis-pro-por'-shon*). General term to indicate that the ratio between the size of the fetal head and the size of the maternal pelvis is abnormally large.

**dissection** (*dis-sek'-shon*). The separation by cutting of parts of the body.

**disseminated** (*di-se-mi-nā-ted*). Scattered. *D. lupus erythematosus*. Also called systemic lupus erythematosus (SLE). A 'collagen disease' producing lesions throughout the body. *D. sclerosis*. Usually called multiple sclerosis. A demyelinating disease giving rise to variable neurological symptoms.

**dissociation** (*di-sō-si-ā'-shon*). Abnormal mental state in which the patient fails to recognize certain, frequently unpalatable, facts relating to himself.

**dissolution** (*dis-so-lū'-shon*). Decomposition.

**distal** (*dis-tal*). Situated away from the centre.

**distichiasis** (*dis-ti-kī'-a-sis*). A double row of eyelashes, causing irritation and inflammation of the eye.

**distillation** (*dis-ti-lā'-shon*). The process of vaporizing a substance and condensing the vapour.

**diuresis** (*dī-ū-rē'-sis*). An increased secretion of urine.

**diuretics** (*di-ū-re-tiks*). Drugs which increase the volume of urine secreted.

**diurnal** (*dī-er-nal*). Daily.

**diverticulitis** (*dī-ver-ti-kū-lī'-tis*). Inflammation of a diverticulum.

**diverticulosis** (*dī-ver-ti-kū-lō'-sis*). Presence of numerous diverticula of the intestine.

**diverticulum** (*dī-ver-ti'-kū-lum*). A pouch-like process from a hollow organ, *e.g.* oesophagus, intestine, urinary bladder.

**dizygotic twins** (*dī-zī-go-tik*). Twins developed from the simultaneous fertilization of separate ova.

**DNA.** Deoxyribonucleic acid.

**DNA viruses.** Viruses in which the genetic material is DNA, *e.g.* adenovirus, papovavirus, herpes virus and pox virus.

**dolor** (*dol'-or*). Pain.

**dominant** (*do-mi-nant*). (1) A gene which has the same expression, *i.e.* produces the same effect when heterozygous (the two genes making up the pair are different) as when homozygous (the two genes are the same), is dominant with respect to the allelic genes, *c.f.* recessive. (2) Dominance of the right or left cerebral hemisphere over the other is responsible for left- or right-handedness.

**donor** (*dōnor*). Individual from whom tissue or organ is removed for transfer to another, *e.g.* blood transfusion, grafting.

**dopa reaction** (*dō-pa rē-ak-shon*). Reaction involving the enzymatic oxidation dihydroxyphenylalanine (dopa) to form the pigment melanin.

**dorsal** (*daw-sal*). Relating to the back. *D. root.* Posterior or sensory root. Nerve root carrying sensory fibres which enter the dorsal part of the spinal cord.

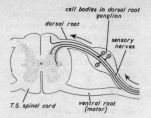

9. *A dorsal root*

**dorsiflexion** (*dor-si-flek-shon*). Bending backwards or in a dorsal direction.

**dorsum** (*daw-sum*). The back.

**double-blind trial** (*du'-bel blīnd trīal*). Clinical trial in which neither physician nor patient knows whether placebo or treatment is administered.

**double recessive** (*du'-bel rē-se'-siv*). Individual who is homozygous for a recessive gene.

**douche** (*doosh*). A shower of water usually used to irrigate a cavity of the body. Hot douche 112°F (44°C); cold douche 60°F (16°C).

**Douglas's pouch** (*dug'-las*). The peritoneal pouch between the back of the uterus and the front of the rectum.

**Down's syndrome** (*downz sin'-drōm*). Mongolism.

**Doyen's clamp** (*doy'-enz klamp*). Straight or curved clamp to close intestinal lumen during anastomosis.

**drainage tubes** (*drā-nāj tūbs*).

Tubes, made of various materials, which are inserted into operation wounds to allow fluids such as blood to drain from the wound.

**drastic** (*dras'-tik*). Strong, severe.

**drip, intravenous** (*drip in-tra-vē'-nus*). The administration into a vein of saline, plasma or blood.

**drive** (*drīv*). In psychology, an urge to satisfy a basic need, such as hunger.

**droplet infection** (*drop-let in-fek'-shon*). Fine droplets of fluid are expelled from the upper respiratory passages during talking or sneezing, etc. These droplets may carry micro-organisms which infect persons inhaling the droplets.

**dropsy** (*drop'-si*). See OEDEMA.

**drug.** Substance used as a medicine. *D. addiction.* A dependence on drugs which is beyond the subject's control. *D. eruption.* Rash due to sensitivity to a drug. *D. reaction.* General reaction to a drug. This may include fever, malaise, joint pains, rashes, jaundice, etc. *D. resistance.* Strains of micro-organisms resistant to the action of antibiotics. The emergence of these resistant strains is now the largest single problem in the treatment of bacterial infection.

**Duchenne's disease** (*dū-shens di-sēz*). Pseudo-hypertrophic muscular dystrophy. A genetically determined abnormality of muscle metabolism (myopathy) first affecting the hip and shoulder girdles.

**Ducrey's bacillus** (*dū-krās ba-si-lus*). *Haemophilus ducreyi*, the organism causing the venereal disease, chancroid.

**duct.** Passage lined by epithelium.

**ductless glands.** See ENDOCRINE.

**ductus** (*duk'-tus*). A duct; a little canal of the body. *D. arteriosus* connects the pulmonary artery and the aorta in fetal life. Occasionally this remains patent.

**dumb-bell tumour.** Neurofibroma of the spinal canal. Part of the tumour is extradural and is connected by a narrow isthmus passing through an intervertebral foramen to a paravertebral position.

**dumping syndrome** (*dum-ping sin'-drōm*). Term applied to symptoms which occasionally follow partial gastrectomy. They are gastric discomfort, cold sweats and palpitations.

**duodenal** (*dū-ōdē-nal*). Belonging to the duodenum.

**duodenostomy** (*dū-ō-de-no'-sto-mi*). Surgical establishment of a communication between the duodenum and another structure.

**duodenum** (*dū-ō-dē'-num*). The first 30 cm (12 in) of the small intestine, beginning at the pyloric orifice of the stomach.

**Dupuytren's contracture.** *See* CONTRACTURE.

**dura mater** (*dū-ra mā-ter*). The outer membrane lining the interior of the cranium and spinal column.

**dwarf** (*dworf*). Individual of stunted growth.

**dys** (*dis*). A prefix meaning bad, difficult, painful, abnormal.

**dysaesthesia** (*dis-es-thē-si-a*). Alteration of sensation.

**dysarthria** (*dis-ar-thri-a*). Impairment of speech.

**dyschezia** (*dis-kē-si-a*). Painful defaecation.

**dyschondroplasia** (*dis-kon-drō-plā'-si-a*). — Multiple enchondromas. Cartilage is deposited in the shaft of some bone(s). The affected bones, often in the hands and feet, are short and deformed.

**dyschromatopsia** (*dis-krō-ma-top'-si-a*). Loss of colour vision.

**dyscoria** (*dis-ko-ri-a*). Abnormality in the shape of the pupil.

**dysdiadokinesis** (*dis-dī-a-dō-kī-nē'-sis*). Inability to carry out rapid alternating move-

ments, such as rotating the hands. A sign of cerebellar disease.

**dysentery** (*di-sen-te-ri*). Inflammation of the large intestine. There are two kinds of dysentery, bacillary and amoebic; the former due to a bacillus, the latter to the *Entamoeba histolytica*.

**dysfunction** (*dis'-funk-shon*). Abnormal or impaired function.

**dyskinesia** (*dis-kī-nē'-si-a*). Impairment of voluntary movement.

**dyslalia** (*dis-lā-li-a*). Mechanical speech defect, *c.f.* dysphasia.

**dyslexia** (*dis-lek'-si-a*). A specific difficulty with the written word, not due to any visual defect, which may cause backwardness in learning to read.

**dysmenorrhoea** (*dis-men-o-re'-a*). A painful or difficult menstruation.

**dysopia** (*di-sō-pi-a*). Defective vision.

**dyspareunia** (*dis-pa-rū-ni-a*). Painful coitus.

**dyspepsia** (*dis-pep-si-a*). Indigestion.

**dysphagia** (*dis-fā-ji-a*). Difficulty in swallowing.

**dysphasia** (*dis-fa-si-a*). Difficulty in speaking.

**dysplasia, polyostotic fibrous** (*dis-plā-si-a   po-li-os-to-tik* *fi-brus*). Metabolic defect in the calcification of bone.

**dyspnoea** (*dis-ne'-a*). Difficult breathing.

**dystaxia** (*dis-tak-si-a*). *See* ATAXIA.

**dystocia** (*dis-to-si-a*). A difficult labour (obstetric).

**dystrophia adiposo-genitalis** (*dis-trō-fi-a a-di-pō-sō-je-ni-tā-lis*). Fröhlich's syndrome. Due to damage to the hypothalamus and is characterized by obesity, sexual infantilism, disturbances of sleep and temperature and diabetes insipidus.

**dystrophia myotonica** (*dis-trō-fi-a mī-ō-tō-ni-ka*). Rare hereditary disease characterized by progressive myotonia and muscular atrophy, cataracts, atrophy of the gonads and baldness.

**dystrophy** (*dis-tro-fi*). Defective structure due to shortage of essential factors.

**dysuria** (*di-sū-ri-a*). Painful micturition.

## E

**ear** (*ē-r*). The organ of hearing. It consists of external, middle and internal ear. The *external ear* comprises the auricle and external auditory canal, and is separated from the middle ear by the tympanic mem-

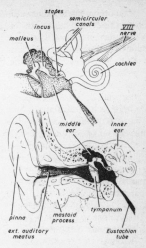

10. *The outer, middle and inner ear; the inset shows the inner ear.*

brane. The *middle ear* is an irregular cavity in the temporal bone. In front it communicates with the Eustachian tube which forms an open channel between the middle ear and the cavity of the nasopharynx. Behind, the middle ear opens into the mastoid antrum, and this in turn communicates with the mastoid cells. There are two openings into the inner ear, both of which are covered with membrane. A string of tiny bones, joined together, extends from the tympanum to the *foramen ovale* of the internal ear. These bones are, from the tympanum, (1) malleus, (2) incus, (3) stapes. The *internal ear* comprises: (*a*) the organ of hearing or cochlea in which are the endings of the auditory nerve, and (*b*) the organ of equilibrium or balance consisting of the three semicircular canals, arranged mutually at right angles.

**ear drum.** The tympanum.

**Eberth's bacillus** (*e-berts ba-si-lus*). The typhoid bacillus.

**ecchondroma** (*e-kon-drō'-ma*). A tumour composed of cartilage.

**ecchymosis** (*e-ki-mō'-sis*). A bruise; an effusion of blood under the skin.

**ECG.** *See* ELECTROCARDIO-GRAM.

**Echinococcus** (*e-kī-nō-ko'-kus*). One of the species of tapeworm. In its adult stage it infests dogs. In its larval stage it produces hydatid cysts in man.

**ECHO virus** (*e-kō vīrus*). Enteropathic cytopathic human orphan virus, *see* ADENOVIRUS. May cause benign lymphocytic meningitis and epidemic myalgia (Bornholm disease).

**echolalia** (*e-kō-la-li-a*). Repetition of everything said.

**eclampsia** (*ek-lamp'-si-a*). Convulsions arising from severe toxaemia of pregnancy.

**ecmnesia** (*ek-mnē-si-a*). A lapse in memory, the memory before and after the lapse being normal.

**ECMO virus** (*ek-mō vīrus*). Enteropathic cytopathic monkey orphan virus. *See* ADENOVIRUS.

**ecology** (*e-ko'-lo-ji*). Biological study of relationships of organisms with environment.

**ecraseur** (*ek-rah'-ser*). Instrument with wire loop used to remove a polypus.

**ECT.** Abbreviation for electroconvulsive therapy.

**ectasis** (*ek-ta-sis*). Distension, as in bronchiectasis when the bronchial tubes are dilated.

**ecthyma** (*ek-thī-ma*). A pustular skin disease, a form of impetigo.

**ectoderm** (*ek'-tō-derm*). The outer layer of the primitive embryo. From it are developed the skin and its appendages, and the nervous system.

**ectogenous** (*ek-to-je-nus*). Originating outside the body.

**ectomy** (*ek'-to-mi*). A suffix denoting removal.

**ectopia** (*ek-tō-pi-a*). Not in the usual place.

**ectopic beat** (*ek-to-pik bēt*).

Contraction of the heart (heart beat) which occurs outside the normal rhythm of the heart.

**ectopic gestation** (*ek-to-pik jes-tā-shon*). Pregnancy in which the fertilized ovum is not situated in the uterus. The ovum may lie in one of the Fallopian tubes or in the abdominal cavity. In course of time the gestation sac is apt to rupture, causing profuse haemorrhage into the abdominal cavity and necessitating immediate operation.

**ectopic viscera** (*ek-to-pik vi-se-ra*). Organs (viscus) which are situated in an abnormal place as a result of a developmental anomaly.

**ectrodactylia** (*ek-trō-dak-ti-li-a*). Absence from birth of one or more toes or fingers.

**ectropion** (*ek-trō-pi-on*). Eversion of the eyelid.

**eczema** (*ek'-ze-ma*). Inflammation of the skin, acute or chronic. There is redness and vesicles may appear which weep and form crusts.

**EDTA.** Ethylenediamine tetra-acetic acid. A chelating agent used especially in the treatment of lead poisoning.

**EEG.** Electroencephalogram.

**effector nerves** (*ef-fek-tor' nervs*). Nerve-endings found in muscles, glands, etc. and which effect the functioning of the organ.

**efferent** (*e'-fe-rent*). Conveying from the centre, *e.g.* the motor nerves which convey impulses from the brain and spinal cord to muscles and glands, *cf.* afferent.

**effervescent** (*ef-fer-ve-sent*). Bubbling. Giving off small bubble of gas.

**effleurage** (*ef-fle-rarj*). Movement performed in physiotherapy. The tips of the fingers or the whole surface of the hand are moved along the course of the blood vessels and lymphatics stimulating the circulation and lymphatic drainage.

**effort syndrome** (*ef-fort sin'-drōm*). A form of anxiety neurosis, characterized by symptoms referable to the heart.

**effusion** (*ef-fū-syon*). Fluid extravasated into serous cavities. *Pleural e.,* fluid in the pleural cavity.

**egocentric** (*e-gō-sen-trik*). Self-centred.

**Eisenmenger's complex** (*ī-sen-men-gers kom-pleks*). A form of cyanotic congenital heart disease, a group of conditions characterized by ventricular septal defect, over-riding of the aorta, right ventricular hypertrophy and pulmonary stenosis, *see*

FALLOT'S TETRALOGY. In Eisenmenger's complex the degree of pulmonary stenosis is minimal.

**ejaculation** (*ē-ja-kū-lā'-shon*). Forcible, sudden expulsion, especially of semen.

**elastin** (*e-las-tin*). Fibrous protein laid down by fibroblasts in connective tissue ground substance. It is structurally similar to collagen and is found particularly in structures which require to withstand mechanical stresses, *e.g.* walls of large arteries. Contrary to earlier opinion, the fibre is considered to be inelastic.

**elastosis** (*e-las-tō'-sis*). Increase in elastic tissue in the skin.

**elation** (*e-lā-shon*). A happy and exalted state of mind.

**elbow** (*el'-bō*). The joint between the arm and fore-

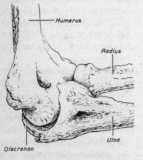

11. *The elbow joint*

arm. The bones forming the joint are the humerus above and the radius and ulna below.

**Electra complex** (*e-lek'-tra com'-pleks*). Female equivalent of Oedipus complex.

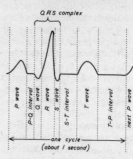

12. *An electrocardiogram (ECG) tracing*

**electrocardiogram** (*e-lek-trō-kar-di-ō-gram*). ECG. Recording of electrical events occurring in the heart muscle. The recording is made by attaching electrodes to the skin and amplifying the electrical signal. The oscillations may be recorded by a pen writer. As the amplitude of the signal will increase as its source approaches the receiving electrode, and decrease as the source recedes, the form of the recording is dependent on factors such as the position of the electrodes in relation to the heart, bulk of heart muscle, etc. A normal ECG tracing from a left-sided lead is shown for one heart beat (normal cardiac cycle). An impulse starts from the sino-atrial node, and passes through the atrial walls causing the atria to contract (P wave), passes through the atrioventricular node and A-V bundle (P-Q interval) to excite the interventricular septum (Q wave), left ventricular wall (R wave) and right ventricular wall (S wave) causing the ventricles to contract. This is followed by an interval (S-T interval) before the muscle becomes recharged (T wave) ready for the next cycle which begins after the atria have filled with blood (T-P or diastolic interval).

**electrocardiophonography** (*e-lek'-trō-kar'-di-ō-fon-o'-gra-fi*). Recording of sound waves from the heart.

**electroconvulsive therapy** (*e-lek-trō-kon-vul-siv the-ra-pi*). Therapy used especially in depressive mental illness, consisting of passing a low amperage electric current between electrodes placed on the side of the head. Ordinarily this would cause a convulsive motor discharge, but the

reaction is 'modified', *i.e.* abolished by general anaesthesia and muscle relaxant drugs administered before the shock is applied.

**electrode** (*e-lek-trōd*). Conducting surface forming a pole to and from which an electric current may flow.

**electroencephalogram** (*e-lek-trō-en-ke-fa-lō-gram*). EEG. Recording of electrical events occurring in the brain obtained from signals received by electrodes placed at various points on the head. The signals are amplified and recorded as with the ECG. The wave forms comprise the average effect of the discharges of thousands of nerves in the cerebral cortex and the brain stem and can therefore be interpreted only at a gross level.

**electrolysis** (*e-lek-tro'-li-sis*). (1) Separation of ions by placing them in an electric field. (2) Destruction of hair follicles by the passage of an electric current.

**electrolytes** (*e-lek-trō-līts*). Substances which ionize in solution.

**electromagnetic spectrum** (*e-lek-trō-mag-ne-tik spek-trum*). Wide range of radiations which are transmitted by photons distributed in a frequency pattern known as electromagnetic waves. The electromagnetic spectrum includes radio waves, light, x-rays and gamma rays.

**electromotive force** (*e-lek-trō-mō-tiv fors*). EMF. The measure of the tendency of an electric current to flow from one point to another. The unit of EMF is the volt.

**electromyography** (*e-lek-trō-mī-o-gra-fi*). EMG. The recording of electrical events occurring in muscle.

**electron** (*e-lek-tron*). A negatively charged atomic particle of mass 0·00055. *E. microscopy*. The use of electrons instead of light to visualize microscopic objects is complex but allows very much greater resolution to be obtained and therefore more details to be seen.

**electroplexy** (*e-lek-trō-plek-si*). *See* ELECTROCONVULSIVE THERAPY.

**electroretinogram** (*e-lek-trō-re'-ti-nō-gram*). Recording of electrical response of retina to light.

**elephantiasis** (*e-le-fan-tī'-a-sis*). Filariasis. A parasitic disease of the lymphatic vessels, causing great enlargement of the limb or limbs affected. It is chronic, and the skin thickens until it somewhat resembles an elephant's hide. The parasite is the *Filaria*.

**elevator** (*e-le-vā'-tor*). (1) A muscle which raises a limb. (2) An instrument used for raising depressed bone, etc.

**elimination** (*e-li-mi-nā'-shon*). The expulsion of poisons or waste products from the body.

**elixir** (*e-lik'-ser*). A term sometimes applied to certain preparations having a sweet taste.

**emaciation** (*e-mā-sē-ā'-shon*). The act of wasting or becoming thin.

**emanation** (*e-ma-nā'-shon*). The act of flowing out. Applied especially to the rays given out by radio-active substances.

**emasculation** (*e-mas-kū-lā'-shon*). Castration of the male.

**embolectomy** (*em-bo-lek-to-mi*). Removal of an embolus.

**embolism** (*em-bo-lism*). Obstruction of blood vessel, usually an artery, by a body, *e.g.* thrombus, fat cells, air, transported in bloodstream.

**embolus** (*em'-bo-lus*). A blood clot or other foreign body in the bloodstream.

**embrocation** (*em-bro-kā'-shon*). Lotion for rubbing on the skin.

**embryo** (*em'-bri-ō*). Animal in process of development from fertilized ovum.

**embryology** (*em-bri-o'-lo-ji*).

Science of the development of the embryo.

**embryoma** (*em-briō'-ma*). *See* TERATOMA.

**embryopathy** (*em-bri-o'-pa-thi*). Disease in, or damage to, embryo by genetic, viral or other agency.

**embryotome** (*em'-bri-ō-tōm*). Instrument for crushing the fetus.

**embryotomy** (*em-bri-o'-to-mi*). Destruction of fetus.

**emesis** (*em'-e-sis*). Vomiting.

**emetic** (*e-me-tik*). Agent which causes vomiting.

**emission** (*e-mi-shon*). Discharge, especially of semen.

**emmetropia** (*em-me-trō'-pi-a*). Normal sight.

**emollients** (*e-mol'-li-ents*). Softening and soothing applications or linaments.

**emotion** (*e-mō-shon*). A response of mind and body to stimuli; such as anger, hate, pleasure or love.

**empathy** (*em-pa-thi*). A form of fantasy when one imagines oneself 'in someone else's shoes' and feels intensely with that person.

**emphysema** (*em-fi-sē-ma*). *Pulmonary e.* The overdistension of the lungs by air. Three types occur: obstructive, compensatory and chronic vesicular emphysema. *Surgical e.* Air bubbles in the subcutaneous tissues following trauma.

**empiricism** (*em-pi'-ri-sizm*). Treatment founded on experience only, not on reasoning.

**emplastrum** (*em-plas'-trum*). A plaster.

**empyema** (*em-pī-ē'-ma*). Collection of pus in a serous cavity.

**emulsion** (*e-mul-shon*). Fine suspension in a fluid of particles of an immiscible fluid, *e.g.* milk is an emulsion of fat in water.

**enamel** (*e-na-mel*). The hard outer coating of the tooth. *See* TEETH.

**enarthrosis** (*e-nar-thrō-sis*). A ball-and-socket joint. *See* p. 203.

**encephalitis** (*en-ke-fa-lī'-tis*). Inflammation of the brain. *See* MENINGITIS. *E. lethargica.* Encephalitis associated with profound disturbance of sleep rhythm.

**encephalocele** (*en-ke-fa-lō-sēl*). Protrusion of brain through the skull.

**encephalography** (*en-ke-fa-lo-gra-fi*). Also called ventriculography. The radiographic examination of the brain after air, which is radiolucent, has been introduced into the cerebral ventricles.

**encephaloid** (*en-ke-fa-loyd*). Resembling the brain.

**encephaloma** (*en-ke-fa-lō'-ma*). A brain tumour.

**encephalomalacia** (*en-ke-fa-lō-ma-lā-si-a*). Softening of the brain.

**encephalomyelitis** (*en-ke-fa-lō-mī-e-lī'-tis*). Inflammation of the brain and spinal cord.

**encephalon** (*en-ke-fa-lon*). The brain.

**encephalopathy** (*en-ke-fa-l-o-pa-thi*). Disease affecting the brain.

**enchondroma** (*en-kon-drō'-ma*). A tumour of cartilage.

**encopresis** (*en-ko-prē-sis*). Faecal incontinence.

**encysted** (*en-sis'-ted*). Enclosed in a sac or cyst.

**endarteritis** (*en-dar-te-rī'-tis*). Inflammation of the intima or lining endothelium of an artery.

**endemic** (*en-de-mik*). Occurring frequently in a particular locality.

**endocarditis** (*endō-kar-dī'-tis*). Inflammation of the endothelial lining of the heart.

**endocardium** (*en-dō-kar-di-um*). The endothelial lining of the heart.

**endocervicitis** (*en-dō-ser-vi-sī-tis*). Inflammation of the mucous membrane lining the canal of the cervix uteri.

**endocolpitis** (*en-do-kol-pī-tis*). Inflammation of the vaginal epithelium.

**endocrine** (*en-dō-krin*). The term used in describing the ductless glands giving rise to an internal secretion. Some of the organs of internal secretion have both an internal and an external secretion, and so may have ducts. The endocrines are: suprarenals, thymus, thyroid, parathyroid, pituitary, pancreas, ovaries and testicles.

**endocrinology** (*en-dō-kri-no'-lo-ji*). Science of the endocrine glands.

**endoderm** (*en-dō-derm*). Germ layer of embryo composed, as is mesoderm, of cells which have migrated from the surface to the interior of the embryo during gastrulation and from which the alimentary tract is largely derived.

**endogenous** (*en-do-je-nus*). Produced within the body.

**endolymph** (*en-dō-limf*). Fluid of the membranous labyrinth of the ear.

**endometrioma** (*en-dō-mē-tri-ō'-ma*). Tumour, from tissue like that of the endometrium but found outside it in myometrium, ovary, uterine ligaments, rectovaginal septum, peritoneum, caecum, pelvic colon, umbilicus and laparotomy scars.

**endometriosis** (*en-dō-mē-tri-ō'-sis*). The presence of endometrioma.

**endometritis** (*en-dō-mē-trī'-tis*). Inflammation of the endometrium.

**endometrium** (*en-dō-mē-tri-um*). The lining membrane of the uterus.

**endoneurium** (*en-do-nū-ri-um*). Connective tissue surrounding nerve.

**endoplasmic reticulum** (*en-dō-plas-mik re-ti-kū-lum*). System of membranes found in the cytoplasm of many cells, *see* CELL.

**end organ** (*end aw-gan*). Collection of cells connected to the peripheral nervous system which act as a transducer, transforming a stimulus into a nerve discharge (receptor) or a nerve discharge into a stimulus, *e.g.* end-plate.

**endoscope** (*en'-dos-kōp*). An instrument for the inspection of the interior of a hollow organ.

**endosteoma** (*en-dos-tē-ō'-ma*). Tumour within a bone cavity.

**endothelioma** (*en-dō-thē-li-ō-ma*). A malignant growth originating in endothelium.

**endothelium** (*en-dō-thē-li-um*). The lining membrane of serous cavities, blood vessels and lymphatics.

**endotoxin** (*en-dō-tok-sin*). An intracellular toxin, *i.e.* retained within the bacteria. When the bacteria are dis-integrated the toxin is liberated.

**endotracheal** (*en-dō-tra-kē'-al*). Within the trachea.

**end-plate** (*end-plāt*). Accumulation of muscle cytoplasm and nuclei in association with the terminal branches of a motor nerve through which the nerve discharge stimulates contraction of muscle.

**enema** (*e-ne-ma*). Passage of liquid into the bowel per rectum.

**enervating** (*en-er-vā-ting*). Weakening.

**engagement of head** (*en-gāj-ment*). Descent of fetal head into the cavity of the pelvis. Normally occurs 2 to 4 weeks before term in the primigravida. In the multigravida may not occur until labour.

**engorgement** (*en-gawj'-ment*). Vascular congestion.

**enophthalmos** (*en-of-thal-mos*). Recession of the eyeball into the orbit.

**enostosis** (*en-os-tō'-sis*). A tumour in a bone.

**ensiform cartilage** (*en-si-fawm kar-ti-lāj*). The sword-shaped process at the lower end of the sternum.

**Entamoeba histolytica** (*en-ta-mē-ba his-tō-li-ti-ka*). The parasite which causes amoebic dysentery.

**enteral** (*en-te-ral*). Intestinal.

**enterectomy** (*en-te-rek-to-mi*).

Excision of part of the intestine.

**enteric fevers** (*en-te'-rik fē-vers*). A term now used to include three separate but closely allied diseases: typhoid, paratyphoid A, paratyphoid B fevers.

**enteritis** (*en-te-rī'-tis*). Inflammation of the small intestine.

**Enterobius vermicularis** (*en-te-rō-bi-us ver-mi-kū-lā-ris*). Threadworm.

**enterocele** (*en-te-rō-sēl*). Hernia containing a piece of bowel.

**enterococcus** (*en-te-rō-ko-kus*). Streptococcus faecalis which occurs as a commensal in the alimentary tract, but is pathogenic in other sites and may cause urinary infections, etc.

**enterocolitis** (*en-te-rō-ko-lī'-tis*). Acute inflammation of the ileum, caecum and ascending colon giving rise to symptoms similar to appendicitis.

**enterokinase** (*en-te-rō-kī'-nās*). An activating enzyme of the succus entericus which converts trypsinogen into trypsin.

**enterolith** (*en'-te-rō-lith*). Stone in the intestines.

**enteropexy** (*en-te-rō-pek'-si*). Suturing of the intestines to the abdominal wall.

**enteroptosis** (*en-te-rop-tō-sis*). Prolapse of the intestines due to stretching of the mesenteric attachment.

**enterorrhaphy** (*en-te-ro'-ra-fi*). The suturing of a rent in the intestine.

**enterospasm** (*en-te-rō-spasm*). Spasm of the intestine. Colic.

**enterostenosis** (*en-te-rō-ste-nō'-sis*). Stricture of the intestines.

**enterostomy** (*en-te-ro'-sto-mi*). Surgically established opening between the small intestine and another surface, *e.g.* gastro-enterostomy, a connection between the stomach and the small intestine. Enterostomies opening on to the anterior abdominal wall are named according to the part of the small bowel involved, thus jejunostomy, ileostomy.

**enteroteratoma** (*en-te-rō-te-ra-tō-ma*). Also known as a raspberry tumour. It consists of prolapsed mucosa appearing at the umbilicus from an unobliterated vitello-intestinal duct.

**enterotomy** (*en-te-ro-to-mi*). Incision into the small intestine.

**enteroviruses** (*en'-te-ro-vī'-ru-sez*). Viruses which can be isolated from intestinal tract, *e.g.* poliomyelitis, Coxsackie and ECHO viruses.

**entropion** (*en-tro'-pi-on*). Inversion of the margin of the eyelid.

**enucleation** (*e-nū-klē-ā'-shon*). (1) Removal of the nucleus. (2) Removal of a central structure, *e.g.* tumour, without its surrounding structures. Usually only possible with encapsulated structures.

**enuresis** (*e-nū-rē-sis*). Incontinence of urine. *Nocturnal e.*, Bedwetting at night.

**environment** (*en-vīr-on-ment*). The external influences which surround a person or thing.

**enzyme** (*en-zīm*). Protein which acts as a catalyst. There are many different kinds of enzyme which increase the reactivity of certain substances, *see* SUBSTRATE, with varying degrees of specificity. Enzymes are essential in order for metabolism to occur at body temperature, since most of the chemical reactions taking place in the body would occur at an imperceptibly slow rate in the absence of enzymes to activate the substrate. The precise mechanism of enzyme action is not yet known.

**eosin** (*ē'-o-sin*). An acid dye used extensively for staining histological sections.

**eosinophilia** (*ē-ō-si-nō-fi-li-a*). (1) Property of being stained by acid dyes such as eosin which combine with basic groups in the tissue. (2) Term used to denote an increase above the normal 2 to 5 per cent in the numbers of poly-morphonuclear leucocytes in the blood which stain deeply with eosin.

**ependyma** (*e-pen'-dī-ma*). The lining membrane of the cerebral cavities and spinal canal.

**ependymoma** (*e-pen-dē-mō'-ma*). A tumour arising from ependymal cells.

**ephedrine** (*e-fe-drin*). Alkaloid from the plant *Ephedra vulgaris* which potentiates the action of adrenaline.

**ephelis** (*e-fe-lis*). A freckle.

**epiblepharon** (*e'-pi-ble'-fa-ron*). Epicanthus.

**epicanthus** (*e-pi-kan-thus*). Projection of the nasal fold to the eyelid.

**epicardium** (*e-pi-kar-di-um*). Visceral layer of the pericardium.

**epicondyle** (*e-pi-kon'-dīl*). Bony eminence as upon the femoral condyles.

**epicranium** (*e-pi-krā-ni-um*). The integuments which lie over the cranium.

**epidemic** (*e-pi-de-mik*). An infectious or contagious disease attacking a number of people in the same neighbourhood at one time.

**epidemiology** (*e-pi-dē-mi-o'-lo-ji*). The study of the distribution of disease.

**epidermis** (*e-pi-der-mis*). The outermost layer of the skin. *See* SKIN.

**epidermophytosis** (*e-pi-der-mō-fī-tō'-sis*). An infection of the skin by fungi, the hands and feet being principally affected. Often termed 'Athlete's Foot' as it is frequently contracted in public gymnasia or swimming baths.

**epididymis** (*e-pi-di'-di-mis*). A long convoluted tube through which sperm pass between the testis and the vas deferens. It forms a mass at the upper pole of the testis.

**epididymitis** (*e-pi-di-di-mī'-tis*). Inflammation of the epididymis.

**epididymo-orchitis** (*e-pi-di-di-mō-aw-kī'-tis*). Inflammation of the epididymis and testes.

**epidural analgesia** (*e-pi-dū-ral a-nal-jē'-si-a*). *See* CAUDAL ANALGESIA.

**epigastrium** (*e-pi-gas'-tri-um*). Surface marking on anterior abdominal wall over region occupied by stomach. *See* ABDOMEN.

**epiglottis** (*e-pi-glot'-tis*). The flap of cartilage which guards the entrance to the glottis or windpipe. *See* LARYNX.

**epilation** (*e-pi-lā'-shon*). Removal of hair with destruction of the hair follicle.

**epilepsy** (*e-pi-lep'-si*). A disorder of the brain marked by the occurrence of convulsive fits. *Idiopathic e.* Typical epilepsy. In many cases the fit is preceded by a warning or aura. This is usually a sensory disturbance. The two main types are: (1) petit mal, momentary loss of consciousness with no convulsion; (2) grand mal, loss of consciousness, tonic and clonic convulsions. *Jacksonian e.* Local spasm, *e.g.* of one limb or one side of the body, due to irritation of the cerebral cortex. It is important to observe in which group of muscles the movements first commence in order that the cerebral lesion may be located.

**epileptiform** (*e-pi-lep'-ti-form*). Like the convulsions of epilepsy.

**epiloia** (*e-pi-loy'-a*). Also called tuberous sclerosis. Inherited defect characterized by sebaceous adenoma of the face, multiple gliomas in the brain, and tumours of the heart, kidneys and retina. Fits are the earliest signs of the disease and mental deficiency usually follows.

**epimenorrhoea** (*e-pē-me-nor-*

*rē'-a*). Menstrual periods of frequent recurrence.

**epinephrine** (*e-pi-nef'-rin*). See ADRENALINE.

**epineurium** (*e-pi-nū-ri-um*). The sheath of a nerve.

**epiphora** (*e-pif'-o-ra*). An excessive flow of tears.

**epiphysis** (*e-pi'-fi-sis*). The separately ossified end of growing bone separated from the shaft, diaphysis by a cartilaginous plate (epiphyseal

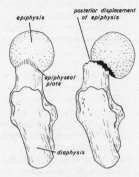

posterior displacement of epiphysis

epiphysis

epiphyseal plate

diaphysis

*13. Epiphysis*

plate). As the bone lengthens more ossified tissue is formed on the diaphyseal side of the epiphyseal cartilage and more cartilage is formed on the epiphysis side. When growth is completed the epiphysis and the diaphysis fuse. *Slipped e*. This affects the upper femoral epiphysis

in late childhood. The cause is unknown.

**epiphysitis** (*e-pi-fi-sī'-tis*). Inflammation of an epiphysis.

**epiplocele** (*e-pi-plō-sēl*). A hernia containing omentum.

**epiploon** (*e'-pi-plō-on*). Omentum.

**episcleritis** (*e-pi-skle-rī'-tis*). Inflammation of the outer layers of the sclera. *See* EYE.

**episiotomy** (*e-pi-si-o'-to-mi*). Incision of the perineum just at the end of the second stage of labour, sometimes performed to avoid extensive laceration of the perineum.

**epispadias** (*e-pi-spa'-di-as*). A congenital malformation in which the urethra opens on the dorsum of the penis.

**epistaxis** (*e-pi-stak'-sis*). Bleeding from the nose.

**epithelial casts** (*e-pi-thē-li-al karsts*). Filaments of renal epithelium found in the urine in certain diseases, when examined under the microscope. They are chiefly cylindrical, are finely granular, and the cells have large nuclei. If in considerable quantity, they signify nephritis, or some other disease of the kidneys.

**epithelioma** (*e-pi-thē-li-ō'-ma*). Tumour of epithelium.

**epithelium** ‾ (*e-pi-thē'-li-um*). Sheet of coherent cells forming the lining of tubes, cavities and surfaces, except if derived embryologically from mesoderm, when it is termed endothelium or mesothelium. Epithelia are classified according to thickness of the sheet and the shape or function of the cells composing them. Epithelium may be mucous, keratinizing, simple (one cell thick), stratified (many cells thick), squamous (flat cells), cubical and columnar (tall cells).

**epitrochlea** (*e-pi-tro'-kli-a*). The inner round projection at the lower end of the humerus.

**epulis** (*e-pū'-lis*). Tumour on the gums.

**erasion** (*e-rā'-zhon*). Scraping.

**Erb's paralysis** (*erbs pa-ra'-li-sis*). The muscles of the upper arm are paralysed due to a lesion of the fifth and sixth cervical nerve roots. May result from excessive traction on the arm during labour. It hangs limply, rotated internally from the shoulder, elbow extended, forearm pronated and palm of hand turned outwards.

**erectile tissue** (*e-rek'-til tis-sū*). Specialized vascular tissue which becomes rigid when filled with blood, *e.g.* penis.

**erector** (*e-rek-tor*). A muscle which raises a part.

**ergograph** (*er'-gō-grarf*). An instrument for recording the amount of work done by muscular action.

**ergosterol** (*er-go-ste-rol*). A sterol found in fats and present in the skin which is converted into vitamin D by irradiation with ultraviolet light.

**ergotism** (*er-go-tism*). Poisoning by alkaloids present in the fungus *Claviceps purpurea* which is found in cereals. One of the alkaloids, ergometrine, is used in obstetrics to control postpartum haemorrhage; another, ergotamine, is used in the treatment of migraine.

**erosion** (*e-rō-zhon*). Ulceration. *Cervical e.* Vaginal epithelium is replaced by columnar epithelium growing down from the cervical canal. As the secretion of the vagina is acid, this epithelium tends to ulcerate and bleed.

**erotic** (*e-ro-tik*). Pertaining to sexual love.

**eructation** (*e-ruk-tā'-shon*). Flatulency, with passage of gas from stomach through the mouth.

**eruption** (*e-rup'-shon*). A breaking out on the skin.

**erysipelas** (*e-ri-si-pe-las*). Acute streptococcal infection of the skin.

**erysipeloid** (*e-ri-si-pe-loyd*). Also called erythema serpens (fish-handler's disease). It is caused by *Erysipelothrix rhusiopathiae* entering a puncture wound in the skin and resembles erysipelas in clinical appearance.

**erythema** (*e-ri-thē-ma*). Red skin, due to vasodilatation in the dermis. *E. multiforme*. Lesions consisting of raised red lesions of varying size and shape which may blister. The cause is unknown but it may represent an abnormal immune response. *E. nodosum*. Red tender skin nodules on the legs which may occur in conjunction with certain conditions such as tuberculosis and sarcoidosis.

**erythrasma** (*e-ri-thras-ma*). An infection of the skin due to a fungus.

**erythroblast** (*e-ri-thrō-blast*). Nucleated cell which is normally found in the bone marrow and which gives rise to a mature red blood cell.

**erythroblastosis fetalis** (*e-rith-rō-blas tō-sis fē-tā-lis*). *See* HAEMOLYTIC DISEASE OF THE NEWBORN.

**erythrocyanosis** (*e-ri-thrō-sī-a nō-sis*). Swelling and blueness of the legs due to vascular spasm.

**erythrocytes** (*e-ri-thrō-sīts*). Red blood cells.

**erythrocyte sedimentation rate** (*e-rith'-rō-sīt se'-di-men-tā-sho̅n r̆at*). *See* ESR.

**erythrocythaemia**. *See* POLY-CYTHAEMIA.

**erythrocytopaenia** (*e-ri-thrō-sī-tō-pē-ni-a*). Diminished number of red blood cells.

**erythrocytosis** (*e-rith-rō-sī-tō-sis*). *See* POLYCYTHAEMIA.

**erythrodermia** (*e-ri-thrō-der-mi-a*). Red skin. The whole body surface is involved in an inflammatory vasodilatation.

**erythromelalgia** (*e-ri-thrō-me-lal-ji-a*). Severe pain associated with extreme dilatation of arteries, especially those supplying the limbs.

**erythropoiesis** (*e-ri-thrō-poy-ē-sis*). The manufacture of red blood cells.

**Esbach's albuminometer** (*es'-baks al-bū-mi-no-me-ter*). A graduated tube used to estimate the quantity of albumin in urine.

**eschar** (*es'-kar*). A dry healing scab on a wound; generally the result of the use of caustic. Also the mortified part in dry gangrene.

**Esmarch's method** (*es'-mar-ches*). A bloodless method for operations. An india-rubber bandage is tightly applied to the limb, beginning at the extremity, and when it has reached above the point of operation a tourniquet is applied and the bandage removed.

**esoteric** (*ē-sō-te'-rik*). For the initiate only.

**esotropia** (*e-sō-trō-pi-a*). Converging squint.

**ESR.** Erythrocyte sedimentation rate. The rate at which red blood cells stick together and sediment to the bottom of a graduated tube. The ESR provides a crude index of the circulating globulins since it is by becoming coated with globulins that the red blood cells are enabled to stick together. In infective conditions which cause a rise in blood globulins, *e.g.* rheumatoid arthritis the rate of erythrocyte sedimentation is increased.

**essentiae** (*es-sen-shi-ē*). Essences; strong solutions of one part volatile oil in five of rectified spirits. Usually given in a few drops on sugar.

**essential oil** (*es-sen-shal oyl*). A volatile oil distilled from an odoriferous vegetable substance, *e.g.* oil of cloves.

**ethmoid** (*eth'-moyd*). A bone of the nose through which the olfactory nerves pass.

**ethnology** (*eth-no-lo-ji*). The science of the races of mankind.

**etiology** (*e-ti-o'-lo-ji*). The science of the causation of disease. *Syn.* aetiology.

**EUA.** Examination under anaesthesia.

**eugenics** (*ū-je-niks*). The study and cultivation of conditions that will improve the human race.

**eunuch** (*ū-nuk*). Castrated human male.

**euphoria** (*ū-fo-ri-a*). Exaggerated sense of well-being.

**euploid** (*ū-ployd*). Having the normal number of chromosomes.

**Eustachian tube** (*ū-stā-shi-an tūb*). The canal from the throat to the ear. *See* EAR.

**euthanasia** (*ū-tha-nā'-si-a*). A painless death procured by the use of drugs.

**evacuation** (*ē-va-kū-ā'-shon*). Discharge of excrement from the body. *See* MOTIONS.

**evaporating lotions** (*e-va-po-rā-ting lō-shons*). Used to procure local coldness. Lead lotion, or eau-de-Cologne and water, are most common.

**eventration** (*ē-ven-trā'-shon*). Protrusion of the intestines.

**eversion** (*e-ver'-shon*). Folding outwards.

**evisceration** (*e-vi-se-rā'-shon*). Removal of the abdominal contents.

**evocation** (*e-vo-kā'-shon*). The indication of a specific direction of development of an embryonic tissue by some agent.

**evolution** (*e-vo-lū'-shon*). Cumulative alteration in the characteristics of a population occurring progressively during the course of successive generations as opposed to the theory of special creation.

**evulsion** (*ē-vul'-shon*). A tearing apart.

**Ewing's tumour** (*ū-wings tū-mer*). Malignant tumour of bone occurring in young adults.

**exacerbation** (*eg-zas-er-bā'-shon*). An increase in the severity of symptoms; a paroxysm of disease.

**exanthemata** (*ek-san-thē-ma'-ta*). Diseases accompanied by specific rashes.

**exchange transfusion** (*eks-chānj trans-fū-shon*). Transfusion of the newborn in which the whole circulatory volume of the infant's blood is removed and replaced by donor blood. This procedure may be necessitated by severe haemolysis of the baby's blood in cases of Rhesus group incompatibility (*see* BLOOD GROUPING) when the Rh positive blood from the baby is replaced by Rh negative blood.

**excipient** (*ek-si'-pi-ent*). The substance used as a medium for giving a medicament.

**excision** (*ek-si'-zhon*). A cutting out.

**excitability** (*ek-sī-ta-bi-li-ti*). (1) Reaction to a stimulus. (2) A state of being unduly excited.

**excitement** (*ek-sīt'-ment*). Increased activity of an organ or organism.

**excoriation** (*eks-ko-rē-ā'-shon*). Abrasions of the skin.

**excrement** (*eks-kre-ment*). Faecal matter.

**excrescence** (*eks-kres'-sens*). An unnatural protruding growth.

**excreta** (*ek-skrē'-ta*). The natural discharges from the body; urine, faeces, sweat.

**exenteration** (*ek-sen-te-rā-shon*). Removal of all contents. *E. of orbit*. Removal of all the contents of the bony orbit. *E. of pelvis*. Removal of pelvic contents and transplantation of ureters on to the sigmoid colon.

**exfoliation** (*eks-fō-li-ā'-shon*). Loss of flakes of material from a surface.

**exfoliative cytology** (*eks-fō-li-a-tiv sī-to-lo-ji*). Study of cells desquamated from epithelia. *See also* CERVICAL SMEAR.

**exhibitionism** (*ek-si-bi-shi-o-nism*). Extravagant behaviour to attract attention.

**exhumation** (*ek-sū-mā'-shon*). Disinterment of a body.

**exogenous** (*ek-so'-je-nus*). Due to an external cause.

**exomphalos** (*ek-som'-fa-lus*). Umbilical hernia of congenital origin.

**exophthalmos** (*ek-sof-thal-mos*). Protrusion of the eyeball. May accompany enlargement of the thyroid gland.

**exostosis** (*ek-sos-tō'-sis*). A tumour growing from bone.

**exotoxin** (*ek-sō-tok-sin*). Toxin released from exterior of an organism, *cf*. endotoxin.

**expectorant** (*ek-spek-to-rant*). A drug which increases expectoration.

**expectoration** (*ek-spek-to-rā'-shon*). The coughing up of sputum.

**exploration** (*ek-splo-rā-shon*). Operative surgical investigation.

**expression** (*ek-spre'-shon*). (1) Intensity with which the effects of a gene are realized in the phenotype. (2) The act of expulsion. (3) Facial appearance.

**exsanguinate** (*ek-san-gwi-nāt*). To make bloodless.

**extension** (*ek-sten-shon*). (1) Traction applied to a fractured limb to hold bones in correct relative position. (2) Unbending of flexed joint as opposed to flexion.

**extensor** (*ek-sten-sor*). A muscle which extends a part.

**external conjugate** (*ek-ster-nal con-jū-gāt*). *See* CONJUGATE.

**external os.** The opening of the cervix into the vagina.

**external version** (*ek-ster-nal ver-shon*). A method of changing the lie or presentation of the fetus by manipulation of the uterus through the abdominal wall.

**extirpate** (*ek-ster-pāt*). To remove completely.

**extra.** Latin for outside.

**extracapsular** (*ek-stra-kap-sū-la*). Outside a capsule.

**extracellular** (*ek-stra-se'-lū-la*). Outside the cells but within the organism. *E. fluid*. Fluid, within the organism, not contained in cells.

**extract** (*ek-strakt*). Preparation obtained by removing substances from a part or organ.

**extrapyramidal** (*ek-stra-pi-ra-mi-dal*). Motor nerve tracts and associated centres which do not directly communicate with the main motor pathway (pyramidal tract). It is a very complex system with many functions, one of which is to regulate muscle tone.

**extrasystoles** (*ek-stra-sis-to-lēs*). Systolic contraction of the heart the impulse for which originates in a focus other than the sinuatrial node, and is therefore outside the normal chain of events in the cardiac cycle.

**extra-uterine gestation** (*ek-stra-ū'-te-rīn jes-tā'-shon*). Pregnancy outside the uterus. *See* ECTOPIC GESTATION.

**extravasation** (*ek-stra-va-sā-shon*). Escape of fluid from its proper channel into surrounding tissue.

**extremity** (*ek-stre-mi-ti*). The end part of any organ. A limb.

**extrinsic** (*ek-strin'-sik*). External. From without. *E. factor. See* CASTLE'S FACTORS.

**extrovert** (*ek-strō-vert*). Outward turned personality, *cf.* introvert.

**exudation** (*ek-sū-dā'-shon*). Oozing; slow escape of liquid.

**eye** (*ī*). The organ of vision.

**eye strain** (*ī strān*). Headache due to effort required to focus on near objects when the refractive properties of the lens (*see* EYE) are defective.

**eye teeth** (*ī tēth*). The canine teeth.

# F

**face presentation** (*fās pre-sen-tā'-shon*). The advance of the fetus face first into the pelvis during labour. It is usually due to some degree of pelvic contraction. The majority of such cases are delivered naturally.

**facet** (*fa-set*). A small, smooth, flattened surface of bone.

**facial** (*fā-shi-al*). Relating to the face. *F. nerve*. Seventh cranial nerve supplying the salivary glands and superficial muscles of the face. *F. paralysis*. Paralysis of the muscles of the face caused by injury or disease involving the facial nerves.

**facies** (*fa-si-ēs*). The appearance of the face, *e.g.* adenoid facies with open mouth and vacant expression.

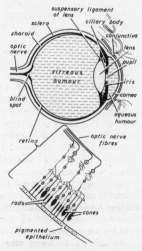

14. The eye

**factor 5 and 7 deficiency.** Deficiency of factor 5 or factor 7 in the blood may cause a clinical syndrome similar to haemophilia.

**facultative** (*fa-kul-ta-tiv*). Able to live under varying conditions.

**faeces** (*fē'-sēs*). The discharge from the bowels. Common abnormalities to be noted are (1) *Colour*. Black may indicate the presence of altered blood or the patient may be taking iron. Green stools occur in enteritis, clay-coloured stools in jaundice. (2) *Consistency*. Loose watery stools occur in diarrhoea, hard dry stools in constipation. Foreign bodies such as worms may be present. Unaltered blood may be due to haemorrhoids. Mucus and blood may be due to colitis or intussusception.

**faecolith** (*fē-kō-lith*). Stone-like body composed of compacted faeces.

**Fahrenheit** (*fa-ren-hīt*). Temperature scale formerly used in the graduation of most clinical thermometers in use in the United Kingdom. Normal body temperature is 98·6°F. For conversion to Celsius, *see* p. 13.

**faint** (*fā-nt*). Syncope.

**falciform** (*fal'-si-form*).
Sickle-shaped. Applied to certain ligaments and other structures.

**Fallopian tubes** (*fa-lō-pi-an*). Two trumpet-like canals, about 8 cm (3 in) long, passing from the ovaries to the uterus. *See* UTERUS AND SALPINGITIS.

**Fallot's tetralogy** (*fa-lōz te-tra-lo-ji*). A group of congenital heart defects consisting of dextra-position of the aorta, right ventricle hypertrophy, intraventricular septal defect and stenosis of the pulmonary artery.

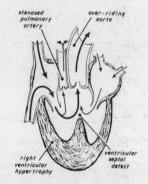

*15. Fallot's tetralogy*

**fall out** (*fawl owt*). Particulate matter containing radioactive material which falls from clouds containing the debris of atomic explosion.

**falx cerebri** (*falks se-re-brē*). The fold of dura between the two cerebral hemispheres.

**familial** (*fa-mi-li-al*). Affecting several members of one family.

**familial periodic paralysis** (*fa-mi-li-al pār-i-o-dik para'-li-sis*). Periodic muscular weakness due to acute extra-cellular potassium deficiency.

**fanaticism** (*fa-na-ti-sizm*). Zeal for some belief or cause carried to excess.

**Fanconi syndrome** (*fan-kō-ni sin'-drōm*). Inherited disorder in which there is a failure of reabsorption of phosphate, amino-acids and sugar by the proximal renal tubules resulting in the appearance of these substances in the urine. The kidneys are also unable to produce an acid urine. The resulting clinical features are thirst, polyuria and rickets followed by chronic renal failure.

**fantasy** (*fan'-ta-si*). A world of imagination controlled by the whim of the individual.

**faradism** (*fa-ra-dism*). An induced low frequency asymmetrical alternating current used to stimulate muscle where the nerve supply is intact.

**farmer's lung** (*fah'-mers lung*). Occupational disease due to inhalation of spores from mouldy hay.

**fascia** (*fa-shi-a*). Sheet of connective tissue, *e.g. Superficial fascia* which is connective tissue separating the dermis from underlying structures. *Deep fascia*: condensations of connective tissue investing muscles and forming compartments for certain structures.

**fascicle** (*fa-sikl*). A little bundle of fibres.

**fat.** (1) Material extractable by fat solvents such as ether. In this sense it includes a large group of chemicals, *e.g.* steroids, carotenoids and phospholipids. (2) True or neutral fat is a compound of glycerol and a certain group of organic aliphatic acids known as fatty acids.

**fat embolism** (*fat em-bo-lism*). *See* EMBOLISM.

**fatigue** (*fa-tēg*). Tiredness.

**fatty degeneration** (*fa-ti dē-ge-ne-rā'-shon*). Term applied to the appearance of certain cells which as a result of damage take on an appearance of having droplets of fat in their cytoplasm.

**fauces** (*faw'-sēs*). The short passage between the back of the mouth and the pharynx.

**favism** (*fā-vism*). Acute haemolysis caused in sensitive individuals by a

substance in the fava bean.
Those who are sensitive have
a deficiency of glucose-6-
phosphate dehydrogenase in
their red blood cells.

**favus** (*fā-vus*). A type of ringworm infection.

**febrile** (*fe'-bril*). Relating to
fever.

**fecundation** (*fe-kun-dā'-shon*).
Impregnation. Fertilization.

**fecundity** (*fe-kun'-di-ti*). Power
of producing young.

**feeble minded** (*fē-bl min-ded*).
Subnormal mentality. No
longer an official classification.

**Fehling's solution** (*fā-lings
so-lū-shon*). Solution which
changes colour on reduction.
Formerly used to detect
reducing substances (sugars)
in the urine.

**fel.** Bile.

**Felty's syndrome** (*fel-tis sin-
drōm*). Syndrome characterized by leukopaenia and
enlargement of the spleen
associated with chronic
rheumatoid arthritis. A
generalized hyperpigmentation of the skin is sometimes
present. The cause of the
syndrome is unknown.

**female** (*fē-māl*). Applied to the
sex that bears young.

**femoral artery** (*fe-mo-ral
ar-te-ri*). The artery of the
thigh, from the groin to the
knee.

**femoral canal** (*fe-mo-ral ka-
nal*). The small canal internal
to the femoral vein. The site
of a femoral hernia.

**femur** (*fē-mur*). The thigh
bone.

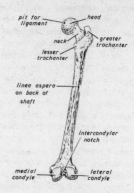

pit for ligament — head
neck
greater trochanter
lesser trochanter
linea aspera on back of shaft
intercondylar notch
medial condyle
lateral condyle

16. *The femur*

**fenestra** (*fe-nes-tra*). A window, term applied to certain
apertures.

**fenestration** (*fē-nes-trā-shon*).
Making an artificial window;
an operation performed in
certain types of deafness.

**fermentation** (*fer-men-tā'-
shon*). Decomposition of
organic material by enzymes
present in certain organisms,
*e.g.* yeasts and bacteria.

**fertility** (*fer-ti-li-ti*). Ability to
produce young, *cf.* infertilty.

**fertilization** (*fer-ti-lī-zā'-shon*).
Union of male and female

germ cells whereby reproduction takes place.

**fester** (*fes'-ter*). Inflammation, with collection of pus.

**fetal.** WHO approved spelling for foetal.

**fetishism** (*fe-ti-shi-sm*). Substitution of a symbolic object for the normal goal of union with a number of the opposite sex, as fulfilment of the sexual instinct.

**fetus** (*fē'-tus*). Unborn child. Old spelling, foetus, now replaced.

**fever** (*fē-ver*). Elevation of body temperature above normal.

**fibre** (*fī-ber*). A thread-like structure.

**fibrillation** (*fī-bri-lā'-shon*). Unco-ordinated contraction of heart muscle. May affect the atria only (atrial fibrillation) or the ventricles (ventricular fibrillation). Because fibrillation prevents efficient contraction of the heart muscle it is rapidly fatal when it affects the ventricles. When only the atria are involved the ventricles beat separately at their own rate.

**fibrin** (*fī-brin*). Long chain protein which forms a fibrous gel matrix as a basis for a blood clot. It is formed from the soluble plasma protein, fibrinogen, by the action of thrombin. *F. foam*: preparation of human fibrin used as haemostatic pack.

**fibro-adenoma** (*fī-brō-a-denō'-ma*). A tumour composed of mixed fibrous and glandular elements.

**fibroblast** (*fī-brō-blast*). Fibrocyte. Branched cell found throughout connective tissue which synthesizes collagen and elastin.

**fibrocartilage** (*fī-brō-kar-ti-lāj*). Cartilage with fibrous tissue.

**fibrochondritis** (*fī-brō-kon-drī'-tis*). Inflamed fibrocartilage.

**fibrocystic disease** (*fī-brō-sis-tik di-sēz*). Mucoviscidosis. A disease due to a defect in salt retention in mucous and sweat glands. As a result the mucopolysaccharide secretions, *e.g.* in the respiratory tract and from the pancreas, become excessively viscous resulting in the formation of retention cysts which become fibrosed, hence the term, fibrocystic disease.

**fibro-elastosis** (*fī-brō-ē-las-tō'-sis*). A rare disorder affecting principally the heart in which an excess of collagen and elastin is formed under the endocardium. This impairs the efficiency of the heart with resultant cardiac enlargement and cardiac failure. Occasionally the heart valves are also involved.

**fibroid** (*fī-broyd*). See FIBRO-MYOMA.

**fibroma** (*fī-brō-ma*). Benign tumour of fibrous tissue.

**fibromyoma** (*fī-brō-mī-ō'-ma*). A tumour composed of mixed muscular and fibrous tissue. Especially common in the uterus, and commonly spoken of as 'fibroids'.

**fibrosarcoma** (*fī-brō-sar-kō'-ma*). Malignant tumour of fibroblasts.

**fibrosis** (*fī-brō-sis*). Decomposition of fibrous connective tissue and usually occurring in regions which have been damaged by some trauma.

**fibrositis** (*fī-brō-sī'-tis*). Inflammation of connective tissue, although the term is not only used in this strict sense.

**fibula** (*fī'-bū-la*). The thin bone on the outer side of the leg.

**field of vision** (*fēld of vi-zhon*). The area which can be seen without movement of the eye. See PERIMETER.

**filament** (*fi-la-ment*). Thread-like piece of fibre.

**Filaria** (*fi-la-ri-a*). Parasitic thread-like worm which may cause lymphatic obstruction. See ELEPHANTIASIS.

**filiform** (*fi-li-fawm*). Thread-like. *F. bougie.* A slender bougie.

**filipuncture** (*fi-li-punk-tūr*). A method of treating aneurysm by inserting a fine wire thread. This acts as a foreign body, and the blood inside the sac clots.

**filter** (*fil-ter*). Device used for removing a certain range of material while allowing others to pass through. The selectiveness of the filter is dependent on its properties. Thus, optical filters made from different types of glass pass only light in certain parts of the spectrum. Fluid filters, according to their pore-size, are used to remove viruses, bacteria or other suspended impurities. Gas filters remove certain gases from air passed through them by adsorption of the gas on to special material.

**filtration** (*fil-trā-shon*). Passage through a filter.

**filum** (*fē-lum*). A structure resembling a thread. *F. terminale.* The tapering end of the enlargement of the lumbar spinal cord.

**fimbria** (*fim-bri-a*). A fringe, especially the fringe-like end of the Fallopian tube.

**finger** (*fing'-ger*). One of the digits of the hand.

**fingerprinting** (*fing'-ger-printing*). Method of protein analysis by enzymatic breakdown to peptides followed by two-dimensional separation by chromatography.

**first intention** (*ferst in-ten'-shon*). A surgical term for aseptic healing of a wound by bringing the edges directly together.

**first stage** (*ferst stāj'*) (**of labour**). The act of parturition from the first pains up to the full dilation of the cervix.

**fissure** (*fis-sūr*). A split or cleft.

**fissure in ano** (*fis-sūr in ā-nō*). Small ulcerated cleft in the mucous membrane of the anus.

**fistula** (*fis-tū-la*). Pathological communication between two epithelial surfaces or cavities, *e.g.* rectovaginal fistula.

**fit.** Convulsion usually with associated loss of consciousness.

**fixation** (*fik-sā'-shon*). (1) Process used in making permanent preparations of tissues by killing the cells with the least structural distortion. Chemicals such as formaldehyde and gluteraldehyde are fixatives. (2) Focussing the eyes on an object. (3) In psycho-analytic terms being emotionally attached to another person or object.

**flaccid** (*flak-sid*). Soft, lacking rigidity.

**flagellum** (*fla-jel'-lum*). Fine, thread-like structure projecting from surface of certain cells, *e.g.* spermatozoa, which by a lashing movement propels the cell, *cf.* cilia.

**flame photometer** (*flām fō-to'-me-ter*). Apparatus used to measure very small quantities of metals by the brightness of their characteristic flame.

**flap.** A piece of skin cut to fold over a wound or amputation stump.

**flatfoot.** Flattening or total loss of the arches of the foot. It then rests completely on the ground, giving characteristic appearance and walk.

**flatulence** (*fla-tū-lens*). Distension of the alimentary tract by gas.

**flatus** (*flā-tus*). Gas in the intestine.

**flea** (*flē*). The human flea is *Pulex irritans*. It is without wings and sucks blood, giving rise to irritation and sepsis.

**flexion** (*flek'-shon*). Being bent; the opposite of extension.

**Flexner bacillus** (*flek-sner ba-si-lus*). One of the Shigella group of pathogenic bacteria which cause bacillary dysentery.

**flexor** (*flex-sor*). A muscle which causes flexion.

**flexure** (*flek'-shur*). A bend. A

curvature of an organ, *e.g.
hepatic f.* bend of the colon
beneath the liver.

**floating ribs** (*flō'-ting ribz*). The
two lower pairs of ribs.

**flooding** (*flu-ding*). Excessive
bleeding from the uterus.

**fluctuation** (*fluk-tū-ā-shon*). A
wavelike motion felt on palpation of an abscess or a cyst
containing fluid.

**fluke** (*flook*). Any of the tre-
matode class of worm.

**fluorescein** (*flo-re-sēn*). A coal-
tar derivative which stains
cornea a vivid green if there
is any loss of surface
epithelium, *e.g.* in an abrasion or ulcer.

**fluorescence** (*flo-re-sens*).
Emission of light at a
wavelength which is different
from that of the incident
light. The emitted light has a
lower energy, *i.e.* is of longer
wavelength from the inci-
dent irradiation which is
absorbed.

**fluorescent screen** (*flo-re-sent
skrēn*). A screen coated with
materials which fluoresce
when exposed to x-rays.

**fluoridation** (*flo-ri-dā'-shon*).
The addition of fluoride, such
as when added to drinking
water.

**fluorine** (*flo-rēn*). A halogen
element. If added in minute
quantities to drinking water it
causes a reduced incidence of

dental decay. The ideal
amount of water is 1 p.p.m.

**fluoroscopy** (*flo-ro-sko-pi*).
Use of fluorescent screen to
view x-ray images.

**flutter** (*flu-ter*). Rapid regular
contraction of the atrial
muscle of the heart. The rate
reaches about 300 beats per
minute. Because of the
recovery time required by the
ventricular myocardium
between successive beats, it
only responds to every
second or third atrial contraction, *i.e.* 2:1 or 3:1. *See*
HEART BLOCK.

**flying squad** (*flī-ing skwod*).
Emergency clinical unit
which can travel rapidly to
domiciliary cases.

**focus** (*fō'-kus*). Point of maximum intensity.

**foetor** (*fē'-tur*). Strong unpleasant smell.

**fetus papyraceus** (*fē-tus pa-pi-
rā-sē-us*). A fetus which has
been retained within the
uterus for months after its
death, and has undergone a
kind of natural mummi-
fication.

**Foley catheter** (*fō-li kā'-the-
ter*). Self-retaining catheter,
kept in position by small bal-
loon.

**folic acid** (*fō-lik a-sid*). Pteroy-
glutamic acid, part of the vitamin B complex found in
liver, yeast, spinach, etc.

Essential for blood formation.

**folie à deux** (*fo'-li ah der*). Delusion shared by two persons.

**follicle** (*fo-li-kl*). (1) Hair follicle. A pit-like structure in the epidermis in which the hair grows and which receives the duct of sebaceous glands. (2) Ovarian follicle. Also called Graafian follicle. A fluid-filled vesicle in the ovary containing a maturing ovum which at ovulation is discharged by rupture of the follicle. The ovaries contain many ripening follicles which are under the control of the pituitary glands, *see* FOLLICLE STIMULATING HORMONE, but normally only one ruptures at each ovulation. The epithelium of the follicle produces oestrogens. After ovulation the follicle becomes a corpus luteum.

**follicle stimulating hormone** (*fo-li-kl sti-mū-lā-ting hor-mōn*). FSH. Hormone secreted by the anterior lobe of the pituitary gland. In the female it stimulates the growth of ovarian follicles and the production of oestrogens. In the male it promotes the development of spermatozoa in the testis.

**follicular keratosis** (*fo-li-kū-la ke-ra-tō-sis*). Hyperkeratosis in the region of hair follicles (phrynoderma) seen in vitamin A deficiency, Darier's disease and a number of uncommon skin conditions.

**follicular tonsillitis** (*fo-li-kū-la ton-si-lī-tis*). Acute tonsillitis in which beads of pus are exuded from the pits of the undulant epithelium.

**fomentation** (*fō-men-tā-shon*). A poultice: hot wet application to the skin.

**fomites** (*fō-mīts*). Articles like clothing or bedding which have been in contact with a patient ill with a contagious disease.

**fontanelle** (*fon-ta-nel'*). A soft space in the skull of an infant before the skull has completely ossified. The anterior fontanelle, or bregma, is where the coronal, frontal and sagittal sutures meet. The posterior fontanelle is where the lambdoid and sagittal sutures meet. The anterior fontanelle should be closed by 2 years of age. Delay is a sign of rickets.

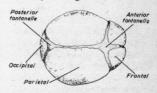

*17. The fontanelles*

**food poisoning.** Diarrhoea and/ or vomiting from eating infected food. Symptoms may be caused by the preformed toxins of *Staphylococcus aureus* or *Clostridium welchii* or from infection by organisms of the *Salmonella group* or rarely by *Botulinus* toxin. Infected foods are usually meat products or confectionery containing eggs, which have been allowed to remain in warm rooms. Another source of infection may be the unwashed hands of those handling food.

**foot.** That part of the leg below the ankle.

**foot and mouth disease.** Virus disease well known in cattle which occasionally affects man causing blistering and ulceration of the buccal mucosa and similar lesions on the hands and feet especially round the nails.

**foot drop.** Inability to keep a foot bent at right angles to the leg. The toes and foot drop and walking becomes difficult. Caused by pressure of bedclothes, or inadequate support to under side of foot when leg is in a splint for a long time, or from paralysis of the muscles which produce dorsiflexion of the ankle.

**foramen** (*fo-rā-men*). An open-

ing. *F. magnum*. Opening in the back of the skull through which the spinal cord passes. *F. ovale*. Opening between the right and left atria in the fetus which allows oxygenated venous blood from the placenta to pass into the left side of the heart and thus bypass the pulmonary circulation. Normally it closes at birth when the pressure in the left atrium rises. *Optic f.*, where the optic nerve enters the skull. Also *Jugular f.*, etc.

**foramen magnum syndrome.** Syndrome due to pressure on the spinal cord and lower cranial nerve nuclei in the medulla. A deformity of the neck and base of the skull results in compression of the cord as it passes through the foramen magnum.

**forceps** (*faw-seps*). Surgical pincers used for lifting and moving instead of using the fingers.

**forceps delivery** (*faw-seps de-li-ve-ri*). Method of assisting the delivery of an infant by applying special forceps to the head.

**forebrain** (*faw-brān*). Cerebrum.

**foreign body** (*fo-ren bo-di*). General term to include any material in the body which is not normally found in that site. Thus a nail in the stomach or in the foot would be regarded as a foreign body (FB).

**forensic medicine** (*fo-ren-sik*). Medicine in so far as it has to do with the law.

**foreskin** (*faw-skin*). The prepuce, or skin covering the end of the penis.

**formication** (*for-mi-kā'-shon*). A sensation as of ants creeping over the body. Used almost entirely to denote tingling sensation in a nerve recovering from pressure or injury, and therefore after nerve injury it is a sign of regeneration.

**formula** (*faw-mū-la*) (pl. **formulae**). A prescription. Statement of constituents which form a compound.

**formulary** (*faw-mū-la-ri*). A collection of formulae for medical preparations such as those found in the British Pharmacopoeia.

**fornix** (*faw-niks*) (pl. **fornices**). An arch. Applied to various anatomical structures, but especially to the roof of the vagina.

**fossa** (*fo-sa*). Little depressions of the body, such as *f. lacrimalis*, the hollow of the frontal bone, which holds the lacrimal gland. *Iliac f.* Concavities of the iliac bones of the pelvis.

**Fothergill's operation** (*fo'-ther-gilz*). Repair of the anterior and posterior vaginal walls and amputation of the cervix.

**fourchette** (*foor-shet*). A thin fold of skin behind the vulva.

**fovea** (*fō-ve-a*). Shallow depression in the retina where there is an absence of rods and a concentration of cones, *see* EYE, and where there are no intervening nerves and blood vessels. It is the site of maximum visual stimulation and the region on which the image is focused when the eyes are fixed on an object.

**Fowler's position** (*fow-lers pō-si-shon*). Position in which the patient is propped up in bed in such a way as to promote drainage of fluid in the peritoneum into the pelvis.

**Fox-Fordyce disease** (*foks for'-dīs di-zēz*). Itching papular eruption in women affecting the axillary, public and perineal regions and round nipples.

**fractional distillation** (*frak'-sho-nel dis'-ti-lā-shun*). Type of distillation in which substances are separated by their differing boiling-points.

**fractional test meal** (*frak-sho-nal test mēl*). A method of investigation, now largely superseded by the penta-gastrin test meal, whereby samples of gastric contents are withdrawn and analysed at intervals after a standard meal.

**fracture** ( *frak-tūr* ). A break in a bone. The symptoms are—pain, swelling, deformity, loss of function, unnatural mobility, shortening, crepitus. A fracture may

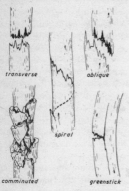

*transverse*   *oblique*

*spiral*

*comminuted*   *greenstick*

18. *Types of fractures*

be: (1) *Simple or closed*, not connected with an external wound. (2) *Compound or open*, communicating with the surface. (3) *Greenstick*, when the bone is fractured half through on the convex side of the bend as in a green twig. Only seen in children. (4) *Comminuted*, where bone

is broken into more than two pieces. (5) *Impacted*, where one fragment is driven into the other. (6) *Complicated*, where fracture is combined with injury to another important structure, *e.g.* artery, nerve, or organ. The type of break may be: (1) *Transverse*, due to direct violence applied at point of fracture. (2) *Oblique*, due to indirect violence when a force applied at a distance causes the bone to break at its weakest point. (3) *Spiral*, when a limb is violently rotated. (4) *Depressed*, only of skull, when bone is driven inwards: it may be *gutter-shaped* with sharp depressed edge, or *pond-shaped* with sloping edge; the latter is only in infants and due to birth injury. *See* COLLES' FRACTURE, POTT'S FRACTURE, SPLINTS, SPONTANEOUS FRACTURE.

**fraenum** ( *frā'-num* ). A small membranous fold attached to certain organs, and acting as a check. *F. linguae*. That under the tongue.

**fragilitas ossium** ( *fra-ji-li-tas o-si-um* ). Abnormal brittleness of the bones.

**framboesia** ( *fram-bē-zi-a* ). *See* YAWS.

**Franschetti's syndrome** ( *fran-ske-tiz sin'-drōm* ). Mandibular-facial dystosis.

**free association.** In psycho-analysis, when the patient gives the first word which a stimulus brings to his mind, or a train of ideas.

**Frei test** (*frī test*). Skin test for lymphogranuloma inguinale in which a small quantity of the heat-inactivated virus is injected into the dermis. If positive a red papule appears in 48 hours at the site of injection.

**Freiberg's disease** (*frī-bergs di-sēz*). Sclerosis of the head of the second or third metatarsal with flattening of the articular surface and swelling and tenderness of the affected joint.

**fremitus** (*fre'-mi-tus*). A vibration perceived by palpation, always applied to a vibration in the chest.

**Freudian** (*froy-di-an*). According to Freud's teaching. He taught that psychological disorders often resulted from unconscious sexual impressions during childhood. These he brought to consciousness through psychoanalysis. Dreams he said were the wish-fulfilment of repressed desires.

**Freund's adjuvant** (*froyndz a'-jū-vent*). Mixture injected with aqueous antigen preparations to increase immune response.

**Frey's syndrome** (*frays - sin'-drōm*). *See* AURICULO-TEMPORAL SYNDROME.

**friction** (*frik'-shon*). (1) A circular movement in massage performed with the tips of the fingers or thumb as deeply as possible over joints; the object being to break down adhesions. (2) The sound heard in auscultation when two dry, roughened surfaces rub together as in pleurisy.

**Friedreich's ataxia** (*frēd-rīks a-tak-si-a*). Inherited degenerative disease of the nervous system in which the posterior and lateral columns of the spinal cord, the cerebellum and occasionally the optic nerves are involved. The onset is in the first or second decade and the condition is progressive. It is characterized by unsteady gait, clumsiness, weakness and dysarthria together with other neurological disturbances.

**frigidity** (*fri-ji-di-ti*). Lack of sexual desire.

**Fröhlich's syndrome** (*frer-liks sin'-drōm*). A disorder with obesity, sexual infantilism, disturbances of sleep and temperature regulation and diabetes insipidus due to damage of the pituitary and hypothalamus.

**frontal** (*frun'dtal*). Relating to the forehead.

**frontal bone** (*frun'-tal bōn*). One of the bones of the skull. *F. sinus. See* SINUS.

**frostbite** (*frost-bīt*). Injury of the skin or a part from extreme cold. There is redness, swelling and pain and necrosis may result.

**fructose** (*frŭk-tōz*). Fruit-sugar.

**fructosuria** (*frŭk-tō-sū-ri-a*). Fructose, the sugar present in fruits, may be extracted in large quantity from the urine if a considerable amount of fruit has been eaten. If the urine is tested for sugar the fructose gives a positive result and may lead to a mistaken diagnosis of diabetes mellitus.

**frustration** (*fru-strā'-shon*). Disappointment experienced by a person who is thwarted and prevented by circumstances from achieving some desired object.

**FSH.** *See* FOLLICLE STIMULATING HORMONE.

**FTA test.** Fluorescent antibody test for syphilis.

**fugue** (*fū'g*). A fleeing from reality as in hysteria. The patient has no recollection of his actions during this time.

**full time or term.** The fetus is said to be at term when it is 20 to 21 in (50–53 cm) long and has finger-nails and toe-nails reaching to the ends of the digits. Such a child should weigh anything from 7 lb (3·2 kg) upwards, and have been developing in the uterus for not less than 40 weeks.

**fulminating** (*ful-mi-nā-ting*). Severe and rapid in its course.

**fumigation** (*fū-mi-gā'-shon*). Sterilization of rooms by disinfectant vapour.

**function** (*funk'-shon*). The normal special work of an organ.

**functional disorder** (*funk-sho-nal di-sor-der*). Subjective sensation of malfunctioning of an organ or organs when there is no evidence of organic disease.

**fundus** (*fun'-dus*). The enlarged part of a hollow organ farthest removed from the orifice; thus the fundus oculi is the interior of the eye behind the lens and pupil, visible with an ophthalmoscope; the fundus uteri is the top of the uterus.

**fungi** (*fun-gī*) (sing. **fungus**). A subdivision of Thallophyta including moulds, mushrooms, rusts, yeasts, etc. Simple plants which lack chlorophyll and are either saprophytic or parasitic. A few fungi cause disease in man. Fungi are used as a source of protein and vitamins, certain enzymes, used in baking and brewing, etc. and antibiotics, notably penicillin.

**fungicide** ( *fun-gi-sīd* ). Any substance used for the destruction of fungi.

**funiculitis** ( *fū-ni-kū-lī'-tis* ). Inflammation of the spermatic cord.

**funnel chest.** Also called pectus excavatum. A developmental deformity in which the sternum is depressed and the ribs and costal cartilages curve inwards.

**furuncle** ( *fu'-rung-kl* ). A boil.

**furunculosis** ( *fu-run-kū-lō'-sis* ). The appearance of one or more boils.

**fusiform** ( *fū'-zi-form* ). Spindle-shaped.

# G

**Gaertner bacillus** ( *gārt-ner ba-si-lus* ). *See* SALMONELLA.

**gag.** An instrument for keeping the mouth open.

**gait** ( *gāt* ). Manner of walking.

**galactagogue** ( *ga-lak-ta-gog* ). An agent that causes an increased flow of milk.

**galactocele** ( *ga-lak'-tō-sēl* ). A cyst of the breast containing milk.

**galactorrhoea** ( *ga-lak-to-re'-a* ). Excessive flow of milk.

**galactosaemia** ( *ga-lak-tō-zē-mi-a* ). A metabolic disorder characterized by presence of galactose in the bloodstream.

**galactose** ( *ga-lak-tōz* ). A hexose sugar which, in combination with glucose, forms the disaccharide lactose which is present in breast milk.

**gall** ( *gawl* ). Also called bile. The secretion of the liver; it accumulates in the gall bladder.

**gall bladder** ( *gawl bla-der* ). The membranous sac which holds the bile. *See* BILE DUCT.

**gallop rhythm** ( *ga-lop rithm* ). Term applied to a particular cadence heard on auscultation of the heart in cases of severe left ventricular failure when as the result of tachycardia there is summation of the sounds of the atrial contraction and of the blood distending the hypotonic ventricles. This gives a third 'beat' which is heard in diastole.

**gallstone** ( *gawl-stōn* ). Calculus in the gall bladder. If the stone passes into the cystic or common bile duct there is great pain, and if in the common bile duct, jaundice. *See* COLIC.

**galvanism** ( *gal-va-nism* ). Therapeutic use of direct electric current, *i.e.* continuous or

# GAL 158

interrupted. Now rarely used for treatment.

**galvanometer** (*gal-va-no-me-ter*). Instrument to measure the flow of very small electric currents.

**gamete** (*ga-mēt*). A sexual reproductive cell, *e.g.* sperm, ovum.

**gametocyte** (*ga-mē-tō-sīt*). A cell which undergoes meiosis to form gametes.

**gamma globulin** (*ga-ma glo-bū-lin*). Protein fraction of plasma, rich in antibodies against infection.

**gamma rays** (*gam'-a rāz*). Electromagnetic waves of extremely short wavelength; similar to x-rays, but shorter. Employed for dry, cold sterilization of any articles which would be destroyed by moisture or heat. Also used in radiotherapy.

**gammopathy** (*ga-mo'-pa-thi*). Excess of immunoglobulins in plasma.

**ganglion** (*gan-glē-on*). (1) A collection of nerve cells forming a semi-independent nerve centre. They are found in the sympathetic nervous system and in other parts of the nervous system. (2) Surgically, a chronic synovial cyst generally connected with a tendon sheath; most common site, back of hand, near the wrist.

**ganglionectomy** (*gan-glē-ō-nek-to-mi*). Excision of a ganglion.

**gangrene** (*gan-grēn*). Massive necrosis of tissue as the result of reduced blood supply. *Dry g.* This results from severe arterial insufficiency. *Wet g.* This is due to concurrent interference in the venous drainage. *Gas g.* Infection by anaerobic organisms, *e.g.*, *Clostridium welchii.*

**Gardiner-Brown's test** (*gard'-ner brownz test*). Tuning fork test of bone condition in aural disease.

**gargle** (*gar'-gl*). A liquid medicine for washing out the throat.

**gargoylism** (*gar-goy-lism*). Hurler's syndrome. A defect of skeletal development in which the skull is grossly deformed and the digital bones are bulbous, the hands assuming a claw-like appearance. There is often associated congenital heart disease and intellectual impairment.

**gas gangrene** (*gas gan'-grēn*). *See* GANGRENE.

**Gasserian ganglion** (*gas-sā-ri-an gan-gli-on*). A ganglion of the sensory root of the fifth cranial nerve, deeply situated in the skull. It is sometimes operated on for the relief of intractable trigeminal neuralgia.

**gastrectomy** (*gas-trek-to-mi*). Removal of the stomach.

**gastric** (*gas'-trik*). Relating to the stomach. *G. aspiration*. Also called *G. suction*. Performed post-operatively after operations on the alimentary tract to prevent dilatation of the stomach. A Ryle's tube is passed and the contents aspirated at frequent intervals or continuously. *G. juice*. The digestive fluid of the stomach. *G. lavage*. Washing out the stomach: a procedure used in the treatment of poisoning.

**gastric ulcer** (*gas-trik ul-ser*). Ulceration of the mucosa lining the stomach. Acute ulceration may be caused by ingested substances, *e.g.* aspirin. Chronic ulceration may be due to reduced capacity of the epithelium to withstand the acid gastric secretion or to a tumour of the epithelium.

**gastrin** (*gas-trin*). A hormone released by cells in the wall of the pyloric antrum, when it is distended. This stimulates the secretion of gastric juice by the secretory cells in the rest of the stomach.

**gastritis** (*gas-trī-tis*). Inflammation of the epithelium lining the stomach.

**gastrocele** (*gas'-trō-sēl*). Hernia of the stomach.

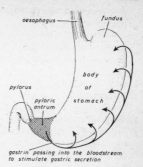

*gastrin passing into the bloodstream to stimulate gastric secretion*

*19. Gastrin*

**gastrocnemius** (*gas-tro-nē-mi-us*). A large muscle of the calf of the leg.

**gastrocolic reflex** (*gas-trō-ko-lik rē-fleks*). Reflex peristaltic contractions in the colon occurring as the result of filling the stomach.

**gastroduodenostomy** (*gas-trō-dū-ō-de-nos-to-mi*), **gastroenterostomy** (*en-te-ros'-to-mi*), **gastrojejunostomy** (*je-jū-nos'-to-mi*). The operation of making an artificial passage direct from the stomach to the duodenum or the jejunum.

**gastroenteritis** (*gas-trō-en-te-rī-tis*). Inflammation of the stomach and intestines.

**gastrogastrostomy** (*gas-trō-gas-tros'-to-mi*), **gastrolysis** (*gas-tro'-li-sis*), **gastroplasty** (*gas'-trō-plas'-ti*). Operations for the cure of hourglass contractions of the stomach.

**gastro-intestinal tract** (*gas-trō-in-tes-tī-nal trakt*). The gut including the mouth, oesophagus, stomach, small and large intestine, rectum and anus and the associated structures.

**gastropexy** (*gas-trō-pek-si*). Fixing a displaced stomach to the abdominal wall by surgery.

**gastroptosis** (*gas-trop-tō-sis*). Downward displacement of the stomach.

**gastroscope** (*gas'-tro-skōp*). An instrument for inspecting the cavity of the stomach. It has a light at the end and is passed per oesophagus.

**gastrostomy** (*gas-tros'-to-mi*). Making an artificial opening into the stomach through which the patient is fed by pouring nourishment through a tube directly into the stomach. Performed for stricture, usually malignant, of the oesophagus.

**gastrotaxis** (*gas'-trō-tak'-sis*). Haemorrhage from the stomach.

**gastrulation** (*gas-trū-lā'-shon*). Embryological term used to describe the complex movements of cells of the embryo in which the cells which give rise to the internal organs migrate inside the embryo.

**Gaucher's disease** (*gō-shāz di-sēz*). A recessively inherited disorder of lipid metabolism in which cells of the reticulo-endothelial system become filled with the phospholipid kerasin. It forms one of the group of conditions known as the *lipoidoses* or lipid storage diseases.

**gauze** (*gawz*). Open mesh material used in surgical dressings.

**gavage** (*ga-vahj*). Forced feeding.

**Geiger-Müller counter** (*gī-ger moo-ler kown-ter*) or **Geiger counter.** Machine which detects and registers radioactivity.

**gelatin** (*je-la-tin*). Denatured collagen obtained by boiling connective tissue.

**gemmellus** (*je-mel'-lus*). Twin, the name of two muscles in the buttock.

**gene** (*jĕn*). The unit of material of inheritance which consists of deoxyribonucleic acid (DNA). The gene is a part of a chromosome which is responsible for one function, *e.g.* the blueprint for the arrangement of amino-acids in one protein. The place the gene occupies in the chromosome is known as its *locus* and variants of the gene which arise by mutation and

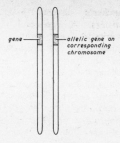

gene — allelic gene on corresponding chromosome

20. *A gene*

which occupy the similar position in corresponding chromosomes are known as allelomorphs, *i.e.* genes occupying similar positions are allelic to each other.

**general paralysis of the insane.** Also called GPI. Dementia due to involvement of the brain in syphilis.

**generation** (*je-ne-rā-shon*). (1) Reproduction. (2) Specific group of individuals resulting from a mating: thus $F_1$ generation (first filial generation) offspring resulting from mating of parental generation ($P_1$); $F_2$ generation (second filial generation) offspring resulting from crossing the members of $F_1$ generation among themselves.

**genetic** (*je-ne-tik*). Pertaining to generation.

**genetics** (*je-ne-tiks*). Study of heredity and its variations.

**geniculate bodies** (*je-ni-kū-lāt bo-dis*). Posterior nuclei of the thalamus. The fibres of the visual pathway relay in the lateral geniculate bodies.

**genitalia** (*je-ni-tā-li-a*). The generative organs.

**genotype** (*je-nō-tīp*). The genetic make-up of an individual, *i.e.* the set of alleles inherited by the individual.

**gentian violet** (*jen-shan vi-ō-let*). An antiseptic dye, used as a paint or lotion, strength 1 in 100 to 1 in 1,000.

**genu** (*je-nū*). The knee.

**genu-pectoral position** (*je-nū-pek-to-ral pō-si-shon*). The knee–chest position, the patient resting upon the knees and chest.

**genu valgum** (*je-nū val-gum*). Knock-knee, a deformity in which the knees are bent inwards. *G. varum*, bow-legged.

**geriatrics** (*je-ri-a-triks*). The study of disease among the elderly.

**germ** (*jerm*). A microbe, bacillus.

**German measles** (*jer-man mē-sels*). *See* RUBELLA.

**germicide** (*jer-mi-sīd*). An agent that destroys micro-organisms.

**gerontology** (*je-ron-to-lo-ji*). The study of ageing.

**Gesell's development charts** (*je-sels*). Charts showing the expected motor activity, manipulation, adaptive behaviour, language, social and play reactions in children at certain ages.

**gestation** (*jes-tā'-shon*). Pregnancy. *G. sac.* The fetus with its enveloping membranes, decidua, etc. The contents of a pregnant uterus.

**Gey's solution** (*gāz sō-loo'-shon*). Solution of mixture of inorganic salts and glucose used as basis for tissue culture medium.

**Ghon's focus** (*gōns fŏ-kus*). Small focus of infection found in primary infection by tubercle bacillus.

**gigantism** (*jī-gan-tism*). *See* ACROMEGALY.

**Gigli's saw** (*jēl-yēs*). An instrument for sawing through bone.

**Gilliam's operation** (*gi-li-amz o-pe-rā-shon*). Operation for uterine retroversion, in which the round ligaments are shortened or sutured to the rectus muscle sheath.

**Gillies needle-holder** (*gil'-ēz nē-del hōl-der*). Combined scissors and fine suture needle holder. *G.'s operation.* (1) plastic repair of cicatricial ectropion; (2) to correct cleft palate repair failure.

**gingival** (*jin-ji-val*). Relating to the gums.

**gingivitis** (*jin-ji-vī-tis*). Inflammation of the gums.

**ginglymus** (*jin'-gli-mus*). A hinge joint such as elbow or knee.

**girdle** (*ger-dl*). Band encircling the body. A term used to describe distribution of cutaneous nerve supply to the thorax. *G. pain.* Pain in this distribution.

**glabella** (*gla-bel'-la*). Triangular space between the eyebrows.

**glairy** (*glār-ē*). Slimy, albuminous.

**gland.** (1) Cell or collection of cells which produce specialized substance(s) to be secreted outside the organ into the bloodstream (endocrine gland) or on to an epithelial surface (exocrine gland). (2) Term, accepted by common usage, applied to lymph nodes.

**glanders** (*glan'-ders*). A virus disease of horses which is occasionally transmitted to man.

**glandular fever** (*glan-dū-la fē-ver*). *See* INFECTIOUS MONONUCLEOSIS.

**glans.** Bulbous extremity of the penis and clitoris.

**glaucoma** (*glaw-kō'-ma*). A disease of the eye with hardening of the globe, due to an increase in the intraocular pressure; acute forms of this disease if untreated may lead to complete loss of sight in a few days.

**glenoid** (*gle'-noyd*). A cavity, a term applied to the socket of the shoulder joint.

**glioma** (*glī-ō-ma*). A tumour composed of neuroglia, nerve connective tissue. It may develop in the brain or spinal cord.

**gliomyoma** (*glī-ō-mī-o'-ma*). A tumour composed of nerve and muscle tissue.

**Glisson's capsule** (*gli-sonz kap'-sūl*). The connective tissue capsule of the liver, enveloping the portal vein, hepatic artery, hepatic ducts.

**globulin** (*glo-bū-lin*). Group of proteins widely distributed in the body with numerous specialized functions. One group, the gamma globulins, are antibodies.

**globus hystericus** (*glō-bus histe'-ri-kus*). Hysterical choking feeling as of a ball in the throat.

**glomerulonephritis** (*glo-me-rū-lō-nef-rī-tis*). One of the causes of acute nephritis syndrome. The exact pathogenesis is not known, but lesions in the glomeruli of the kidneys are frequently associated with streptococcal infection in the throat or elsewhere.

**glomerulus** (*glo-me-rū-lus*). The filtration unit of a nephron. It consists of a coil of fine capillaries apposed to an expansion of urinary epithelium.

**glomus tumour** (*glō-mus tū-mer*). Tumour formed from specialized muscle cells which surround blood vessels (pericytes). These are particularly frequent in sites where arteriovenous shunts are situated in the skin, *e.g.* at tips of fingers and toes.

**glossal** (*glos'-sal*). Relating to the tongue.

**glossectomy** (*glo-sek-to-mi*). Surgical removal of the tongue.

**glossitis** (*glos-sī'-tis*). Inflammation of the tongue.

**glossodynia** (*glos-sō-di-ni-a*). Pain in the tongue sometimes associated with trigeminal neuralgia but often of unknown origin.

**glossopharyngeal** (*glos-sō-fa-rin-jē-al*). Relating to tongue and pharynx. *G. nerve* is the ninth cranial nerve.

**glossoplegia** (*glos-sō-plē-ji-a*). Paralysis of the tongue.

**glottis** (*glot'-tis*). The aperture between the vocal cords in the larynx.

**glucaemia** (*glū-sē'-mia*). Presence of glucose in blood.

**glucocorticoids** (*glū-kō-kor-ti-koyds*). Steroid hormones, secreted by the adrenal cortex, which control carbohydrate metabolism.

**glucose** (*glū-kōs*). Dextrose. A hexose sugar, *i.e.* containing six carbon atoms, which is widely distributed in nature in disaccharides like sucrose and lactose and polysaccharides such as starch. Glucose is the currency of energy production in metabolism.

**glucose tolerance test.** Test performed in cases suspected of

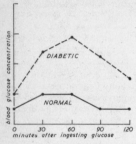

*21. Glucose tolerance test chart*

diabetes, occasionally in other instances. A glucose load is taken, usually by mouth, and the concentration of glucose in the blood is estimated at intervals afterwards. The results are expressed as a graph.

**glue ear.** Accumulation of fluid in middle ear.

**gluteal** (*glū'-tē-al*). Pertaining to the buttock.

**gluten** (*glū-ten*). A protein constituent of certain cereals which acts as an antigen in coeliac disease.

**gluteus** (*glū-te'-us*). *G. maximus, G. medius, G. minimus.* The three large muscles of the buttock.

**glycaemia** (*glī-sē'-mia*). Presence of sugar in blood.

**glycerin** (*gli-se-rin*). Clear, viscous fluid produced as a by-product in the manufacture of soap.

**glycine** (*glīsēn*). An amino-acid.

**glycogen** (*glī-kō-jen*). A polysaccharide composed of hexose sugars connected in branching chains.

**glycogenesis** (*gl'-kō-je-ne-sis*). The formation of glycogen from glucose.

**glycogenolysis** (*glī'-kō-je-nō-lī-sis*). Breakdown of glycogen.

**glycogen storage disease.** Inherited disorder in which there is a deficiency of enzyme(s) involved in the breakdown of glycogen. As a result the tissues of the body become infiltrated with glycogen.

**glycolysis** (*glī-kō-lī-sis*). Breakdown of glucose.

**glycoside** (*glī-kō-sid*). Substance which on hydrolysis yields a sugar, usually glucose, and one or more other substances.

**glycosuria** (*glī-kō-sū-ri-a*). Sugar in the urine.

**gnathic** (*nath'-ik*). Relating to the jaw or cheek.

**goblet cells** (*go-blet sels*). Pear-shaped cells in certain epithelia which secrete mucin.

**goitre** (*goy-ter*). Enlargement of the thyroid.

**gold therapy.** Used in treatment of rheumatoid arthritis.

**Golgi apparatus** (*gol-gē a-pa-rā-tus*). Microscopic system consisting of a number of membrane-surrounded vacuoles. It is considered a possible site of synthesis of cellular membranes. *See* CELL.

**gomphosis** (*gom-fō-sis*). Joint when bony eminence fits into a socket.

**gonadal dysgenesis** (*gō-na-dal dis-je-ne-sis*). Turner's syndrome. This is the result of a chromosomal abnormality in which one of the sex chromosomes is missing. The chromosome complement is designated 44 + XO. The clinical features include failure of sexual development, stunted growth and associated deformities such as webbed neck, congenital heart disease, etc.

**gonadotrophic** (*gō-na-dō-trō-fik*). Promoting the activity of the gonads.

**gonadotrophins** (*gō-na-dō-trō-fins*). Hormones which stimulate the gonads, *e.g.* FSH, LH.

**gonads** (*gō-nads*). Reproductive glands: ovary of the female, testis of the male.

**Gonin operation** (*gō-nin o-perā-shon*). Operation for retinal detachment.

**gonococcus** (*go-nō-ko-kus*). The microbe causing gonorrhoea. It is a Gram negative intracellular diplococcus. *See* BACTERIA.

**gonorrhoea** (*go-no-rē-a*). Venereal disease caused by the gonococcus. May be transmitted to the newborn as it passes through an infected birth canal (ophthalmia neonatorum), and to children by means of infected towels and linen.

**Goodpasture's syndrome** (*good'-pah-stūrs sin'-drōm*). Pneumonitis with haemoptysis followed by glomerulonephritis and uraemia.

**gouge** (*gowj*). A grooved instrument of steel used to scoop out dead bone.

**gout** (*gowt*). Inherited defect of purine metabolism in which uric acid is in excess in the tissues. During acute attacks it is characterized by painful swelling of a joint, classically the big toe.

**GPI.** *See* GENERAL PARALYSIS OF THE INSANE.

**Graafian follicles** (*grah-fi-an*). *See* FOLLICLE.

**Graefe's knife** (*grāfs nīf*). Scalpel used in ophthalmic surgery.

**graft** (*grahft*). To induce union between tissues which are normally separate. The parts may be transferred from one place to another in the same individual (autograft) or from one individual (donor) to another (recipient) of the same species (homograft) or of a different species (heterograft).

**gram** (*gram'*). Metric unit; 30 grams equivalent to 1 oz avoirdupois approx.

**Gram's stain.** Bacteria which resist decolorization by alcohol after staining with methyl violet and Gram's solution are termed Gram positive, *e.g.* staphylococci, pneumococci. Those which are decolorized by alcohol are termed Gram negative, *e.g.* E. coli, gonococci.

**grand mal** (*gro mal*). *See* EPILEPSY.

**granular** (*gra'-nū-la*). Composed of grains or granulations.

**granular layer** (*gra-nū-la lār*). Region in keratinizing epithelia where the cytoplasm of the cells appears granular.

**granulation tissue** (*gra-nū-lā-shon ti-shoo*). Newly formed vascular connective tissue formed at surface of wounds.

**granule** (*gra-nūl*). Small particle or grain.

**granuloma** (*gra-nū-lō-ma*). A tumour composed of granulation tissue.

**graph** (*grahf*). A diagrammatic record of given information.

**gravel** (*gra'-vel*). A popular term for small concretions formed in the kidney or bladder.

**Graves' disease.** *See* HYPERTHYROIDISM.

**gravid** (*gra-vid*). Pregnant.

**Grawitz tumour** (*grah-wits*). A malignant epithelial tumour of the kidney.

**greenstick fracture.** *See* FRACTURE.

**grey matter.** Tissue of the CNS in which are situated numerous cell bodies of nerves, dendritic processes, glial cells, etc.

**Griffith's types** (*gri'-fiths tīps*). Strains of *Streptococcus pyogenes* classified according to surface antigens.

**grippe.** Influenza.

**Grocco's sign** (*gro'-kōz sīn*). Paravertebral triangle of dullness to percussion on side opposite a pleural effusion.

**groin** (*groyn*). Junction of the thigh and abdomen.

**growing pains.** Pain of uncertain origin which may

accompany phases of rapid growth in children. There is a danger of overlooking acute rheumatism.

**guaiacum** (*gwī-a-kum*). Sometimes used to detect presence of blood in the urine.

**Guillain-Barré syndrome** (*gwē-ya-ba-rā sin'-drōm*). Acute infective polyneuritis in which there is both motor and sensory loss. The most characteristic feature is the great rise of protein content while the cell count of the cerebrospinal fluid remains normal.

**guillotine** (*gil'-lō-tēn*). An instrument for excising the tonsils.

**guinea worm** (*gi-nē werm*). Nematode worm which may infest man. The female migrates into the subcutaneous tissues.

**gullet** (*gul'-let*). The oesophagus.

**gumma** (*gum'-ma*). A soft tumour occurring in the tertiary stage of syphilis. This may ulcerate. The characteristics of a gummatous ulcer are: it has a vertical, punched-out edge, the surrounding tissues are healthy, the base is formed by a 'wash-leather' slough; it is painless and very slow to heal. *See* SYPHILIS.

**gustatory** (*gus-ta-to-ri*). Pertaining to taste.

**gut.** The intestine.

**Guthrie test** (*guth'rē test*). Screening test on babies for several inborn errors of metabolism including phenylketonuria.

**gutta.** A drop.

**guttatim.** Drop by drop.

**gutter splints.** For limbs, made of wood, tin or some malleable metal, and grooved to fit the limb, and often lined with felt.

**gynaecology** (*gī-nē-ko-lo-ji*). The study and practice of the management and treatment of disorders affecting female organs, *e.g.* ovaries, uterus, vagina.

**gynaecomastia** (*gī-nē-kō-mas-ti-a*). Enlargement of the breasts in the male.

**gyrus** (*jī'-rus*). A convolution, such as the convolutions of the brain.

# H

**habit** (*ha-bit*). Constant and often involuntary action established by frequent repetition.

**habitat** (*ha-bi-tat*). The natural abode of an animal or plant.

**haem** (*hēm*). (1) Prefix pertaining to blood. (2) Tetrapyrrollic ring containing an atom of ferrous iron. When combined with protein globin forms haemoglobin.

**haemagglutinin** (*hē-ma-glü-ti-nin*). Antibodies present in the blood which combine with red blood cells of a different blood group and cause agglutination. *See* BLOOD GROUPING.

**haemangioma** (*hē-man-jē-ō'-ma*). Abnormal growth of blood vessels.

**haemarthrosis** (*hē-mar-thrō'-sis*). Effusion of blood into a joint cavity.

**haematemesis** (*hē-ma-te-me-sis*). Vomiting blood.

**haematin** (*hē-ma-tin*). The oxidized product of haem.

**haematinic** (*hē-ma-ti-nik*). A substance which increases the amount of haemoglobin in the blood, *e.g.* iron.

**haematocele** (*hē-ma-to-sēl*). A swelling or cyst containing blood.

**haematocolpos** (*hē-ma-tō-kol'-pos*). Collection of menses in the vagina due to the presence of a septum.

**haematocrit** (*hē-ma-tō-krit*). Packed cell volume (PCV). It is a measurement of the proportion of the circulating blood occupied by red blood cells.

**haematology** (*hē-ma-to'-lo-ji*). The study of the blood.

**haematoma** (*hē-ma-tō'-ma*). A swelling composed of blood. A bruise.

**haematometra** (*hē-ma-to-mē'-tra*). Accumulation of blood in the uterus.

**haematomyelia** (*hē-ma-tō-mī-ē-li-a*). Haemorrhage into the spinal cord.

**haematoporphyrin** (*hē-ma-tō-por'-fi-rin*). *See* PORPHYRINS.

**haematorrachis** (*hē-ma-tō-ra'-kis*). Haemorrhage into the extramedullary region of the spinal cord.

**haematosalpinx** (*hē-ma-tō-sal'-pinks*). Distension of the Fallopian tube with blood.

**haematoxylin** (*hē-ma-īok-si-lin*). Basic dye prepared from logwood. It stains acid groups in tissue, particularly nucleic acids, and is much used in histology.

**haematozoa** (*hē-ma-to-zō-a*). Protozoan parasites in the bloodstream.

**haematuria** (*hē-ma-tū-ri-a*). Blood in the urine.

**haemochromatosis** (*hē-mō-krō-ma-tō-sis*). Also known as 'bronzed diabetes'. An inherited defect in the metabolism of iron with resultant deposition of iron in tissues thus interfering with their function. Diabetes mellitus, hyperpigmentation of the skin and cirrhosis of the liver are associated clinical features.

**haemoconcentration** (*hē-mō-kon-sen-trā'-shon*). Concentration of the blood.

169 **HAE**

**haemocytometer** (*hē-mō-sī-to'-me-ter*). Instrument to measure the average diameter of red blood cells.

**haemodialysis** (*hē-mō-dī-a'-li-sis*). Passage of circulating blood through dialysing apparatus, *e.g.* artificial kidney, to restore normal balance of chemical components.

**haemoglobin** (*hē-mō-glō-bin*). Respiratory pigment in red blood cells composed of an iron-containing group (haem) and a complex protein (globin). In combination as haemoglobin it has the property of forming a reversible combination with oxygen.

**haemoglobinometer** (*hē-mō-glō-bi-no-me-ter*). Instrument to measure the amount of haemoglobin in the blood.

**haemoglobinuria** (*hē-mō-glō-bi-nū-ri-a*). Haemoglobin, freed by lysis of red blood cells, in the urine.

**haemolysin** (*hē-mō-lī'-sin*). Agent causing the breakdown of the red cell membrane.

**haemolytic** (*hē-mō-li-tik*). Having the power to destroy red blood cells. *H. anaemia*, resulting from destruction of red cells as in forms of poisoning, or by the action of antibodies. *H. disease of the newborn*. Jaundice in a Rhesus positive infant caused by red cell destruction by anti-Rhesus antibodies generated in the Rhesus negative mother's circulation during pregnancy. *See* BLOOD GROUPING.

**haemopericardium** (*hē-mō-pe-ri-kar-di-um*). Blood in the pericardium.

**haemoperitoneum** (*hē-mō-pe-ri-tō-ne-um*). Blood in the peritoneal cavity.

**haemophilia** (*hē-mō-fi-li-a*). A congenital tendency to haemorrhage, the clotting power of the blood being deficient. It occurs only in males, but is transmitted through the females of the family.

**haemophiliac** (*hē-mō-fi-li-ak*). A person suffering from haemophilia.

**Haemophilus influenzae** (*hē-mō-fi-lus in-flū-en-zē*). Bacterium often isolated among organisms causing secondary infection in virus diseases of the respiratory tract. They do not cause influenza.

**haemophthalmia** (*hēm-of-thal'-mi-a*). Haemorrhage into the eye.

**haemopoiesis** (*hē-mō-poy-ē-sis*). The process of formation of the blood cells, particularly the red blood cells. In the fetus, haemopoiesis occurs in the spleen and liver, in the adult, in the bone marrow.

**haemopoietin** (*hē-mō-poy-ē-tin*). Complex of vitamin B$_{12}$ and intrinsic factor which stimulates haemopoiesis.

**haemoptysis** (*hē-mop-ti-sis*). Coughing up blood.

**haemorrhage** (*hē-moř-āj*). A flow of blood. It may be: *arterial*, occurring in spurts, and bright red in colour; *venous*, occurring in a steady stream and dark in colour; *capillary*, oozing from a large wound surface. Haemorrhage may be (1) *primary*, at time of injury; (2) *reactionary*, within 24 hours of injury due to a rise in the blood pressure; (3) *secondary*, usually within seven to ten days of injury, due to sepsis. Haemorrhage may be *visible* or *concealed*, into one of the cavities of the body and not appearing at the surface. The symptoms of concealed haemorrhage are pallor of skin and mucous membranes, quick, sighing respiration, rapid, small, weak pulse, restlessness, subnormal temperature, coldness, sweating and collapse. *Inevitable h.* Bleeding due to placenta praevia.

**haemorrhagic disease of newborn** (*hē-mo-ra-jik di-sēz*).
Congenital abnormality of vitamin K metabolism which results in deficiency of prothrombin in the blood. As a result haemorrhages occur in the body following even slight trauma.

**haemorrhoidectomy** (*hē-mo-roy-dek'-to-mi*). Surgical removal of haemorrhoids.

**haemorrhoids** (*he-mo-royds*). Varicose rectal veins.

**haemostasis** (*hē-mō-stā-sis*). The prevention of haemorrhage or the measures taken for its arrest.

**haemostatic** (*hē-mō-sta'-tik*). An agent to arrest a flow of blood.

**haemothorax** (*hē-mō-tho'-raks*). Escape of blood into the cavity of the chest.

**hair ball** (*hār bawl*). Also called trichobezoar. It is a rare cause of intestinal obstruction. Persons swallowing hair are frequently feeble-minded.

**hair-follicle** (*hār fo-likl*). See FOLLICLE.

**half-blue baby.** Infant with cyanosis of head and arms, usually due to transposition of aorta and pulmonary artery with patency of ductus arteriosus.

**half-life.** The time in which the total radiation emitted by a radioactive substance is reduced by decay to half its original value. It is a constant for each isotope and is independent of the quantity.

**halitosis** (*ha-li-tō'-sis*). Foul breath.

**hallucination** (*ha-lū-si-nā-shon*). The patient perceives something for which there is no sensory stimulus, *i.e.* the sights and sounds are entirely imaginary, *cf.* delusion.

**hallucinogen** (*ha-loo'-si-no-jen*). Drug causing hallucinations.

**hallux** (*ha-luks*). The great toe. *H. rigidus*. Literally a rigid big toe caused by destruction

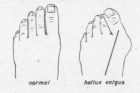

normal          hallux valgus

22. *Hallux valgus; a normal toe shown for comparison*

and ankylosis of the metatar-sophalangeal joint. *H. valgus*. Displacement of the great toe towards the other toes.

**halogens** (*ha-lo-jens*). Non-metallic elements of the series fluorine, chlorine, bromine, iodine. They are anionic in solution and combine with metals to form salts.

**hamartoma** (*ha-mar-tō-ma*). A term used to classify tumours arising from the overgrowth of developing tissues. The original Greek meant missing the target with the javelin'. Missing the target in development gives rise to benign lesions such as vascular naevi and neurofibromas.

**hamate bone** (*ha-māt bōn*). One of the wrist bones.

**hammer toe** (*ha-mer tō*). A deformity of a toe in which there is permanent dorsal flexion of the first phalanx and plantar flexion of the second and third phalanges.

**hamstrings.** The tendons traversing the popliteal region.

**Hand-Schüller-Christian disease** (*hand-shū-ler-cris-ti-an di-sēz*). Granulomas containing cholesterol are found affecting chiefly the skull; the orbit and pituitary gland may be affected. The aetiology is unknown. General symptoms may include hyper-cholesterolaemia, spleno-megaly, eczema, polyuria and exophthalmos.

**Hanot's disease** (*ha-nōs disēz*). Also called primary biliary cirrhosis. A form of cirrhosis of the liver in which the fibrosis is situated mainly round the ductules of the biliary system. The cause is frequently obscure but mucoviscidosis of the intra-hepatic ducts is recognized as one.

**haploid** (*hap-loyd*). Having a set of unpaired chromosomes in the nucleus, characteristic of gametes, *i.e.* sperm cells, ova.

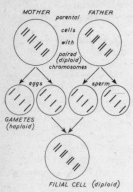

MOTHER    FATHER
parental cells with paired (diploid) chromosomes

eggs    sperm

GAMETES (haploid)

FILIAL CELL (diploid)

*23. Haploid*

**hapten.** Substance which itself cannot induce antibody production but is antigenic when combined with a protein.

**hard chancre** (*hard kan-ker*). *See* CHANCRE.

**hare lip.** Defect of development in which there is a failure of fusion between the central and lateral maxillary buds leaving a fissure in the upper lip. It is frequently associated with various degrees of cleft palate.

**Harrison's sulcus** (*ha-ri-sons sul-kus*). A groove extending from the level of the ensiform cartilage towards the axillae. It is present in rickets.

**Hartmann's pouch** (*hart-mans powch*). A pouch at the neck of the gall bladder in which gallstones may become impacted.

**Hartmann's solution** (*hart-mans so-lū-shon*). A saline solution containing sodium lactate. Used in acidosis and also in severe haemorrhage before blood is cross-matched for transfusion.

**Hartnup disease** (*haht'-nup di-sēz*). Pellegra-like skin rash with periodic ataxia and constant amino-aciduria (hereditary).

**Hashimoto's disease** (*ha-shi-mō-tōs di-sēz*). A chronic thyroiditis due to autoimmunity to thyroglobulin. It causes myxoedema.

**hashish** (*ha-shēsh*). Extract of Indian hemp.

**Hassall's capsules** (*ha-sals kap-sūls*). Bodies which have the appearance of epidermal inclusion cysts which are found in the thymus gland.

**haustrations** (*how-strā-shons*). Sacculations of colon seen on x-ray.

**haustus** (*hows'-tus*). A draught of medicine.

**Haverhill fever** (*hā-ver-hil fēver*). Epidemic disease. *Streptobacillus moniliformis* causes fever, polyarthritis and erythromatous rash.

**Haversian canals** (*ha-ver-si-an ka-nals*). The minute canals which permeate bone. *See* BONE.

**hay fever** (*hā fē-ver*). Allergic rhinitis caused by exposure of sensitized respiratory epithelium to certain dusts and pollens.

**headache** (*he-dāk*). Pain in the head.

**Heaf test.** A method used for testing immunity to tuberculosis before doing BCG.

**healing** (*hē-ling*). Any procedure which cures. The repair of broken tissue.

**health** (*helth*). A state of well-being with mind and body functioning at their optimum.

**heart** (*hart*). A hollow muscular organ situated in the anterior chest to the left of the mid-line. It pumps the blood round the circulatory system and is derived from a modification of blood vessels and is thus lined by endothelium (endocardium), folds of which form the heart valves. The heart muscle is modified to conduct electrical

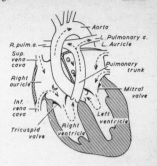

24. *Blood flow through the heart*

impulses. The heart is contained in a serous membranous bag known as the pericardium.

**heart block** (*hart blok*). State of partial or complete prevention of the passage of the cardiac impulse through the atrio-ventricular bundle. *See also* ELECTROCARDIOGRAM.

**heartburn.** Burning sensation at lower end of the oesophagus, due to acid regurgitation from the stomach.

**heart failure.** *See* CARDIAC FAILURE.

**heart-lung machine.** Machine used in cardiac surgery to oxygenate the blood.

**heart murmurs** (*hart mermers*). Adventitious sounds heard on auscultation of the heart resulting from altered haemodynamics, in which the flow of blood through the heart becomes turbulent and exceeds a certain critical velocity. These conditions may occur when there is narrowing or incompetence of valves, abnormal communications between chambers of the heart, or where there is a hyperdynamic circulation as in hyperthyroidism and severe anaemia.

**heart sounds** (*hart sownds*). The normal heart sounds are shown diagrammatically in the Fig. The first heart sound 'lub' is due to the closure of the right and left atrioventricular valves (shown as

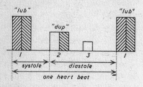

*25. Diagram of the heart sounds*

differently shaded components in the diagram) which occurs at the beginning of the ventricular contraction (*systole*). The second sound 'dup' is due to the closure of the aortic and pulmonary valves. Very occasionally a third sound is heard due to rapid filling of the atria. *Abnormal heart sounds* may be due to

exaggeration or distortion of the normal sounds, *e.g.* 'splitting' of the components of the first or second sounds or the production of adventitious new sounds. *See* HEART MURMURS.

**heart transplant.** *See* TRANSPLANTATION.

**heat exhaustion** (*hēt eg-zaws'-shon*). Condition caused by great heat when patient has rapid pulse, dyspnoea and abdominal cramp due to excessive sweating and loss of sodium chloride.

**heat stroke.** Hyperpyrexia due to failure of temperature-regulating mechanisms of the body.

**hebephrenia** (*hēb-frē-ni-a*). *See* SCHIZOPHRENIA.

**Heberden's disease** (*he-ber-dens di-sēz*). Generalized form of osteoarthritis in which there is symmetrical involvement of joints of the hands, knees, jaw and spine. It occurs in postmenopausal women and is characterized by osteophytes on the dorsal surface of the terminal phalanges (Heberden's nodes).

**Heberden's nodes** (*he-ber-dens nōds*). Small bony nodules which form at the sides of the finger joints in osteoarthritis.

**hedonism** (*hē-do-nism*). Excessive devotion to pleasure.

**Hegar's dilators** (*hā-gars dī-lā-tors*). A series of graduated metal bougies for dilating the cervix and uterus.

**Hegar's sign** (*hā-gars sīn*). Spongy feel of the cervix in pregnancy.

**HeLa cells** (*hē-la selz*). Malignant squamous epithelial cells originating from carcinoma of cervix uteri. Used as medium for growth of viruses in tissue culture.

**heliotherapy** (*hē-li-ō-the-ra-pi*). Treatment by exposure to sunlight.

**helium** (*hē-li-um*). An inert gas, used in certain respiratory tests.

**helix** (*hē-liks*). Literally twisted. Used to describe (1) the configuration of certain molecules, *e.g.* DNA, keratin and (2) the outer rim of the external ear.

**Heller's operation.** Division of muscle between stomach and oesophagus in cases of dysphagia in cardiospasm.

**helminthagogue** (*hel-min'-tha-gog*). Medicine to expel worms.

**helminthiasis** (*hel-min-thī-a-sis*). Infestation with worms.

**helminthology** (*hel-min-tho'-lo-ji*). Study of worms.

**hemeralopia** (*he-me-ra-lō-pi-a*). Partial blindness: patient is not able to see in bright daylight.

**hemianopia** (*he-mi-an-ō-pi-a*). Loss of sight in half of the visual field.

**hemiatrophy** (*he-mi-a-tro-fi*). Atrophy of one side of the body only.

**hemiballismus** (*he-mi-ba-lis-mus*). Violent athetoid movements of one side of the body due to brain damage.

**hemicolectomy** (*he-mi-kō-lek-to-mi*). Surgical removal of half the colon, thus right or left hemicolectomy.

**hemicrania** (*he-mi-krā-ni-a*). Headache on one side of the head. *See* MIGRAINE.

**hemiparesis** (*he-me-pa-rē-sis*). Paralysis of one side of the body.

**hemiplegia** (*he-mi-plē-ji-a*). Paralysis of one side of the body. The lesion is in the opposite side of the brain.

**hemispheres** (*he-me-sfārs*). Usually cerebral hemispheres, the two sides of the forebrain.

**hemizygous** (*he-mi-zī-gus*). Genetic constitution of male as regards sex-linked traits.

**Henoch's purpura** ((*hē-noks per-pū-ra*). A form of syndrome caused by sensitivity reaction of the vascular endothelium. Blood leaks out of the damaged vessels causing purpuric spots in the skin and other variable symptoms according to which organs are affected. In the *Henoch type* there is abdominal pain. The *Schönlein type* is associated with joint involvement. Often both types co-exist.

**hepar.** The liver.

**heparin** (*he-pa-rin*). A sulphur-containing polysaccharide which is stored by mast cells. It has the property of preventing blood from clotting, *i.e.* it is an anti-coagulant.

**hepatectomy** (*he-pa-tek'-to-mi*). Excision of the liver.

**hepatic** (*he-pa-tik*). Relating to the liver.

**hepatic coma** (*he-pa-tik kō-ma*). Coma resulting from poisoning of the brain cells by ammonia. The ammonia is formed by commensal organisms in the intestine but is normally detoxicated, *i.e.* changed into urea, by the liver. In severe liver disease, or if the blood from the gut bypasses the liver, detoxication of ammonia fails to occur.

**hepatic flexure** (*he-pa-tik flek-sūr*). The right-hand bend of the colon, under the liver.

**hepaticostomy** (*he-pa-ti-kos'-to-mi*). Operation to make a fistula in the hepatic duct.

**hepatic portal system.** System of veins which carry the blood from the intestine to the liver so that, with the exception of neutral fats, all the materials absorbed from the gut go straight to the liver.

**hepatitis** (*he-pa-tī-tis*). Inflammation of the liver.

**hepatization** (*he-pa-tī-zā-shon*). Conversion into a liver-like substance. A term used to describe the lungs in lobar pneumonia.

**hepatocele** (*he-pa-tō-sēl*). Hernia containing hepatic tissue.

**hepatojugular reflux** (*he-pa-tō-jū-gū-la rē-fluks*). Test sometimes useful in determining marginal congestive cardiac failure. Pressure is applied over the liver and the venous return to the heart increased with a consequent rise in the right atrial pressure which is reflected by distension of the veins of the neck when the patient is reclining at 45°.

**hepatolenticular degeneration** (*he-pa-tō-len-ti-kū-la dē-je-ne-rā-shon*). Wilson's disease. A recessively inherited defect of copper metabolism in which copper is deposited in the body causing cellular damage. It is characterized by degeneration of the basal ganglia, cirrhosis of the liver and pigmented rings on the cornea (Kayser-Fleisher rings).

**hepatoma** (*he-pa-tō-ma*). Neoplasm of liver cells.

**hepatomegaly** (*he-pa-tō-me-ga-li*). Enlargement of the liver.

**hepatosplenomegaly** (*he-pa-tō-sple-nō-me-ga-li*). Enlargement of the liver and the spleen.

**hereditary** (*he-re-di-ta-ri*). Transmitted from one's ancestors.

**heredity** (*he-re'-di-ti*). The transmission of genetic characteristics.

**hermaphrodite** (*her-ma-frō-dīt*). Abnormality of development in which an individual has tissue capable of producing both male and female gametes. It is associated with ambiguity of secondary sexual characteristics and the individual is generally sterile.

**hermetic** (*her-me-tik*). Protected from the air. Airtight.

**hernia** (*her-ni-a*). Protrusion of an organ from its normal position, most common in the case of the bowel. *Inguinal h.* is through the inguinal canal. *Femoral h.* through the femoral ring. *Scrotal h.* is hernia descending into the scrotum, and *umbilical h.* is hernia at the navel. A hernia not amenable to manipulation is termed *irreducible*. If the blood supply to this is interfered with it is termed *strangulated*. *H. cerebri* is protrusion of the brain through a wound in the skull. *Ventral h.* Hernia of the ventral surface of the body such as an umbilical or *incisional h.*, the latter is through an old scar.

**hernioplasty** (*her-ni-ō-plas-ti*). Operation for hernia when the weak structures are repaired.

**herniorrhaphy** (*her-ni-or-ra-fi*). Operation to repair a hernia.

**herniotomy** (*her-ni-o-to-mi*). Dividing the constricting band of a strangulated hernia and returning the protruding part.

**heroic** (*he-rō'-ik*). Severe treatment of the kill-or-cure type.

**herpangina** (*herp-an-jī-na*). Mild epidemic throat infection in children. Vesicles and later ulcers on and around tonsils, probably caused by Coxsackie viruses.

**herpes** (*her-pēs*). Vesicular eruption due to infection by a virus. *Herpes simplex* virus may reside in epidermal cells without causing any reaction but under certain circumstances, for example associated with a cold, an immunological reaction to the virus occurs with blistering and ulceration of the skin known as 'cold sores'. *Herpes zoster* virus is closely related, if not identical with, the chicken-pox virus and attacks sensory nerves producing pain and vesiculation in the distribution of the nerves (shingles).

**herpetic** (*her-pe-tik*). Relating to herpes.

**Herxheimer reaction** (*herks-hī-mer rē-ak-shon*). Exacerbation of syphilitic lesions for a short period following the commencement of penicillin therapy. It is thought that the killing of the spirochaete initially causes a massive release of endotoxin.

**Hess's test.** Test used in the differential diagnosis of purpura. A cuff is inflated on the arms so that the veins are obstructed, thus raising the pressure in the capillaries: If the capillaries are weak blood seeps out forming small purpuric spots when the cuff is released.

**heterogeneous** (*he-te-rō-jē-nē-us*). Differing in kind or in nature.

**heterograft** (*he-te-rō-grahft*). *See* GRAFT.

**heterologous** (*he-ter-o'-lo-gus*). Derived from a different species.

**heterophoria** (*he-te-rō-fo-ri-a*). Latent squint. A squint which

develops only when the patient is tired or in ill health.

**heterotropia** (*he-te-ro-trō-pi-a*). Squint.

**heterozygous** (*he-te-rō-zī-gus*). Having two different allelomorphs in the corresponding loci of a pair of chromosomes, *cf.* homozygous. The phenotype of the heterozygote may correspond to one allelomorph (dominant gene) or may be intermediate between the two alleles.

**hiatus** (*hī-ā-tus*). An opening or space. *H. hernia.* Hernia of the stomach through the diaphragm at the oesophageal opening.

**hibernation** (*hī-ber-nā-shon*). Winter sleep. Artificial hibernation (hypothermia) is now widely employed in surgery.

**hiccup** (*hi-kup*). Repeated spasmodic inspiration associated with sudden closure of the glottis which gives rise to the characteristic 'hic' sound. It may be produced by irritation of the diaphragm but in most cases the cause is unknown.

**hidradenitis** (*hī-dra-de-nī-tis*). Inflammation of the sweat glands.

**hidrosis** (*hī-drō-sis*). Sweating.

**hilar** (*hī-la*). Relating to the hilum.

**hilum** (*hī-lum*). Site at which the pedicle of an organ is attached.

**hindbrain** (*hīnd-brān*). Embryological component which becomes the medulla and cerebellum.

**hip.** The upper part of the thigh.

**hip joint.** Ball and socket joint between the head of the femur and the acetabulum. *Congenital dislocation of h.j.* Abnormality of development in which the head of the femur does not articulate with the acetabulum.

**Hippocrates** (*hi-po-kra-tēz*). Greek physician (400 BC) regarded as the founder of medicine as a science.

**Hirschprung's disease** (*her-sh-proongs di-sēz*). Developmental abnormality in which there is a defect in the nerve supply to part of the terminal colon which acts as an obstruction and results in dilatation and hypertrophy of the more proximal segment (congenital megacolon).

**hirsutes** (*her-sū-tes*). Abnormal growth of hair.

**His, bundle of.** *See* AURICULO-VENTRICULAR BUNDLE.

**histamine** (*his-ta-mēn*). An organic base which is released from tissues, esp. mast cells, following injury. It increases the permeability of blood vessels and thus acts as the initiator of the inflammatory reaction.

**histidine** (*his-ti-din*). An amino-acid.

**histiocyte** (*his'-ti-ō-sīt*). Macrophage-like cell in connective tissue.

**histochemistry** (*hi-stō-ke-mi-stri*). Study of the distribution of enzymes and chemicals in tissues by means of special staining methods.

**histogenesis** (*hi-stō-je-ne-sis*). The differentiation of tissues.

**histology** (*hi-sto-lo-ji*). The morphological study of tissues.

**histolysis** (*his-to'-li-sis*). Degradation of tissue.

**hives** (*hīvs*). Urticaria.

**hobnail liver** (*hob-nāl li-ver*). The gross appearance of a cirrhotic liver.

**Hodgkin's disease.** A neoplasm of lymphatic tissue, i.e. the lymphocyte-histiocyte system. Clinical features of the disease are lymph node enlargement, splenomegaly, anaemia and fever.

**Holger-Nielsen method** (*hōl-ger nēl-sen me'-thod*). A method of artificial respiration used occasionally if the face is too badly injured for the mouth to mouth method.

**Holmes's syndrome.** Disturbance, especially of space perception, after cerebral palsy.

**Homan's sign** (*hō-mans sīn*). Physical sign of deep vein thrombosis in the leg. Pain is felt in the calf when the toes are dorsiflexed.

**homeopathy** (*hō-mē-o'-pa-thi*). Medicine worked on the system of cures such as those started by Hahnemann. Homeopathic medicines are mostly given in infinitesimal doses.

**homeostasis** (*hō-mē-ō-stā'-sis*). Maintenance of a stable system.

**homeothermic** (*hō'-mē-ō-ther'-mik*). Maintaining constant body temperature.

**homicide** (*ho-mi-sīd*). Killing a person.

**homogeneous** (*hō-mō-jē'-ne-us*). Having the same nature.

**homograft** (*hō-mō-grahft*). *See* GRAFT.

**homolateral** (*hō-mō-la-te-ral*). Ipsilateral. On the same side.

**homologous** (*ho-mo'-lō-gus*). Of the same type. Identical in structure.

**homosexuality** (*hō-mō-sek-sū-a-li-ti*). Psychological abnormality in which sexual attraction is towards members of the same sex.

**homozygous** (*ho-mō-zī-gus*). Having the same gene in the corresponding loci on paired chromosomes, *cf.* heterozygous.

**hookworm.** *See* ANKYLOSTOMA.

**hordeolum** (*hor-dē-ō'-lum*). A stye on the eyelid.

**hormone** (*hor'-mōn*). A substance produced in one organ, which excites functional activity at a distant site. *H. replacement therapy* or HRT, is the use of a hormone or combination of hormones to counteract the hormone imbalance during and after the climacteric.

**Horner's syndrome** (*sin'-drōm*). Unilateral small pupil, ptosis and vasodilatation of the cheek with absence of sweating, due to damage to the sympathetic nerves in the neck.

**horseshoe kidney.** Developmental abnormality of the

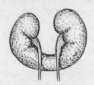

*26. A horseshoe kidney*

kidney in which the left and right kidneys are joined.

**host** (*hōst*). Organism on which a parasite lives.

**hour-glass contraction.** A condition of the uterus in prolonged labour. *See* RETRACTION RING.

**hour-glass stomach.** A stomach divided by a constriction or spasm into two separate cavities seen after a barium meal x-ray. It may be due to a temporary spasm or the result of fibrosis of a gastric ulcer.

**housemaid's knee.** Inflammation of the bursa patellae, caused by constant kneeling on hard substances. *See* PATELLAR BURSAE.

**Houssay animal** (*hoo'-sā a'-ni-mal*). Dog with pancreas and pituitary removed. *H. phenomenon.* Remission of diabetes mellitus after destruction of pituitary.

**Houston's folds** (*hoos-tonz*). Three oblique folds in the mucous membrane of the rectum.

**humanized milk.** Cow's milk with reduced fat and increased sugar.

**humerus** (*hū-me-rus*). The bone of the upper arm.

**humidity** (*hū-mid'-it-i*). Moisture. State of being moist.

**humour** (*hū-mer*). A fluid, thus *aqueous h.* and *vitreous h.* of eye.

**hunger pain.** A sympton of peptic or duodenal ulcer. The pain is relieved on taking food.

**hunger stools.** Frequent small greenish stools passed by underfed infants.

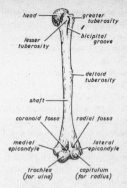

27. *The anterior view of left humerus*

**Huntington's chorea** (*ko-rē-a*). Inherited defect which results in the onset in middle age of chorea and progressive dementia. *See also* CHOREA.

**Hurler's syndrome.** *See* GARGOYLISM.

**Hürthle cell adenoma** (*hur-tel sel a-de-nō'-ma*). Tumour of thyroid consisting of large, eosinophilic, foamy polygonal cells, thought to be derived from thyroid epithelium.

**Hutchinson's teeth.** A condition of the upper central permanent incisors: the cutting edge is smaller than the base, and therefore the teeth are peg-shaped. The edge is deeply notched, a sign of congenital syphilis.

**hyaline** (*hī-a-lin*). Transparent like glass. Hyaline cartilage is smooth and pearly. It covers the articular surfaces of bones.

**hyaline membrane.** Eosinophilic material found in the air passages of the newborn. It is probably derived from amniotic fluid and may cause collapse of the lungs in the so-called 'pulmonary syndrome of the newborn'. The primary cause, however, is failure of the pulmonary circulation. Also known as respiratory distress syndrome.

**hyaloid membrane** (*hī'-a-loyd mem'-brān*). The glassy membrane which encloses the vitreous humour of the eye.

**hybrid** (*hī-brid*). Offspring resulting from gametes which are genetically unlike.

**hydatid** (*hī-da-tid*). Cyst formed by the larvae of certain tapeworms.

**hydatidiform mole** (*hī-da-ti-di-form mōl*). Cyst formed from the degeneration of the chorion. It may give rise to chorion epithelioma.

**hydragogue** (*hī-dra-gog*). Substance which attracts water, *i.e.* it is osmotically active.

**hydramnios** (*hī-dram-ni-os*). Excess of amniotic fluid.

**hydrarthrosis** (*hī-dra-thrō'-sis*). Collection of fluid in a joint.

**hydrate** (*hī-drāt*). Combination with water.

**hydroa aestivale** (*hī-drō-a ī-sti-va-lē*). Form of porphyria in which the skin is sensitive to light. Blisters result from exposure to the sun.

**hydrocarbon** (*hī'-drō-kar'-bon*). A compound formed of hydrogen and carbon.

**hydrocele** (*hī-drō-sēl*). Swelling containing clear fluid. Most often applied to watery swelling of scrotum.

**hydrocephalus** (*hī-drō-ke-fa-lus*). Excess of cerebrospinal fluid causing pressure on the brain.

**hydrocortisone** (*hī-drō-kor-ti-sōn*). The major glucocorticoid secreted by the adrenal.

**hydrolysis** (*hī-dro-li-sis*). Breakdown of complex substance(s) with the addition of water to give simpler substances.

**hydroma** (*hī-drō'-ma*). Literally, watery swelling.

**hydrometer** (*hī-dro-me-ter*). An instrument for determining the specific gravities of liquids.

**hydrometria** (*hī-drō-mē'-tri-a*). Collection of fluid in the uterus.

**hydronephrosis** (*hī-drō-nef-rō-sis*). Distension of the pelvis and calyces of the kidney due to obstruction to the ureter. Prolonged back pressure results in atrophy of the renal substance.

**hydropathic** (*hī-drō-pa-thik*). Relating to cure by means of water; as by baths.

**hydropericardium** (*hī-drō-pe-ri-kar'-di-um*). Fluid in the pericardial sac, *i.e.* pericardial effusion.

**hydroperitoneum** (*hī-drō-pe-ri-tō-nē-um*). Peritoneal effusion, *i.e.* ascites.

**hydrophobia** (*hī-drō-fō-bi-a*). *See* RABIES.

**hydropneumothorax** (*hī-drō-nū'-mō-tho-raks*). Fluid and air in the pleural cavity.

**hydrops** (*hī-drops*). Oedema. *H. fetalis.* Generalized oedema associated with severe haemolytic anaemia in the fetus due to Rhesus incompatibility.

**hydrorhachis** (*hī-dro-ra-kis*). Abnormal accumulation of cerebrospinal fluid in the spinal canal.

**hydrosalpinx** (*hī-drō-sal'-pinx*). Distension of the Fallopian tube by clear fluid.

**hydrotherapy** (*hī-drō-ther'-a-pi*). Use of water in treatment.

**hydrothorax** (*hī-drō-thaw'-rax*). Fluid in the cavity of the chest.

**5-hydroxytryptamine** (*fīv hī-drok-si-trip-ta-mēn*). Serotonin. Substance which acts as a chemical transmitter in brain synapses. It is also elaborated by argentaffin cells of the gastrointestinal tract and stimulates smooth muscle.

**hygiene** (*hī'-jēn*). The science of the preservation of health.

**hygroma** (*hī-grō-ma*). Cyst in the neck resulting from abnormal development of the lymphatic system.

**hygrometer** (*hī-gro-me-ter*). An instrument for measuring the moisture in the atmosphere.

**hygroscopic** (*hī-grō-sko-pik*). Having the property of absorbing moisture from the air, *e.g.* common salt.

**hymen** (*hī'-men*). A fold of membrane at the entrance to the vagina.

**hymenotomy** (*hī-men-o'-to-mi*). Incision of hymen.

**hyoid** (*hī'-oyd*). Shaped like a V; the name of a bone at the root of the tongue.

**hyper** (*hī-per*). A prefix denoting excessive, above, or increased.

**hyperacidity** (*hī-per-a-si-di-ti*). Excess acid.

**hyperactivity** (*hī-per-ak-ti-vi-ti*). Overactivity.

**hyperaemia** (*hī-per-ē-mi-a*). Excess of blood in a part.

**hyperaesthesia** (*hī-per-es-thē-si-a*). Excess of sensitiveness in a part.

**hyperalgesia** (*hī-per-al-gē-si-a*). Excessive sensibility to pain.

**hyperasthenia** (*hī-per-as-thē-ni-a*). Great weakness.

**hyperbaric** (*hī-per-ba-rik*). A pressure greater than atmospheric pressure.

**hyperbilirubinaemia** (*hī-per-bi-li-rū-bi-nē-mi-a*). Excess of bilirubin in the blood. Normal level of serum bilirubin is less than 20 μmol/litre.

**hypercalcaemia** (*hī-per-kal-sē-mi-a*). Excess of calcium in the blood.

**hypercapnia** (*hī-per-kap-ni-a*). Excess of carbon dioxide in the blood.

**hyperchlorhydria** (*hī-per-klor-hī-dri-a*). Excess of hydrochloric acid in the gastric juice.

**hyperchromia** (*hī-per-krō-mi-a*). Excessively coloured.

**hypercholesterolaemia** (*hī-per-kō-les-te-rol-ē-mi-a*). Excess of cholesterol in the blood.

**hyperemesis** (*hī-per-em'-e-sis*). Excessive vomiting. *H. gravidarum*, of pregnancy.

**hyperexcitability** (*hī-per-ek-sī-ta-bi-li-ti*). Ease of excitation as of a nerve or muscle fibre.

**hyperextension** (*hī-per-eks-ten-shon*). Extension beyond the normal range of a joint.

**hyperflexion** (*hī-per-flek-shon*). Flexion beyond the normal range.

**hyperglycaemia** (*hī-per-glī-sē-mi-a*). Excessive sugar in the blood; occurs in diabetes mellitus.

**hypergonadism** (*hī-per-gō-na-dism*). Excessive secretion of sex hormones causing precocious puberty and premature fusion of the epiphyses.

**hyperhydrosis** (*hī-per-hī-drō'-sis*). Excess of perspiration.

**hyperkalaemia** (*hī-per-ka-lē-mi-a*). Excess of potassium in the blood.

**hyperkeratoses** (*hī-per-ke-ra-tō-sēs*). Lesions on the skin in which there is excessive production of keratin.

**hyperkinesis** (*hī-per-kī-nē'-sis*). Excessive movement.

**hyperlipaemia** (*hī-per-lip-ē-mi-a*). Familial increase in serum triglycerides with abdominal crises and liability to early coronary artery atheroma.

**hypermetropia** (*hī-per-me-trō-pi-a*). Long sight, a visual affection. The opposite of myopia. Corrected by wearing a biconvex lens.

**hypermnesia** (*hī-perm-nē-zi-a*). An exaggeration of memory involving minute details of a past experience. It may occur in mentally unstable individuals after a shock.

**hypermotility** (*hī-per-mō-ti-li-ti*). Increased motor activity.

**hypermyotonia** (*hī-per-mī-ō-tō-ni-a*). Increase in muscle tone.

**hypernatraemia** (*hī-per-na-trē'-mia*). Excess of sodium in blood.

**hypernephroma** (*hī-per-ne-frō'-ma*). Malignant tumour of kidney.

**hyperonychia** (*hī-per-ō-ni-ki-a*). Thickening of the nails.

**hyperostosis** (*hī-per-os-tō'-sis*). Hypertrophy of bony tissue.

**hyperparathyroidism** (*hī-per-pa-ra-thī-roy-dism*). Excessive secretion of parathormone, usually from an adenoma of one of the parathyroid glands.

**hyperphagia** (*hī-per-fā-ji-a*). Eating to excess.

**hyperphoria** (*hī-per-fo-ri-a*). Elevation of one visual axis above the other.

**hyperpiesis** (*hī-per-pī-ē-sis*). See HYPERTENSION.

**hyperpituitarism** (*hī-per-pi-tū-i-ta-rism*). Excess secretion of hormones from the anterior pituitary, especially somatotrophin or growth hormone. See ACROMEGALY.

**hyperplasia** (*hī-per-plā-si-a*). Excessive growth of tissue.

**hyperpnoea** (*hī-per-pnē-a*). Overbreathing.

**hyperpyrexia** (*hī-per-pī-rek-si-a*). High fever, arbitrarily above 40·5°C (105°F).

**hypersecretion** (*hī-per-se-krē-shon*). Excessive secretion.

**hypersensitive** (*hī-per-sen-si-tiv*). Excessive sensitivity.

**hypersplenism** (*hī-per-sple-nism*). A condition in which there is enlargement of the spleen associated with inhibition of maturation of cells in the bone marrow. It is thought that the spleen secretes some inhibitory factor.

**hypertension** (*hī-per-ten-shon*). Blood pressure above the normal limits, *i.e.* above 140/95 resting BP. Hypertension may be *primary* or *essential, i.e.* cause unknown or *secondary* to arterial obstruction, renal disease, endocrine disturbances and other factors.

**hyperthecosis** (*hī-per-thē-kō'-sis*). Hyperplasia of cortical stroma of ovary, sometimes with inclusion of lutein-containing cells.

**hyperthermia** (*hī-per-ther-mi-a*). Raised body temperature.

**hyperthymia** (*hī-per-thī-mi-a*). An overactive state of mind with a tendency to perform impulsive actions.

**hyperthyroidism** (*hī-per-thī-roy-dism*). Excessive secretion of thyroid hormones.

**hypertonia** (*hī-per-tō-ni-a*).

Excessive tonicity, as in a muscle or an artery.

**hypertonic** (*hī-per-to-nik*). High tone. (1) Increased tone of muscle. (2) Having a higher osmotic pressure than body fluids, *cf.* isotonic, hypotonic saline.

**hypertrichosis** (*hī-per-tri-kō'-sis*). Excessive growth of hair, or growth of hair in unusual places.

**hypertrophy** (*hī-per-tro-fi*). Increase in size in response to demand on the structure, *cf.* hyperplasia.

**hyperventilation** (*hī-per-ven-ti-lā-shon*). Overbreathing.

**hypnosis** (*hip-nō-sis*). Condition resembling sleep in which conscious control of behaviour is reduced. The state is brought about voluntarily in the subject by 'suggestion'.

**hypnotic** (*hip-nō-tik*). (1) Relating to hypnotism. (2) Drug producing sleep.

**hypo** (*hī-pō*). Prefix denoting below.

**hypoaesthesia** (*hī-pō-es-thē-si-a*). Diminished sense of feeling in a part.

**hypocalcaemia** (*hī-pō-kal-sē-mi-a*). Diminished amount of blood calcium.

**hypochlorhydria** (*hī-pō-klor-hī-dri-a*). Deficiency of hydrochloric acid in the gastric juice.

**hypochondria** (*hī-pō-kon'-dri-a*). An anxiety state about health, the patient suffering from many imaginary ills.

**hypochondriac** (*hī-pō-kon'-dri-ak*). Person suffering from many and varied ills for which no organic cause may be found.

**hypochondrium** (*hī-pō-kon-dri-um*). Surface anatomy nomenclature relating to the region of the anterior abdominal wall beneath the ribs.

**hypochromic** (*hī-pō-krō-mik*). Deficient in colour. Usually applies to red blood cells in which there is a reduced haemoglobin content, hence *hypochromic anaemia*.

**hypodermic** (*hī-pō-der-mik*). Beneath the skin; used of injections.

**hypodermoclysis** (*hī-pō-der'-mo-kli'-sis*). Continuous infusion of saline fluid under the skin.

**hypofibrinogenaemia** (*hī-pō-fī-bri-nō-je-nē-mi-a*). Condition in which there is a deficiency of fibrinogen in the blood.

**hypogastric** (*hī-pō-gas'-trik*). Pertaining to the hypogastrium.

**hypogastrium** (*hī-pō-gas-tri-um*). *See* ABDOMEN for surface anatomy terminology.

**hypoglossal** (*hī-pō-glo-sal*).

Beneath the tongue. *H. nerves*. Twelfth pair of cranial nerves.

**hypoglycaemia** (*hī-pō-glī-sē-mi-a*). Deficiency of sugar in the blood.

**hypogonadism** (*hī-pō-gō-na-dism*). Defective development of the ovaries or testicles.

**hypokalaemia** (*hī-pō-ka-lē-mi-a*). Reduced potassium content of blood.

**hypomania** (*hī-pō-mā-ni-a*). Mild form of the affective disorder, mania, in which there is abnormal elation of mood and great energy.

**hypomotility** (*hī-pō-mō-ti-li-ti*). Decreased movement.

**hyponatraemia** (*hī-pō-na-trē'-mi-a*). Reduction of blood sodium concentration.

**hypoparathyroidism** (*hī-pō-pa-ra-thī-roydism*). Diminished function of parathyroid glands.

**hypophoria** (*hī-pō-fo-ri-a*). Depression of one visual axis below the other.

**hypophosphataemia** (*hī-pō-fos-fa-tē-mi-a*). Reduced inorganic phosphate content of blood.

**hypophosphatasia** (*hī-pō-fos-fa-tā-si-a*). Abnormally low amount of alkaline phosphatase in the blood. *Congenital h*. Inherited deficiency of alkaline phosphatase in the bone cells. As a result there is a failure of the bones to calcify adequately and the serum calcium concentration may rise and there may be anorexia, vomiting and wasting. The amount of alkaline phosphatase in the serum is greatly reduced.

**hypophysectomy** (*hī-pō-fi-sek-to-mi*). Operation to remove the pituitary gland.

**hypophysis cerebri** (*hī-pō-fi-sis se-re-brē*). Pituitary gland.

**hypopiesis** (*hī-pō-pī-ē'-sis*). *See* HYPOTENSION.

**hypopituitarism** (*hī-pō-pi-tū-i-ta-rism*). Condition resulting from insufficiency of pituitary secretion.

**hypoplasia** (*hī-pō-plā-si-a*). Tendency to grow to a size smaller than normal.

**hypoproteinaemia** (*hī-pō-prō-ti-nē-mi-a*). Too little protein in the blood.

**hypoprothrombinaemia** (*hī-pō-prō-throm-bin-ē'-mi-a*). Deficiency of prothrombin in the blood.

**hypopyon** (*hī-pō'-pi-on*). Pus in the anterior chamber of the eye.

**hyposecretion** (*hī-pō-se-krē'-shon*). Too little secretion.

**hypospadias** (*hī-pō-spā-di-as*). Malformation of lower wall of the urethra, so that the urethra opens on the under-surface of the penis.

**hypostasis** (*hī-pō-stā-sis*). Deposit: passive congestion.

**hypostatic pneumonia** (*hī-pō-sta-tik nū-mō-ni-a*). Due to congestion at bases of lungs, often caused by allowing elderly patients to lie flat on their backs for long periods.

**hypotension** (*hī-pō-ten-shon*). Low blood pressure.

**hypothalamus** (*hī-pō-tha-la-mus*). A special area of grey matter in the floor of the third ventricle of the brain. Linked with the pituitary gland and also with the thalamus and the autonomic nervous system.

**hypothenar eminence** (*hī-pō-thē-na e-mi-nens*). Prominence on the palm below the little finger.

**hypothermia** (*hī-pō-ther-mi-a*). State of being abnormally cold. *Artificial h.* Technique used in conjunction with major heart surgery, etc., in which the blood is cooled by passing it through a heat exchanger. The body temperature is lowered to about 85°F (29·44°C), at which level the oxygen requirements of tissues, especially the brain cells, are greatly reduced. This enables the circulation to be stopped for a time.

**hypothesis** (*hī-pō'-the-sis*). A suggested explanation of some happening or phenomenon.

**hypothrombinaemia** (*hī-pō-throm-bin-ē'-mi-a*). Deficiency of thrombin in the blood.

**hypothyroidism** (*hī-pō-thī'-roy-dism*). Insufficiency of thyroid secretion.

**hypotonia** (*hī-pō-tō-ni-a*). Deficient tone, especially of muscle.

**hypotonic** (*hī-pō-to-nik*). (1) Lacking in tone. (2) Of salt solution: having an osmotic pressure less than that of physiological saline (0·9 per cent NaCl).

**hypovitaminosis** (*hī-pō-vi-ta-mi-nō-sis*). Suffering from lack of vitamins in food intake.

**hypoxia** (*hī-pok-si-a*). Lacking oxygen.

**hystera** (*hīs'-te-ra*). The uterus or womb.

**hysterectomy** (*his-te-rek-to-mi*). Removal of the womb by operation. *Sub-total h.* is removal of all the womb except the cervix. *Pan h.*, total hysterectomy. *Vaginal h.*, womb removed per vaginam.

**hysteria** (*his-tār-i-a*). A functional neurosis in which there is a reaction, never fully conscious on the part of the patient, to obtain relief from stress by the exhibition and experience of symptoms of illness.

**hysterocele** (*his-te-rō-sēl*). Hernia involving the uterus.

**hysterography** (*his-te-ro'-gra-fi*). Radiological examination of uterus.

**hysteromyoma** (*his'-te-rō-mī-ō'-ma*). Uterine fibroid.

**hysteromyomectomy** (*his-te-rō-mī'-ō-mek-to-mi*). Excision of uterine fibroid.

**hysteropexy** (*his-te-rō-pek'-si*). Suturing of the uterus to the abdominal wall to prevent prolapse.

**hysteroptosis** (*his-te-rop-tō-sis*). Uterine prolapse.

**hysterosalpingography** (*his-te-rō-sal'-pin-go'-gra-fi*). X-ray examination of uterus and Fallopian tubes following the introduction of a contrast medium.

**hysterotomy** (*his-te-ro-to-mi*). Incision into the uterus. The term usually excludes caesarean section.

**hysterotrachelorrhaphy** (*his-te-rō-tra-ke-lo-ra-fi*). Repair of a lacerated cervix uteri.

# I

**iatrogenic** (*ī-at-rō-jen'-ik*). Applied to disorder resulting from treatment.

**ichthyosis** (*ik-thi-ō-sis*). Inherited defect of keratinization in which the skin is dry and scaly. The so-called acquired ichthyosis is similar in appearance but due to defective nutrition.

**icterus** (*ik'-te-rus*). Jaundice.

**idea** (*ī-dār*). A mental image.

**identical twins.** Monozygotic twins, *i.e.* derived from the same fertilized ovum.

**identification** (*ī-den-ti-fi-kā-shon*). (1) Recognition. (2) Psychiatric emotional attachment to an individual resulting in transposition of behavioural characteristics.

**idiocy** (*i-di-o-si*). Before the Mental Health Act, 1959, idiots were officially categorized as having an intelligence quotient of less than 20. The present official legal term is *severely subnormal* which covers mental defectives with an IQ of less than 50 who were imbeciles and idiots in the old classification. High-grade defectives with IQs of 50 to 75 are classed as *subnormal* and were previously termed feeble minded. In psychiatric terminology all cases with an IQ of less than 75 are termed cases of *amentia*.

**idiopathic** (*i-di-ō-pa-thik*). Without apparent cause.

**idiosyncrasy** (*i-di-ō-sin'-kra-si*). Individual character or property. Generally used in connection with unusual or unexpected response to drugs.

**idiot** (*i-di-ot*). *See* IDIOCY.

**ileectomy** (*ī-lē-ek-tom-i*). Excision of the ileum.

**ileitis** (*ī-lē-ī-tis*). Inflammation of the ileum. *Regional i.* Crohn's disease. Characterized by localized regions of non-specific chronic inflammation of the terminal portion of the ileum. Occasionally other parts of the intestine are also affected. The cause is not known.

**ileocaecal valve** (*ī-lē-ō-sē-kal valv*). Valve at the junction of the large and small intestines.

**ileocolitis** (*ī'-le-ō-kō-lī'-tis*). Inflammation of ileum and colon.

**ileocolostomy** (*ī-lē-ō-ko-los-to-mi*). Surgical anastomosis between the ileum and the colon.

**ileoproctostomy** (*ī-lē-ō-prok-tos-to-mi*). Surgical anastomosis between the ileum and the rectum.

**ileorectal** (*ī'-lē-ō-rek'-tal*). Relating to the ileum and the rectum.

**ileostomy** (*ī-lē-os-to-mi*). Fistula constructed so that the ileum opens on to the anterior abdominal wall to act as an artificial anus.

**ileum** (*ī-le-um*). The lower portion of the small intestine between the jejunum and caecum. *See* BOWEL.

**ileus** (*ī'-le-us*). Obstruction of the bowel. Paralytic ileus caused by paralysis of the muscle. It may be a complication of abdominal operations, particularly if the bowel has been extensively handled. It may be due to peritonitis.

**iliac crest** (*i-li-ak krest*). The crest or highest portion of the ilium.

**iliac spine** (*i-li-ak spīn*). The tubercle at the anterior end of the iliac crest.

**iliococcygeal** (*i-lē-ō-kok-si-jē-al*). Relating to the ilium and the coccyx, *e.g.* iliococcygeal ligament: ligament passing between the ilium and the coccyx.

**ilium** (*i'-li-um*). The upper part of the innominate bone.

**illegitimate** (*i-le-ji-ti-mat*). Born out of wedlock.

**illusion** (*il-lū'-zhon*). A deceptive appearance. The misinterpretation of a sensory image.

**image** (*i-māj*). A mental picture of an external object. *I. intensifier.* Apparatus to increase brightness of fluoroscopic image in x-ray screening.

**imbalance** (*im-ba-lans*). Lack of balance.

**immobility** (*i-mō-bi-li-ti*). The state of being fixed.

**immune response** (*i'-mūn res-pons'*). Immunological reaction to antigenic stimulus.

**immunity** (*i-mū'-ni-ti*). State of resistance to infection due to the presence of antibodies capable of combining with antigen(s) carried by the infecting organism and thus damaging the invader or neutralizing enzymes or toxins released by the organism. As well as viruses, bacteria and other parasites, the body regards cells from a different individual, *i.e.* different genotype, as infecting organisms. Hence the difficulties of homografting kidneys, etc. *see* GRAFT. In a wider, and less common, usage of the term, immunity implies all mechanisms, such as impermeability of the skin, antiseptic properties of sebum, disinfection of food by stomach acid, etc. which enable the body to resist infection.

**immunization** (*i-mū-nī-zā'-shon*). Process of increasing the state of immunity, either by contact with the infecting organism or some variant of it, which is *active immunization*. In *passive immunization* there is receipt of antibody. Active immunization is the principle behind vaccination against smallpox, inoculation, against diphtheria, tetanus, etc. Passive immunization is temporary: the fetus is passively immunized by antibodies from the maternal blood and these enable the newborn baby to resist infection for about 6 weeks after birth.

**immuno-assay** (*i'-mū-nō-a'-sā*). Quantitative estimation of proteins, *e.g.* hormones, by serological methods.

**immunocyte** (*i'-mū-nō-sīt*). Cell capable of proliferation and antibody production if stimulated by antibody.

**immunodiagnosis** (*i'-mū-nō-dī-ag-nō'-sis*). Diagnosis by immunological methods.

**immunodiffusion** (*i'-m-ū-nō-di-fū'-shon*). Analysis of antigens or antibodies by diffusion through gel. Precipitate forms where known and unknown substances meet.

**immuno-electrophoresis** (*i'-mū-nō-e-lek-trō-for-ē'-sis*). Analysis of antigens by combination of electrophoresis and immunodiffusion.

**immunofluorescence** (*i'-mū-nō-flū-or-es'-ens*). Microscopic demonstration of antigens and antibody by fluorescent dye technique.

**immunogenic** (*i-mū-nō-je'-nik*).

Generating an immune response.

**immunoglobulins** (*i'-mū-nō-glo'-bū-linz*). Group of globulins able to react as antibodies.

**immunology** (*i-mū-no'-lo-ji*). Scientific study of immunity.

**immunosuppression** (*i'-mū-nō-su-pre'-shon*). Deliberate inhibition of normal immune response, especially to permit successful organ grafting.

**immunotransfusion** (*i'-mū-nō-trans-fū'-shon*). Blood transfusion from a donor who has been immunized against infection from which recipient suffers.

**impaction** (*im-pak-shon*). Wedging or jamming together, *e.g. impacted fracture* where the bony fragments are jammed together. *Impacted wisdom tooth*, where there is insufficient room in the jaw to accommodate the erupting tooth, which becomes jammed.

**impalpable** (*im-pal'-pa-bl*). Not capable of being felt.

**imperforate** (*im-per'-fo-rāt*). Completely closed.

**impetigo** (*im-pe-tī-gō*). Acute infection of the skin. Most commonly caused by the staphylococcus or streptococcus.

**implantation** (*im-plan-tā-shon*). The act of setting in; grafting.

*I., dermoid*. Cyst due to the accidental implantation of epidermis into the dermis.

**implants** (*im-plants*). Pellets of drugs such as testosterone which are inserted under the skin from where they are slowly absorbed.

**impotence** (*im'-pō-tens*). Absence of power or desire for sexual intercourse.

**impregnation** (*im-preg-nā'-shon*). The act of becoming pregnant; the fertilization of an ovum by a spermatozoon.

**impulse of the heart.** Sensation of a stroke felt on placing the hand on the cardiac region, occurring as the ventricles contract.

**inanition** (*i-na-ni-shon*). Exhaustion from want of food.

**inarticulate** (*i-nar-ti-kū-lāt*). (1) Without joints. (2) Unable to speak clearly.

**incarcerated** (*in-kar-se-rā-ted*). Imprisoned. Term applied to a hernia which cannot be reduced.

**incest** (*in'-cest*). Sexual intercourse between near relatives.

**incidence** (*in-si-denz*). Occurrence, such as of a disease.

**incipient** (*in-si'-pi-ent*). Beginning.

**incision** (*in-si-zhon*). Act of cutting into with a sharp instrument.

**incisors** (*in-sī-sers*). Chisel-shaped cutting teeth at the front of the mouth. *See* DENTAL FORMULA.

**inclusion bodies** (*in-klū-zhon bo-dis*). Extraneous material found in the cytoplasm of cells. The term does not include material in phagocytosis or pinocytosis vacuoles and is almost exclusively applied to bodies formed by accumulations of virus material.

**incoherent** (*in-kō-hā-rent*). Disconnected.

**incompatible** (*in-kom-pa-ti-bl*). Incapable of admixture, *e.g.* incompatible transfusion.

**incompetence** (*in-kom-pe-tens*). Incapable of natural function, *e.g.* aortic incompetence in which the aortic valve of the heart does not close adequately with the result that blood leaks back into the left ventricle.

**incontinence** (*in-kon-ti-nens*). Absence of voluntary control over the passing of urine or faeces.

**inco-ordination** (*in-kō-or-din-ā-shon*). Inability to perform harmonious muscular movements.

**incrustation** (*in-krus-tā'-shon*). Forming of a scab on a wound.

**incubation** (*in-kū-bā-shon*). Literally to hatch. *I. period.*

Time between infection and the appearance of symptoms when it is assumed the infecting organisms multiply.

**incubator** (*in-kū-bā-tor*). Apparatus used to provide optimum conditions for incubation. Incubators are used for many purposes. (1) Premature babies. (2) Culture of viruses, bacteria and other organisms. (3) To allow enzyme reactions to proceed at optimum temperatures.

**incus** (*in'-kus*). A small anvil-shaped bone of the middle ear. *See* EAR.

**index.** (1) The forefinger. (2) The ratio of measurement of any quantity in comparison with a fixed standard.

**indication** (*in-di-kā-shon*). Circumstances determining a particular form of treatment.

**indicator** (*in-di-kā-tor*). Substance showing a chemical reaction by its change in colour.

**indigenous** (*in-dī'-je-nus*). Native to a particular place.

**indigestion** (*in-dī'-jest'-chon*). Failure of the digestive powers; dyspepsia.

**indolent** (*in-dō-lent*). Slow to heal.

**induction** (*in-duk-shon*). (1) Influence of one embryonic tissue in modifying the development of another. (2)

In obstetrics, the artificial production of labour.

**induration** (*in-du-rā-shon*). Hardening of tissue.

**industrial disease.** A disease due to a person's occupation, such as silicosis found among silica workers, etc. *I. dermatitis.* Contact dermatitis due to material used in industrial processes.

**inebriety** (*in-e-brī'-et-i*). Habitual drunkenness.

**inertia** (*i-ner-sha*). (1) Resistance to change in motion. (2) In psychiatry, extreme apathy. (3) *Uterine i.* Sluggish contraction of the uterus during labour.

**in extremis** (*in eks-trā-mis*). At the point of death.

**infant** (*in-fant*). Baby less than one year old.

**infanticide** (*in-fan'-ti-sid*). Murder of an infant.

**infantile eczema** (*in-fan-tīl ek-se-ma*). Type of eczema affecting infants and children.

**infantile paralysis.** Anterior poliomyelitis, *see* POLIO-MYELITIS.

**infantilism** (*in-fan-ti-lism*). Persistence of childish ways in an adult.

**infarct.** Region of tissue affected by ischaemic changes due to the blocking of the principal artery supplying the part.

**infection** (*in-fek'-shon*). The communication of a disease from one patient to another. *Droplet i.* In the fine spray which is ejected from the mouth on talking, sneezing, coughing.

**infectious disease** (*in-fek'-shus*). A communicable disease.

**infectious mononucleosis** (*in-fek-shus mo-nō-nū-klē-ō-sis*). Glandular fever. Probably a virus infection and characterized by malaise, pyrexia, muscle pains, sore throat, enlargement of the lymph glands and the spleen and an increase in the numbers of mononuclear white blood cells. Occasionally there is enlargement of the liver, jaundice and a rash. *See* PAUL-BUNNELL TEST.

**inferior** (*in-fā-ri-or*). Lower.

**inferior vena cava.** The chief vein of the lower part of the trunk of the body.

**inferiority complex** (*in-fā-ri-o-ri-ti kom-pleks*). A feeling of unjustified inferiority which may show itself by over-confident or aggressive behaviour.

**infertility** (*in-fer-ti-li-ti*). Inability to reproduce. It may affect either the male or female.

**infestation** (*in-fes-tā-shon*). The invasion of the body by parasites such as lice.

**infiltration** (*in-fil-trā-shon*). Penetration of tissue by fluid, cells or other material.

**inflammation** (*in-fla-mā-shon*). The vascular response to tissue damage. It consists of dilatation of blood vessels, increased permeability of vessels to the passage of serum into the tissue and the diapedesis of leucocytes into the site of the damage.

**inflation** (*in-flā-shon*). Blown out and expanded by air or gas.

**influenza** (*in-floo-en'-za*). Virus infection affecting the epithelium of the respiratory tract.

**infra** (*in-fru*). Below.

**infra-red** (*in-fru-red*). Electromagnetic waves with longer wavelength than visible red light, *i.e.* photons with a lesser frequency than the lower end of the visible spectrum. Because it is easily absorbed, *i.e.* not reflected, by bodies, infra-red radiation transfers heat to the absorbing material and is used therapeutically for this purpose.

**infundibulum** (*in-fun-di-bū-lum*). (1) A funnel-shaped orifice or passage. (2) Outgrowth of floor of brain forming part of the pituitary gland.

**infusion** (*in-fū-zhon*). (1) Fluid allowed to flow into a vein (intravenous infusion) or a muscle (intramuscular infusion) by a gravity feed. (2) Crude extract of material using boiling water, *e.g.* tea is an infusion of tea leaves.

**ingestion** (*in-jes'-chon*). Taking in of food or other substances.

**ingrowing toe nail.** Lateral parts of a nail growing into the nail bed often causing discomfort and infection.

**inguinal** (*in-gwi-nal*). Pertaining to the groin. *Inguinal canal*, about 4 cm (1½ in) in length, lies in groin; and is occupied in the male by the spermatic cord, and in the female by the round ligament, with their corresponding vessels and nerves.

**inhalation** (*in-ha-lā-shon*). Volatile medicinal substance which is inhaled.

**inherent** (*in-hār-ent*). Existing or abiding in a person, *e.g.* an inherent property or quality.

**inhibition** (*in-hi-bi-shon*). Literally restraint. The term is used ubiquitously to imply the prevention of some activity, thus psychological inhibition, enzymatic inhibition, nerve inhibition, etc.

**initial** (*i-ni-shal*). Pertaining to the beginning.

**injected** (*in-jek'-ted*). Congested.

**injection** (*in-jek-shon*). Introduction of material under pressure into tissues.

**innate** (*i-nāt*). Inborn, congenital.

**innervation** (*in-ner-vā'-shon*). The supply of nerves or the conveyance of nervous impulses to or from a part. *Reciprocal i.* One set of muscles contracts whilst those opposing it relax.

**innocent** (*i-nō-sent*). Not malignant.

**innocuous** (*i-no'-kū-us*). Harmless.

**innominate artery** (*i-no-mi-nāt ar-te-ri*). The large artery which arises from the arch of the aorta and divides into the right common carotid and right subclavian arteries.

**innominate bone.** Bone forming anterior walls and sides of the pelvic cavity.

**innoxious** (*in-ok'-shus*). Not harmful.

**inoculation** (*i-no-kū-lā-shon*). Introduction of microorganisms into tissues or culture media, etc.

**inorganic** (*i-nor-ga-nik*). Mineral as opposed to living material or its products. The distinction at a refined level is not obvious.

**inquest** (*in-kwest*). A judicial inquiry into the cause of death.

**insanity** (*in-san'-i-ti*). An out-

dated term usually meaning severe mental illness.

**insecticide** (*in-sek-ti-sīd*). A preparation for destroying insects.

**insemination** (*in-se-mi-nā'-shon*). Introduction of semen into the vagina. *Artificial i.* Injection of semen into vagina or uterus. The semen may either be from the legal husband (AIH) or from a donor (AID).

**insertion** (*in-ser'-shon*). The attachment of a muscle to the part it moves.

**insidious** (*in-si-di-us*). Literally cunning. Usually applies to onset of disease in which there are no perceptible signs or symptoms.

**insight** (*in-sīt*). An awareness of one's own mental state and behaviour.

**in situ** (*in-si'-too*). In position.

**insomnia** (*in-som-ni-a*). Sleeplessness.

**inspiration** (*in-spi-rā-shon*). The act of breathing in.

**inspissated** (*in-spi-sā'-ted*). Thickened by evaporation.

**instep.** The longitudinal arch of the foot.

**instillation** (*in-stil-lā'-shon*). Pouring in drop by drop.

**instinct.** An inherited organization of perception, feeling and action, *e.g.* the sight of something which threatens life arouses the emotion of fear and the instinct to flee.

**insufflation** (*in-suf-lā-shon*). Blowing into a structure.

**insula** (*in'-sū-la*). Small part of the cerebral cortex lying deeply in the lateral sulcus.

**insulation** (*in-sū-lā-shon*). Material preventing loss of or access to internally situated structure of heat, light, electrical current, water, etc.

**insulin** (*in-sū-lin*). A polypeptide hormone, secreted by the β-cells of the islets of Langerhans in the pancreas, which exerts control over the metabolism of glucose in the body.

**insulinoma** (*in-sū-lin-ō'-ma*). Adenoma of islets of Langerhans.

**integument** (*in-te-gū-ment*). The skin.

**intellect** (*in-te-lekt*). Reasoning power whereby we can think logically.

**intelligence** (*in-te-li-jenz*). Certain mental ability involving reasoning and recognition of pattern, etc. as distinct from memorization of information or other mental functions.

**intelligence quotient** (*in-te-li-jenz kwō-shent*). A measure of intelligence expressed as a figure where the average is 100.

**intelligence tests.** Tests not based on a person's knowledge but on his ability to learn. *See* INTELLIGENCE.

**intensive care unit.** Specialized hospital ward where acute illnesses are treated.

**intention tremor** (*in-ten-shon tre-mor*). Tremor which occurs only during active movement.

**inter** (*in'-ter*). A Latin prefix meaning 'between' and used with many medical terms, such as *intercostal*, between the ribs; *intermittent* fevers, in which there are regular pauses between the attacks.

**interarticular** (*in-ter-ar-tik'-ū-la*). Between the joints.

**intercellular** (*in-ter-se'-lū-la*). Between cells, *e.g.* intercellular fluid.

**intercourse** (*in-ter-kors*). Communication. *Sexual i.* Coitus.

**intercurrent** (*in-ter-ku'-rent*). Occurring between. *I. infection.* Another infection occurring in a patient already suffering from some other one.

**interference microscopy** (*in-ter-fā-rens mī-kros-ko-pi*). Optical system used to study cells grown in tissue or organ culture.

**interferon** (*in-te-fār-on*). Material elaborated by cells which interferes with the synthesis of nucleoprotein. It thus tends to limit the multiplication of viruses within the cell.

**intermittent.** Occurring at intervals. When applied to the pulse, signifies that some of the beats of the heart fail to reach the wrist.

**intermittent claudication** (*in-ter-mi-tent claw-di-kā-shon*). Literally intermittent limping, due to ischaemia of the muscles of the legs.

**internal** (*in-ter'-nal*). Inside.

**internal os.** The junction of the cavity of the cervix uteri with that of the body of the uterus. *See also* UTERUS.

**internal version.** Version by inserting one hand completely into the uterus, and so changing the presentation or lie of the fetus.

**interosseous** (*in-ter-os-sē-us*). Between two bones.

**interphase** (*in'-ter-fāz*). Period of cell cycle between two successive cell divisions.

**interstitial** (*in-ter-sti-shal*). Between parts, *i.e.* in connective tissue.

**interstitial keratitis** (*in-ter-sti-shal ke-ra-tī-tis*). Manifestation of congenital syphilis consisting of inflammation of the cornea.

**intertrigo** (*in-ter-trī'-gō*). Eczematous condition of deep crevices or folds of skin, due to retention of perspiration.

**intertrochanteric** (*in-ter-trō-kan-te-rik*). Between the trochanters.

**interventricular** (*in-ter-ven-tri-kū-la*). Between the ventricles.

**intervertebral** (*in-ter-ver-te-bral*). Between the vertebrae.

**intestinal malabsorption** (*in-tes-tī-nal mal-ab-sawp-shon*). Malabsorption syndrome. Failure to absorb certain foodstuffs. There are numerous causes. Usually there is a failure to absorb fats and fat-soluble vitamins.

**intestinal obstruction** (*in-tes-tī-nal ob-struck-shon*). Obstruction to the passage of food or faeces through the intestine. It may be due either to a physical blockage or to the absence of peristalsis.

**intestines** (*in-tes'-tinz*). The alimentary canal from the stomach to the anus.

**intima** (*in-ti-ma*). Inner coat of arteries consisting of endothelium and its elastic fibre attachment to the connective tissue of the mesial or middle layer.

**intolerance** (*in-to-le-rans*). Constitutional incapacity to endure or benefit by a remedial agent.

**intra** (*in'-tra*). Within.

**intra-abdominal** (*in-tra-ab-do-mi-nal*). Within the abdominal cavity.

**intra-articular** (*in-tra-ar-ti-kū-la*). Within the capsule of a joint.

**intracellular** (*in-tra-sel-lū-la*). Within a cell.

**intracranial** (*in-tra-krā-ni-al*). Pertaining to the interior of skull.

**intradermal** (*in-tra-der'-mal*). In the dermis.

**intradural** (*in-tra-dū-ral*). Within the dura mater.

**intragastric** (*in-tra-gas'-trik*). In the stomach.

**intrahepatic** (*in-tra-he-pa'-tik*). Within the liver.

**intralobular** (*in-tra-lo'-bū-la*). Within a lobule.

**intramedullary** (*in-tra-me-du'-ler-i*). In the bone marrow.

**intramuscular** (*in-tra-mus-kū-la*). Inside a muscle, *e.g.* intramuscular (IM) injection.

**intranasal** (*in-tra-nā'-sal*). Within the nasal cavity.

**intra-ocular fluids** (*in-tra-o'-kū-la floo-ids*). The fluids inside the eye, *viz.* the aqueous humour and the vitreous humour. The aqueous humour is constantly being formed from the ciliary body and is drained through the canal of Schlemm. If this circulation is impaired the *intra-ocular fluid pressure*

may rise, *see* GLAUCOMA. The normal pressure is 20 to 25 mm Hg.

**intra-osseous** (*in-tra-os-sē-us*). Within a bone.

**intraperitoneal** (*in-tra-pe-ri-to-nē-al*). Pertaining to the peritoneal cavity.

**intrathecal** (*in-tra-thē'-kal*). Pertaining to the lumen of a sheath or canal, usually meaning the spinal canal.

**intratracheal** (*in-tra-tra-kē-al*). Inside the trachea. Thus *intratracheal cannula*. Those used for the administration of anaesthetic are known as *endotracheal* tubes.

**intra-uterine** (*in'-tra-ū-ter-īn*). Within the uterus.

**intra-uterine contraceptive device** (*in'-tra-ū'-te-rin kon'-tra-sep'-tiv de-vis'*). Plastic or copper coated plastic device of varying shapes inserted into the uterus through the cervix to prevent conception. Exact method of action not known. Copper may help its effectiveness.

**intravenous** (*in-tra-vē-nus*). Pertaining to the lumen of a vein.

**intrinsic** (*in-trin-sik*). Inherent, peculiar to a part.

**intrinsic factor.** Castle's antipernicious anaemia substance. Factor present in normal gastric juice which enables the absorption of cyanocobalamin ($B_{12}$) to take place. It is probable that it is an enzyme.

**introitus** (*in-trō-i-tus*). Opening into a viscus. Usually refers to the external opening of the vagina.

**introspection** (*in-trō-spek-shon*). State of mental self-examination.

**introvert** (*in-trō-vert'*). An individual whose attention centres on himself rather than on outside things. Opposite to an extrovert.

**intubation** (*in-tū-bā-shon*). Insertion of a tube into a passage or organ, esp. tracheal intubation.

**intussusception** (*in-tu-sus-sep'-shon*). Condition in which part of the intestine is drawn into a more distal part.

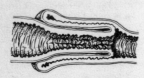

*28. An intussusception*

**inunction** (*in-unk-shon*). Putting ointment on the skin.

**in utero** (*in ū-te-rō*). Within the uterus.

**invagination** (*in-va-ji-nā-shon*). Forming a pouch.

**invasion** (*in-vā-zhon*). Onset.

**inverse** (*in-vers*). Opposite.

**inversion** (*in-ver-shon*). Turning upside down or inside out.

**in vitro** (*in vi-trō*). Literally in glass, *i.e.* in the test-tube as opposed to in life, *cf. in vivo.*

**in vivo** (*in vē-vō*). In the living body.

**involution** (*in-vo-lū'-shon*). (1) A turning in. (2) The shrinking of the uterus and surrounding structures after labour. The uterus, from weighing 2 pounds at labour, shrinks in 8 weeks to the weight of 2 ounces. Arrest of this process is called sub-involution.

**involutional melancholia** (*in-vo-lū-sho-nal me-lan-kō-li-a*). Severe depressive illness in the elderly which usually responds well to antidepressant treatment.

**iodism** (*ī-o-dism*). Iodine poisoning.

**ion** (*ī-on*). An atom or group of atoms carrying an electrical charge.

**ion exchange resin.** Special resins which preferentially take up certain ions, *e.g.* sodium, in exchange for others such as ammonia.

**ionization** (*ī-o-nī-zā-shon*). The process of becoming electrically charged.

**ionizing radiation** (*ī-on-ī-sing rā-di-ā-shon*). High energy radiation capable of producing ions in materials exposed to it.

**ipsilateral** (*ip-si-la'-te-ral*). On the same side.

**IQ.** *See* INTELLIGENCE QUOTIENT.

**iridectomy** (*ir-i-dek'-to-mi*). Cutting off a piece of the edge of the iris to make an artificial pupil to the eye.

**iridocele** (*ī-ri-dō-sēl*). Protrusion of a portion of iris through a wound in the cornea.

**iridocyclitis** (*ī-ri-dō-sī-klī-tis*). Inflammation of the iris and uveal tract.

**iridoplegia** (*ī-ri-dō-plē-ji-a*). Paralysis of the muscle which constricts or dilates the pupil.

**iridotomy** (*ī-ri-do'-to-mi*). An incision into the iris.

**iris** (*ī-ris*). The coloured circle surrounding the pupil of the eye. *See* EYE.

**iritis** (*ī-rī'-tis*). Inflammation of the iris.

**irradiation** (*i-rā-di-ā-shon*). Exposure to electromagnetic waves or atomic particles ($\alpha$, $\beta$ and $\gamma$ rays, neutrons).

**irreducible** (*ir-re-dū'-si-bl*). Incapable of being returned to its proper place by manipulation; usually term applied to a hernia.

**irrigation** (*i-ri-gā-shon*). Washing out.

**irritant** (*i-ri-tant*). Agent causing irritation, *i.e.* resulting in a response.

**ischaemia** (*is-kē-mi-a*). Diminished supply of blood to a part.

**ischaemic contracture** (*is-kē-mik con-trak-tūr*). Volkmann's contracture. Permanent shortening of muscle by fibrosis resulting from impairment of blood supply.

**ischium** (*is'-kē-um*). The lower and hind part of the innominate bone.

**islets of Langerhans** (*ī-lets of Lan-ger-hans*). Endocrine cells scattered in groups or islands within the pancreas, *see also* INSULIN.

**iso-antibodies** (*ī-sō-an-ti-bo-dis*). Terminology used to distinguish types of antibody in the circulation capable of acting against red blood cells. Iso-antibodies are specific for individual red cell antigens, *e.g.* AB or Rhesus antigens.

**isolation** (*ī-sō-lā'-shon*). The act of setting apart; an isolation room or ward is one kept for contagious or infectious diseases, and the doctor and nurse have to follow strict rules to prevent the spread of the disease.

**isomers** (*ī-sō-mers*). Substances having the same chemical composition but unlike physical or chemical properties owing to a difference in the relative positions of the atoms within the molecules.

**isometric** (*ī-sō-met'-rik*). Of equal length. Static.

**isotonic** (*ī-so-to-nik*). Having the same tone. *I. solutions.* These have the same osmotic pressure as physiological saline, 0·9 per cent NaCl.

**isotopes** (*ī-sō-tōps*). Differing forms of the same element with different atomic weights but the same chemical properties. *Radioactive i.* Isotopes with radioactive properties, emitting $\alpha$, $\beta$ or $\gamma$ radiation. Used to diagnose and treat disease.

**isthmus** (*is'-mus*). The neck or constricted part of an organ.

**itching** (*i-ching*). Sensation of irritation of the skin which commonly causes scratching.

**itis** (*ī'-tis*). Suffix meaning inflamed, *e.g.* dermatitis, inflammation of the skin.

**IUD.** Intra-uterine contraceptive device.

# J

**Jacksonian epilepsy** (*jak-sō-ni-an e-pi-lep-si*). *See* EPILEPSY.

**Jackson's membrane.** Peritoneal fold or adhesion between caecum or ascending colon and right abdominal wall. *J.'s sign.* (1) Asthmatoid wheezing sound due to foreign vegetable body in trachea; (2) Froth in pyriform fossa.

**Jacquemier's sign** (*jak-mē-āz sīn*). Blueness of the vaginal walls seen in early pregnancy.

**jaundice** (*jawn-dis*). A syndrome characterized by increased levels of bile pigments in the blood and tissue fluids. These pigments are taken up by the tissues giving rise to a yellow colour of the sclera, skin and mucous membranes. The causes of jaundice are generally classified as obstructive, hepatocellular and haemolytic. Excessive destruction of red blood cells (haemolysis) may be secondary to inherited abnormalities in their metabolism (spherocytosis), or infection, *e.g.* malaria or lysis in antigen-antibody reactions, *e.g.* Rhesus incompatibility, or other causes. Hepatocellular jaundice includes conditions such as infective hepatitis, a virus disease affecting the liver; toxic damage to the liver cells, *e.g.* acute yellow atrophy, and other conditions which reduce the efficiency of the liver in excreting bile pigments. Obstruction to any portion of the biliary tree may result in jaundice. The commonest cause of obstruction is gallstones.

**jaw bone.** *See* MAXILLA.

**jejunectomy** (*jā-jū-nek'-to-mi*). Excision of jejunum or part of it.

**jejunostomy** (*je-jū-nos'-to-mi*). Making an artificial opening into the jejunum.

**jejunum** (*jē-jū'-num*). That portion of the small intestine which lies between the duodenum and the ileum. *See* BOWEL.

**jerk.** A sudden contraction of muscle.

**jigger.** A tropical sand flea (*Dermatophilus penetrans*) which is parasitic in man, burrowing into the toes. Another name is chigoe.

**joint** (*joynt*). Point of contact of two or more bones. An articulation.

**jugular** (*jū-gū-la*). Relating to the neck.

**jugular foramen syndrome** (*fo-rā-men sin'-drōm*). Syndrome characterized by compression of the lower cranial nerves (ninth, tenth and eleventh) by tumours occupying jugular foramen in the skull.

**jugular veins.** Two large veins in the neck which convey most of the blood from the head.

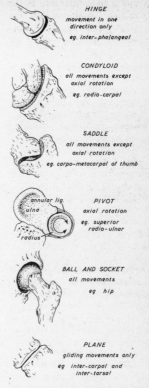

29. *Types of joints*

**Jung.** The founder of one school of psycho-analysis.

**jurisprudence, medical.** *See* MEDICAL.

**justo major** (*jus'-tō mā'-jer*).

Generally and equally enlarged pelvis.

**justo minor** (*jus'tō mī-ner*). Generally and equally contracted pelvis.

**juxta-glomerular apparatus** (*juks'-ta-glom-e-rū'-ler ap-a-rā-tus*). Group of cells forming cuff round afferent renal arteriole at its entry to Bowman's capsule, which probably acts as a stretch receptor to control release of renin when arteriolar tension falls.

**juxtaposition** (*juk-sta-pō-si-shon*). Placed alongside or next to.

## K

**kala-azar** (*ka-la-ā-za*). Visceral leishmaniasis. A disease caused by the protozoon *Leishmania donovani* which is transmitted from man to man by sand-flies. The parasite is found in reticulo-endothelial cells in the liver, spleen, bone marrow and occasionally lymph nodes and causes fever, anaemia and enlargement of the spleen.

**Kayser Fleischer rings** (*kā-ser flī-sher*). Brownish pigmented rings seen in the cornea of patients with Wilson's disease.

**Keller's operation.** Operation to correct hallux valgus.

**keloid** (*kē-loyd*). Overgrowth of connective tissue arising in scars.

**Kennedy's syndrome** (*ke'-ne-diz sin'-drōm*). Frontal lobe tumour involving one optic nerve. Optic atrophy.

**keratectasia** (*ke-ra-tek-tā-si-a*). Protrusion of the cornea.

**keratectomy** (*ke-ra-tek'-to-mi*). Surgical removal of part of the cornea,

**keratin** (*ke-ra-tin*). Fibrillar protein made from closely bonded polypeptide chains. It is produced by epithelial cells and imparts great strength to keratin-containing structures, such as horns, hooves and hair, and protective covering of the skin.

**keratitis** (*ke-ra-tī -tis*). Inflammation of the cornea.

**keratolytics** (*ke-ra-tō-li-tiks*). Agents which break down keratin such as salicylic acid.

**keratoma** (*ke-ra-tō'-ma*). A callosity or horny overgrowth.

**keratomalacia** (*ke-ra-tō-ma-lā-si-a*). Abnormal softening of cornea which may lead to ulceration and blindness. Occurs in association with vitamin A deficiency.

**keratome** (*ke'-ra-tōm*). Scalpel used in ophthalmic surgery.

**keratometer** (*ke-ra-to'-me-ter*).

Instrument for measuring corneal astigmatism.

**keratoplasty** (*ke-ra-tō-pla-sti*). Corneal graft.

**keratosis** (*ke-ra-tō-sis*). Thickening of the horny layer of the skin.

**kerion** (*ke'-ri-on*). A term for crusted ringworm.

**kernicterus** (*ker-nik-te-rus*). Many areas of the brain, particularly the basal ganglia, central cerebellar nuclei, the medulla and hippocampus are stained yellow with bilirubin. The brain cells are damaged. A complication of haemolytic jaundice of the newborn.

**Kernig's sign.** A sign of meningitis. It consists of an inability to extend the knee joint when the thigh is flexed at right angles to the trunk.

**ketogenic diet** (*kē'-tō-je'-nik dī-et*). Diet with high fat content.

**ketonaemia** (*kē-tō-nē-mi-a*). Ketone bodies in the blood.

**ketone** (*kē-tōn*). Chemical compounds containing carbonyl radicle ($C = O$), *e.g.* acetone.

**ketonuria** (*kē-tō-nū-ri-a*). Ketone bodies in the urine.

**ketosis** (*kē-tō'-sis*). Acidosis.

**ketosteroids** (*kē-tō-ste-royds*). Steroid substances which contain carbonyl radicles. Many of the breakdown products of steroid metabolism are excreted in the urine as ketosteroids.

**kidneys** (*kid-nēs*). Bilaterally situated upper abdominal viscera the function of which

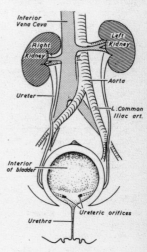

*30. The urinary organs (anterior aspect)*

is to secrete urine. *Artificial k.* Apparatus through which blood is passed and allowed to dialyse, *see* DIALYSIS, across a membrane, usually a coiled tube, placed in a warm bath of saline. This process allows waste products and other materials to be removed from the blood and simulates the function of the kidneys. *Ectopic k.* Kidney which is abnormally situated in the abdominal cavity. *K. failure*. Renal failure is basically the inability of the kidneys to do their job. There may be a number of different reasons for this and renal failure is usually classified as extra-renal and renal. Extra-renal causes are such things as severe haemorrhage or burns, dehydration or other causes of a prolonged and severe drop in blood pressure so that the blood flow to the kidneys is too low for them to function. Renal causes are classed as *acute*, e.g. acute nephritis and *chronic renal failure* which may be the end result of a large number of widely different kidney diseases.

**Kienboek's disease** (*kēn-bōks di-sēz*). An atypical osteochondritis affecting the semilunar bone of the wrist.

**Killian's operation.** For suppuration in the frontal sinus. Removal of part of frontal bone to allow of complete drainage.

**kilogram** (*ki-lō-gram*). A thousand grams, equivalent to 2⅕ lb.

**Kimmelstiel-Wilson syndrome** (*ki-mel-stēl wil-son sin'-drōm*). Nephrotic syndrome

associated with diabetes mellitus.

**kinaesthesis** (*kīn-ēs-thē'-sis*). The sense of muscular movement.

**kinematics** (*kī-ne-ma-tiks*). The study of motion.

**kineplasty** (*kin-nē-plas-ti*). A plastic amputation with the object of making the stump useful for locomotion.

**kinesis** (*kī-nē-sis*). Movement. Usually applied to cells migrating in response to a stimulus.

**kinetics** (*kī-ne-tiks*). The study of movement or change.

**King-Armstrong units.** Used for estimating alkaline phosphatase in blood.

**Kirschner wire** (*ker-shner wīr*). Wire used in orthopaedic surgery to apply skeletal traction to a fractured bone.

**kiss of life.** Mouth-to-mouth artificial respiration.

**Klebsiella** (*kleb-si-e'-la*). Genus of bacteria.

**Klebs-Loeffler bacillus** (*klebs lerf-ler ba-si-lus*). The bacillus of diphtheria. Also known as *Corynebacterium diphtheriae*.

**kleptomania** (*klep-to-mā-ni-a*). Obsessional neurosis which is manifested by compulsive stealing.

**Klinefelter syndrome** (*klīn-fel-ter sin-drōm*). Syndrome resulting from non-disjunction of the X chromosome with the result that the individual inherits an extra X chromosome and has an XXY complement of sex chromosomes. The patient is sometimes of low intelligence and may have eunuchoid characteristics.

**Klumpke's paralysis** (*kloompkers pa-ra-li-sis*). Paralysis of the flexor muscles to the wrist and fingers caused by injury to the eighth cervical and first dorsal nerves.

**knee** (*nē*). The joint between femur and tibia.

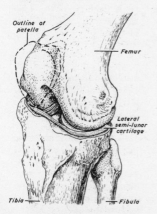

Outline of patella

Femur

Lateral semi-lunar cartilage

Tibia — Fibula

*31. The knee joint*

**knee-cap.** Patella.
**knee-elbow position.** *See* GENU-PECTORAL.

**knee jerk.** A jerk of the leg elicited by tapping on the patellar tendon when the knee is flexed. May be absent or exaggerated in diseases of the nervous system.

**knock-knee.** Genu valgum.

**knuckle** (*nukl*). Dorsal aspect of a phalangeal joint.

**Koch's bacillus** (*koks ba-si-lus*). *Mycobacterium tuberculosis*.

**Kock-Weeks bacillus** (*kok-wēks ba-si-lus*). Micro-organism causing acute conjunctivitis.

**Köhler's disease** (*ker-lers disēz*). Osteochondritis affecting the scaphoid bone in the foot which becomes compressed and sclerotic. It occurs in children.

**koilonychia** (*koy-lō-ni-ki-a*). Spoon-shaped nails found in iron deficiency anaemia.

**Koplik's spots.** Small white spots to be found on the inner surface of the cheeks in measles, often before the skin rash appears.

**Korsakow's syndrome** (*kor'-sa-kovs sin'-drōm*). A confusional state especially as to recent events due to brain injury or toxic causes such as chronic alcoholism. Confabulation is used by the patient in an attempt to cover the memory defect.

**kraurosis vulvae** (*kraw-rō-sis vul-vī*). Senile degeneration of the skin of the vulva.

**Krebs citric acid cycle.** The final common pathway in the degradation of foodstuffs whereby pyruvate is oxidized to give $CO_2$ and water. The energy derived from these reactions is captured by the cell in the form of adenosine triphosphate. The reactions are catalysed by enzymes located in the mitochondria. *K. urea cycle*. Enzyme reactions system where urea is formed in the liver by the union of ammonia with carbon dioxide with the elimination of water.

**Krukenberg's tumour** (*kroo-ken-bergs tū-mer*). A secondary carcinoma in the ovary, the primary usually occurring in the stomach.

**Küntscher nail** (*koon-cher*). An intramedullary nail used to fix fragments of fractured long bone in alignment.

**Kupffer cells** (*koop-fer sels*). Reticulo-endothelial cells which line the sinusoids of the liver.

**Kveim test** (*ke-fīm test*). Intradermal test for sarcoidosis by injection of splenic extract from known sarcoidosis patient.

**kwashiorkor** (*kwa-shi-aw-kor*). Syndrome characterized by wasting, oedema, anaemia and enlargement of the liver and due to lack of adequate protein in the diet. Occurs most commonly when a child is weaned from the breast.

**kyphoscoliosis** (*kī-fō-skō-li-ō-sis*). Combined antero-posterior deformity (kyphosis) and lateral curvature (scoliosis) of spine.

**kyphosis** (*ki-fō-sis*). Antero-posterior curvature of the spine causing hump-back deformity (*see illustration* p. 322).

## L

**labia majora** (*lā-bi-a ma-jo-ra*). (sing. **labium**). Two large folds at the mouth of the pudendum; called also the *labia pudendi*.

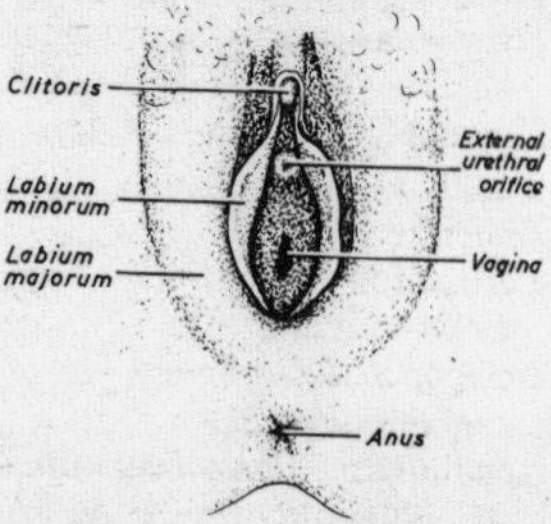


*32. The external genitalia in the female*

**labia minora** (*lā-bi-a mi-no-ra*). Two smaller folds within the majora; called also the *nymphae*.

**labial** (*lā'-bi-al*). Relating to the lips or to the labia.

**labile** (*lā-bīl*). Unstable.

**laboratory** (*la-ba-ra-to-ri*). A place where scientific experiments and investigations are carried on.

**labour** (*lā'-ber*). The progress of the birth of a child. There are three stages. (1) The dilatation of the cervix. (2) The passage of the fetus through the canal and its birth. (3) From the birth of the child to the expulsion of the placenta.

**labyrinth** (*la-bi-rinth*). The internal ear. *See* EAR.

**labyrinthitis** (*la-bi-rin-thī'-tis*). Inflammation of the labyrinth.

**laceration** (*la-se-rā-shon*). A lacerated wound with torn or irregular edges; not clean cut.

**lacrimal** (*lak'ri-mal*). Relating to tears and the glands which secrete them.

**lacrimation** (*lak-ri-mā'-shon*). Flow of tears.

**lactagogue** (*lak'-ta-gog*). Galactagogue.

**lactalbumin** (*lak-tal-bū'-min*). The albumin of milk. A protein.

**lactase** (*lak'-tāz*). An enzyme of the succus entericus which converts lactose into glucose.

**lactate.** A salt of lactic acid.

**lactation** (*lak-tā'-shon*). The process or period of suckling.

**lacteals** (*lak-tē-als*). The lymphatic vessels, which convey the chyle from the intestinal canal.

**lactic acid.** An acid produced by the fermentation of lactose.

**lactiferous ducts** (*lak-ti-fe-rus dukts*). The canals of the mammary glands.

**lactifuge** (*lak'-ti-fūj*). Reduction of milk secretion.

**lactobacillus** (*lak-tō-ba-si-lus*). A non-pathogenic Gram positive bacterium.

**lactogenic** (*lak-tō'-je'-nik*). Promoting the flow of milk. *L. hormone.* Prolactin. A hormone released from the anterior pituitary which causes milk production following parturition.

**lactose** (*lak-tōz*). A disaccharide sugar, composed of glucose and galactose, which occurs in milk.

**lacuna** (*la-kū-na*). A space.

**Laennec's cirrhosis** (*la-neks si-rō-sis*). The commonest type of cirrhosis of liver and frequently attributable to damage to the liver by high consumption of alcohol.

**laevulose.** *See* FRUCTOSE.

**laked** (*lakt*). Describes haemolysed blood.

**lambdoid** (*lam'-doyd*). Like Greek letter λ, chiefly applied to the suture between the occipital and parietal bones.

**lamellae** (*la-me-lē*). Thin sheets of tissue, *e.g.* bone.

**lamina** (*la-mi-na*). A thin layer.

**laminectomy** (*la-mi-nek-to-mi*). Excision of vertebral laminae.

**Lancefield's groups** (*larntsfēlds groops*). A classification of streptococci into groups of which Group A includes the common pathogenic haemolytic streptococcus.

**lancet** (*lahn'-set*). A sharp pointed surgical instrument.

**Landouzy-Dejerine dystrophy** (*lan-doo-zi-de-je-rēn dis-tro-fi*). A type of myopathy also known as facio-scapulo-humeral dystrophy. It is not associated with pseudo-hypertrophy.

**Langerhans' islets.** Small area of special cells in the pancreas. They secrete insulin. *See* INSULIN and DIABETES.

**lanolin** (*lan'-ō-lin*). Purified wool-fat. Used as the basis for various ointments.

**Lansing virus.** A strain of poliomyelitis virus.

**lanugo hair** (*la-nū-gō hār*). Thin unmedullated hair.

**laparoscope** (*la'-pa-ro-skōp*). Endoscope for examining the abdominal cavity.

**laparotomy** (*la-pa-ro-to-mi*). Operation involving the opening of the abdominal cavity, usually as an investigative procedure.

**laryngeal** (*la-rin'-je-al*). Relating to the larynx. *L. stridor*. Gasping respiration due to spasm of the glottis.

**laryngectomy** (*lar-in-jek'-to-mi*). Removal of the larynx.

**laryngismus stridulus** (*la-rin-jis'-mus stri'-dū-lus*). Laryngeal spasm.

**laryngitis** (*la-rin-jī-tis*). Inflammation of the larynx.

**laryngology** (*la-rin-go'-lo-ji*). Study of diseases of the larynx.

**laryngopharynx** (*la-rin-gō-fa-rinks*). The lower part of the pharynx.

**laryngoscope** (*la-rin-gō-skōp*). Instrument for examining a larynx.

**laryngospasm** (*la-rin-gō-spasm*). Spasm of the glottis.

**laryngostenosis** (*la-rin'-gō-ste-nō'-sis*). Stricture of the larynx.

**laryngotomy** (*la-rin-go-to-mi*). Cutting into the larynx for the insertion of a tube.

**laryngo-tracheo-bronchitis** (*la-rin-gō-tra-kē-ō-bron-kī-tis*). Acute viral inflammatory disease affecting the respiratory tract. Often occurs during influenza epidemics and effects principally young children.

**larynx** (*la-rinks*). The upper part of the windpipe from which the voice sounds proceed.

**laser** (*lā-zer*). (Light Amplification by Stimulated

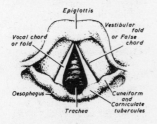

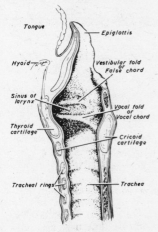

33. *The larynx*

*upper figure =
laryngoscopic view*

*lower figure =
sagital section*

Emission of Radiation.) Source of intense monochromatic light which can be delivered in large but precise amounts to very small areas. Used especially in ophthalmology for detached retina, and experimentally.

**lassitude** (*la-si-tūd*). Feeling of weakness, a frequent feature of debilitating diseases such as anaemia.

**latent** (*lā-tent*). Not visible, lying hidden for a time. *L. period*. Incubation time.

**lateral** (*la-te-ral*). On the side, *cf.* medial. *L. meniscus*. Cartilage between femur and tibia on the outside of the knee. *L. position*. Lying on the side. A position, favoured by some obstetricians, which may be adopted by the mother during delivery.

**laughing gas** (*lar-fing gas*). Nitrous oxide gas. An anaesthetic.

**Laurence-Moon-Biedl syndrome** (*lo-rens-moon-bē-del sin'-drōm*). A genetically determined syndrome characterized by obesity, hypergonadism polydactyly, retinitis pigmentosa and mental deficiency.

**lavage** (*la-varj*). Washing out.

**laxative** (*lak-sa-tiv*). A mild purgative.

**lead poisoning** (*led*). Usually occurs in children due to excessive lead in atmosphere or chewing cots and toys covered with paint containing lead. The symptoms and signs include malaise, colic, peripheral neuropathy, and sometimes encephalitis. Pallor is often marked and a blue line on the gums is characteristic.

**leather-bottle stomach.** Loss of elasticity in the stomach wall resulting from infiltration of neoplastic cells.

**lecithin** (*le-si-thin*). A phospholipid.

**Lederer's anaemia** (*le-de-rers a-nē-mi-a*). A term sometimes given to severe haemolytic anaemias of unknown cause.

**leech** (*lētsh*). Aquatic worm which is able to suck blood from the skin.

**leg.** Anatomically the part of the lower limb from knee to ankle. *White l.* Condition caused by venous thrombosis in the lower limb. Sometimes seen after childbirth.

**Leishman-Donovan body** (*lesh-man do-no-van bo-di*). Eosinophilic bodies representing rounded forms of *Leishmania donovani* found in the cells parasitized in kala-azar.

**Leishmaniasis** (*lesh-ma-nī-a-sis*). *See* KALA-AZAR.

**lens.** Transparent refractile tissue of the eye, *see* EYE, which focuses the image on the retina.

**lente insulin** (*len'-tā in'-sū-lin*). Slowly absorbed insulin preparation.

**lenticular.** Pertaining to a lens.

**lentigo** (*len-tī-go*). A freckle.

**Leon virus** (*lē-on vīrus*). A strain of poliomyelitis virus.

**leontiasis ossea** (*lē-on-tī-a-sis o-sē-a*). A localized form of fibrous dysplasia of bone, causing deformation of the face.

**leproma** (*le-prō-ma*). Swelling in the skin found in certain cases of leprosy.

**leprosy** (*le'-pro-si*). Hansen's disease is an endemic disease of the tropics. It is of low infectivity and is caused by *Mycobacteria leprae*. In the UK leprosy is a notifiable disease.

**leptomeningitis** (*lep-tō-men-in-jī-tis*). Inflammation of the pia mater and arachnoid coverings of the brain, distinguished from pachymeningitis, in which the dura mater is the seat of inflammation.

**leptospira** (*lep-tō-spī-ra*). Type of spirochaete. Notably *L. icterohaemorrhagicae* which causes Weil's disease.

**Leriche syndrome** (*le-rēsh sin'-drōm*). Obstruction to the flow of blood at the lower end of the aorta giving rise to intermittent claudication, and pain in the buttocks.

**lesion** (*lē'-zhon*). Any injury or morbid change in the function or structure of an organ.

**lethal** (*lē-thal*). Deadly, fatal.

**lethargy** (*le-thar-ji*). Drowsiness.

**leucine** (*lū-sin*). An amino-acid.

**leucocyte** (*lū-kō-sīt*). A white blood cell.

**leucocythaemia** (*lū'-kō-sī-thē'-mi-a*). Abnormally increased numbers of white cells in the blood.

**leucocytolysis** (*lū'-kō-sī-to'-li-sis*). Destruction of leucocytes.

**leucocytosis** (*lū-kō-sī-tō-sis*). Increased numbers of white cells in the blood.

**leucoderma** (*lū-kō-der-ma*). A condition in which there are patches of skin which are defectively pigmented, and consequently pale in colour.

**leuco-erythroblastic anaemia** (*lū-ko-e-ri-thrō-blas-tik a-nē-mi-a*). Descriptive term applied to the appearance of nucleated red cells and primitive white cells in the circulation. It is due to neoplastic infiltration of bone marrow.

**leuconychia** (*lū-kō-ni-ki-a*). Curved white lines on the finger-nails showing interrupted nutrition.

**leucopenia** (*lū-kō-pē-ni-a*). Diminution of the number of white cells in the blood.

**leucopoiesis** (*lū-kō-poy-ē-sis*). Formation of white blood cells.

**leucorrhoea** (*lū-kor-re'-a*). A whitish mucoid discharge from the vagina.

**leucotomy** (*lu-ko-to-mi*). Transection of nerve fibres passing to and from a lobe of the brain. Usually *prefrontal leucotomy*, an operation undertaken to relieve certain types of mental disorder in which the prefrontal lobes are surgically isolated from the rest of the brain.

**leukaemia** (*lū-kē-mi-a*). A disease of blood-forming organs, characterized by increase of white cells of the blood. *Lymphatic l.*, that in which large numbers of primitive lymphocytes appear in the blood. *Myeloid l.*, that in which primitive polymorphonuclear leucocytes appear in large numbers. *Monocytic l.*, *Eosinophilic l.*, as for the other forms, but exhibiting monocytes and eosinophils respectively. *See* BLOOD.

**leukoplakia** (*lū-kō-plā-ki-a*). A

smooth glazed white state of the tongue which may precede cancer of that organ. A similar condition of the vulva is also found in women.

**levator** (*le-vā-ter*). A muscle which lifts up a part. *L. ani*: muscle of the pelvis which plays an important part in keeping pelvic viscera in position. *L. palpebrae superioris*: muscle which raises the upper eyelid.

**levulose** (*le-vū-lōs*). Fruit sugar or fructose.

**Lewis blood group system.** System characterized by antigen (Le[a]), present in about 22 per cent of Europeans.

**libido** (*li-bi-dō*). The drive to obtain satisfaction through the senses. Term sometimes used for sexual desire.

**Libman-Sachs endocarditis.** Endocarditis in which the valves of the heart are damaged. The disease is associated with systemic lupus erythematosus.

**lichen** (*lī-ken*). (1) Subdivision of Thallophytes, which are organisms formed from a symbiotic association of algae and fungus. They are found on rocks, trees and bare areas. (2) A term used in dermatology roughly descriptive of the appearance of certain eruptions such as *lichen simplex, see* LICHENIFICATION, and *lichen planus*. The latter has a characteristic appearance consisting of an eruption of diamond-shaped flat violaceous papules.

**lichenification** (*lē-ke-ni-fi-kā-shon*). Also called lichen simplex. Thickening of the epidermis caused by constant friction. Often it occurs on the skin in sites exposed to habitual rubbing or scratching, from which it inherits the original name of neurodermatitis.

**lid retraction.** A sign of hyperthyroidism in which the upper eyelids are raised so as to expose the sclera above the cornea.

**lie of fetus.** The position of the fetus in the uterus is termed its lie, *i.e.* transverse lie, vertical lie.

**Lieberkühn's glands** (*lē'-ber-kūn*). Tubular glands of the small intestine, which secrete the intestinal juice.

**lien** (*lē-en*). The spleen.

**lienculus** (*lē-en'-kū-lus*). An accessory spleen.

**ligament** (*li-ga-ment*). A tough band of fibrous tissue connecting together the bones at the joints.

**ligation** (*li-gā-shon*). The application of a ligature.

**ligatures** (*li-ga-tūrs*). Threads of silk, wire, catgut, fascia, nylon, etc., used to tie arteries, stitch tissue, etc.

**light adaptation.** The contraction response of the pupil of the eye to light incident on the retina. Also termed *light reflex, cf.* dark adaptation.

**lightning pains** (*līt'-ning pānz*). Shooting, cutting pains felt in some cases of tabes dorsalis.

**limbus** (*lim'-bus*). Literally a border; applied to the junction between the sclera and cornea.

**liminal** (*li'-mi-nal*). At the threshold of perception.

**linctus** (*link'-tus*). A syrup. Usually applied to a cough mixture.

**linea alba** (*li-ne-a al-ba*). The white line down the centre front of the abdomen. It is formed by the tendons of the abdominal muscles.

**linea nigra** (*lin'-e-a nē-gra*). A pigmented line seen in pregnant women running in midline from above the umbilicus to the symphysis pubis.

**lineae albicantes** (*lin-e-ē al-bi-kan-tēz*). *See* STRIAE GRAVIDARUM.

**lingual** (*lin-gwal*). Relating to the tongue.

**liniment** (*lin'-i-ment*). A liquid preparation for application to the skin with friction.

**linolenic acid** (*li-nō-le-nik*). A constituent of vegetable fats, essential for health.

**lint.** Loosely woven cotton material, having one side smooth and the other rough. The smooth side is applied next to the skin.

**lipaemia** (*lī-pē-mi-a*). Presence of excess of fat in the blood.

**lipase** (*lī-pās*). Enzyme which splits the esters of fatty acids, *see* FAT.

**lipo-atrophy** (*lī-pō-a-tro-fi*). Loss of subcutaneous fat. A complication which may arise in sites of insulin injections.

**lipochondrodystrophy** (*lī-pō-kon-drō-dis-tro-fi*). Term sometimes used to describe gargoylism or Hurler's syndrome.

**lipodystrophy** (*lī-pō-dis-tro-fi*). A disorder of fat metabolism which most commonly affects women, who show little fat above the waist but are obese about the buttocks and legs.

**lipoidosis** (*li-poy-dō'-sis*). General term for diseases of fat metabolism.

**lipoids** (*li-poyds*). Substances, *e.g.* lecithin, which resemble fats, in being dissolved by organic solvents such as alcohol and ether. They occur in living cells.

**lipoma** (*li-pō-ma*). Tumour of fat cells.

**lipotrophic substances** (*lī-pō-trō-fik*). Substances which mobilize fat from the liver.

**Lippes loop** (*lip'-ēz loop*). One

type of intra-uterine contraceptive device.

**liquor amnii** (*lī-kwor am-nē-ē*). The watery fluid by which the fetus is surrounded.

**liquor folliculi** (*lī-kwor fo-li-kū-lē*). Fluid in a Graafian follicle.

**liquores** (*lī-kwo-rēs*). Solutions of active substances in water. *Liquor calcis saccharatus* lime-water.

**lithagogues** (*li-tha-gogs*). Drugs which expel or dissolve stones.

**lithiasis** (*li-thī-a-sis*). Formation of stone.

**litholapaxy** (*li-thō-lā-pak-si*). Operation for crushing a stone in the bladder and removing the fragments at the same sitting.

**lithopaedion** (*li-thō-pē-di-on*). A calcified fetus in the abdominal cavity.

**lithotomy** (*li-tho-to-mi*). Operation of cutting into a bladder to remove a stone.

**lithotomy position.** Patient supine with thighs and knees flexed. The hips must be abducted.

**lithotrite** (*lith'-ō-trīt*). An instrument for crushing stones in the bladder. It is passed through the urethra.

**lithotrity** (*lith-ot'-ri-ti*). Operation of crushing a stone in the bladder.

**lithuria** (*li-thū-ri-a*). Passing gravel or crystals of uric acid with the urine.

**litmus** (*lit'-mus*). A blue pigment turned red by acids. *L. paper*. Paper impregnated with litmus; used for testing urine and gastric secretion. A red litmus paper is turned blue by an alkali.

**litre** (*lē-ter*). 1,000 ml or 1·7598 pint or 35·196 fluid ounces.

**Little's disease.** Spastic paraplegia or diplegia of infants due to birth injury or faulty development of the brain.

**Littré's hernia** (*lē-trās her-ni-a*). A diverticular hernia.

**liver.** Large organ occupying the upper right portion of the abdomen. It has many important functions including the secretion of bile, the manufacture of serum albumin and the storage of glycogen, etc.

**livid.** Bluish in colour.

**LMP.** Abbreviation for last menstrual period.

**LOA.** Abbreviation for left occipito-anterior presentation of fetus.

**lobar** (*lō'-ba*). Pertaining to a lobe.

**lobe** (*lōb*). Rounded division of an organ.

**lobectomy** (*lō-bek'-to-mi*). Excision of a lobe.

**Lobo's disease** (*lō'-bōz di-sēz*). Keloid tumours of the legs induced by fungus infection.

**lobule** (*lo-būl*). Small lobe.

**localized** (*lō-kal-īzd*). Limited to a certain area; not widespread.

**lochia** (*lō-ki-a*). The vaginal discharge following delivery. For the first day or two is almost pure blood, but in normal cases becomes rapidly brown and then paler and ceases in a few weeks.

**locked twins.** The condition of twins when some part of one absolutely prevents the birth of the other by causing complete impaction.

**lock-jaw.** *See* TETANUS.

**locomotor ataxia** (*lō-kō-mō-tor a-tak'-si-a*). Impaired gait in walking. A chronic disease due to degeneration of parts of the spinal cord and nerves. *See* TABES DORSALIS.

**loculated** (*lo-kū-lā-ted*). Divided into many cavities.

**locum tenens** (*lō-kum te-nens*). A practitioner who temporarily takes the place of another.

**loin** (*loyn*). The lateral portion of the back between the thorax and pelvis.

**longevity** (*lon-gev'-i-ti*). Long life.

**LOP.** Abbreviation for left occipito-posterior presentation of fetus.

**Lorain syndrome** (*lo-rān*). Type of pituitary dwarfism.

**lordosis** (*lor-dō'-sis*). Undue curvature of the spine with the convexity forwards; an exaggeration of the normal curve of the lumbar part of the spine.

**lotion** (*lō-shon*). A medical solution for external use.

**louse** (*lows*). A type of insect. *See* PEDICULUS.

**Lovset's manoeuvre** (*luv-sets ma-noo-ver*). An obstetrical manoeuvre used to deliver breech presentations with extended arms.

**lower motor neurone disease.** Disease affecting the lower motor neurone fibres. These arise from cell bodies in the anterior horn of the spinal cord and pass to the motor end-plates of the muscles which they innervate. Lesions of the lower motor neurones result in paralysis and wasting of the muscles.

**lower uterine segment** (*lō-wer ū'-te-rīn seg'-ment*). That portion of the uterus, consisting of the cervix and the lower end of the body, which undergoes dilatation during labour.

**LSD.** Lysergic acid, a hallucinogen.

**'lub-dup'.** Heart sounds. The first sound is heard when the atrio-ventricular valves close, the second on closure of the semilunar valves.

**lubricant** (*loo-bri-kant*). Any substance, such as an oil, which makes a surface slippery.

**lucid** (*loo'-sid*). Clear.

**Ludwig's angina** (*lood-vigs an-jī-na*). An acute inflammatory condition in the sublingual and submaxillary regions.

**lumbago** (*lum-bā'-gō*). Painful condition of the lumbar muscles, due to inflammation of their fibrous sheaths. May be caused by a displaced intervertebral disc.

**lumbar** (*lum'-ba*). Pertaining to the region of the loins.

**lumbar puncture** (*lum-ba pung-cher*). The operation of tapping the cerebrospinal fluid in the lumbar region.

**lumbar sympathectomy** (*lumba sim-pa-thek-to-mi*). Operation to remove the sympathetic chain in the lumbar region.

**lumen** (*lū-men*). The cavity inside a tube.

**lungs.** The two organs of respiration, situated in the right and left sides of the cavity of the chest.

**lunula** (*lū'-nū-la*). White crescent at the root of the nail.

**lupus erythematosus** (*loo-pus e-ri-the-ma-tō-sus*). A disorder classed with the so-called collagen diseases. A localized form may affect the skin of exposed regions. The generalized form is known as systemic lupus erythematosus (SLE). The clinical manifestations of the disease are very varied. The criterion of diagnosis is the detection of antinuclear factor (ANF) by immunofluorescent techniques. Antibodies to DNA may also be found. LE cells may be present but are found in other diseases as well as SLE.

**lupus pernio** (*loo-pus per-ni-ō*). A form of cutaneous sarcoidosis.

**lupus vulgaris** (*loo-pus vul-ga-ris*). Tuberculosis affecting the skin.

**luteinizing hormone** (*lū-ti-nī-zing*). Hormone of the anterior pituitary gland stimulating the formation of corpus luteum in the ovary.

**Lutembacher's syndrome** (*loo-tem-ba-kers sin'-drōm*). Atrial septal defect associated with mitral stenosis.

**luteotrophin** (*lū-tē-ō-trō'-fin*). Pituitary hormone responsible for subsequent growth and development of the corpus luteum after its formation by the follicle stimulating hormone and the luteinizing hormone.

**luteus** (*loo'-tē-us*). Latin word for yellow. *See* MACULA LUTEA and CORPUS LUTEUM.

**Lutheran blood group system.**

Blood group characterized by possession of antigen Lu<sup>a</sup>, found in about 7 per cent of population in England.

**luxation** (*luk-sā'-shon*). Dislocation of a joint.

**lying-in** (*lī-ing in'*). The puerperium.

**lymph** (*limf*). That part of the blood plasma which has passed through the walls of the capillaries, bathing the tissue cells, giving them nourishment and taking away waste products. It is also found in the lymphatic vessels and serous cavities.

**lymphadenitis** (*lim-fa-de-nī'-tis*). Inflammation of the lymphatic glands.

**lymphadenoid goitre** (*lim-fa-de-noyd goy-ter*). *See* HASHIMOTO'S DISEASE.

**lymphangiectasis** (*lim-fan-jē-ek'-ta-sis*). Dilated state of lymphatic vessels.

**lymphangioma** (*lim-fan-ji-ō'-ma*). Tumour arising from the endothelial cells lining the lymphatic vessels.

**lymphangioplasty** (*lim-fan-jē-ō-pla'-sti*). An operation for the relief of lymphatic obstruction.

**lymphangitis** (*lim-fan-jī-tis*). Inflammation of lymphatic vessels.

**lymphatic leukaemia** (*lim-fa-tik lū-kē-mi-a*). *See* LEUKAEMIA.

**lymphatics** (*lim-fa-tiks*). Small vessels pervading the body, and containing lymph.

**lymphocytaemia** (*lim-fō-sī-tē-mi-a*). Increase of lymphocytes in the bloodstream.

**lymphocytes** (*lim'-fō-sīts*). One of the normal varieties of white blood cells. *Lymphocytosis*, excess of these cells in the blood: found in leukaemia, whooping cough, tuberculosis and lymphadenoma. *Lymphocytopenia*, deficiency of lymphocytes.

**lymphogram** (*lim-fō-gram*). Method of demonstrating the lymphatic system following the injection of contrast medium opaque to x-rays.

**lymphogranuloma inguinale** (*lim-fō-gra-nū-lō-ma in-gwi-nar-lē*). Sexually transmitted disease due to a virus.

**lymphoid** (*lim-foyd*). Having the character of lymph. *L. tissue*. Adenoid tissue.

**lymphoma** (*lim-fō'-ma*). Tumour of lymphatic tissue.

**lymphosarcoma** (*lim-fō-sar-kō'-ma*). A sarcoma originating in lymphatic tissue.

**lysine** (*lī'-sēn*). *See* AMINOACIDS.

**lysins** (*lī-sins*). Antibodies able to dissolve cells. *Haemolysins*, those able to dissolve red blood cells. *Bacteriolysins*, those able to dissolve bacteria.

**lysis** (*lī-sis*). Dissolution.

**lysosomes** (*lī-sō-sōms*). Intracellular vesicles produced probably by the Golgi apparatus in which are segregated a number of hydrolytic enzymes. *See* CELL.

# M

**McArdle's syndrome** (*ma-kahr'-delz sin'-drōm*). Myopathy resulting from absence of enzyme, phosphorylase, from voluntary muscle.

**McBurney's point** (*mak-ber-nis poynt*). On line from umbilicus to anterior superior iliac spine, at outer edge of rectus muscle; corresponds to base of the appendix, and pressure here may cause tenderness depending on the position of the appendix.

**maceration** (*ma-se-rā'-shon*). The softening of a solid by soaking it in a liquid; or of a fetus which has died some time before delivery.

**Mackenrodt's ligaments** (*ma-ken-rōtz li'-ga-ments*). Also called transverse cervical or cardinal ligaments. One of the chief supports of the uterus.

**macrocephalous** (*ma-krō-ke-fa-lus*). Having a large head.

**macrocheilia** (*ma-krō-kī-li-a*). Excessively large lips.

**macrocytes** (*mak'-rō-sīts*). Abnormally large cells, present in the blood in certain types of anaemia.

**macrodactyly** (*mak-rō-dak'-ti-lē*). Enlargement of the fingers.

**macroglobulinaemia** (*mak-rō-glo-bū-li-nē'-mi-a*). Syndrome associated with presence in blood of abnormal globulins of high molecular weight, characterized by multiple haemorrhages, dyspnoea and fatigue, especially in elderly men.

**macroglossia** (*ma-krō-glo-si-a*). Hypertrophy of the tongue.

**macromastia** (*mak'-rō-mas'-ti-a*). Abnormally developed breasts.

**macrophages** (*ma-krō-fā-jes*). Wandering scavenger cells which form part of the reticulo-endothelial system. Their function is to engulf tissue debris and foreign particles. In connective tissue they are termed *histiocytes* and in the blood they are known as *monocytes*. The engulfment of material is termed *phagocytosis*, or *pinocytosis*.

**macroscopic** (*ma-krō-sko-pik*). Visible to the naked eye.

**macrostomia** (*ma-kro-stō-mi-a*). Rare abnormality of development of the mouth due to non-fusion of the mandibular and maxillary processes.

**macula** (*ma-kū-la*). A spot discolouring the skin. *M. lutea*. Central spot of the posterior surface of the retina, just lateral to the optic disc marked by a small depression, and where vision is most acute.

**maculopapular** (*ma-kū-lō-pa'-pū-la*). A rash having both macules and papules.

**Magendie, foramen of** (*ma-jen-dē fo-rā-men*). An opening in the roof of the fourth ventricle through which the cerebrospinal fluid passes into the subarachnoid space.

**main en griffe** (*mun aw grēf*). Claw-like deformity of hand.

**mal.** Sickness. *Mal de mer*: sea sickness. *Grand mal*: major epilepsy. *Petit mal*: minor epilepsy.

**malabsorption** (*ma-lab-sorp-shon*). Reduced ability to absorb substances in the food from causes such as intestinal hurry, loss of absorbing surface as in extensive bowel resections, and diseases affecting the bowel wall including tropical sprue, coeliac disease and idiopathic steatorrhoea.

**malabsorption syndrome** (*ma-lab-sorp-shon sin'-drōm*). Syndrome produced by malabsorption which is characterized by some or all

of the following features: diarrhoea, loss of weight, abdominal distension, anaemia, tetany and vitamin deficiencies.

**malacia** (*ma-lā-ki-a*). Pathological softening.

**maladie de Roger** (*ma-la-dē de ro-ja*). Term sometimes used to describe small ventricular septal defects which do not give rise to symptoms unless some secondary disorder, such as bacterial endocarditis, supervenes.

**maladjustment** (*mal-a-just'-ment*). A state of being not in line, as with a badly set bone. In psychology, development which is not acceptable to the society in which the individual lives.

**malaise** (*ma-lāz*). A general feeling of illness or discomfort.

**malar** (*mā'-lar*). Relating to the cheekbone.

**malaria** (*ma-lār-i-a*). Tropical disease caused by parasite transmitted by Anopheles mosquitoes. There are four varieties of human malaria due to infection respectively by *Plasmodium vivax* (benign tertian malaria), *Plasmodium ovale* (benign tertian malaria), *Plasmodium falciparum* (malignant tertian malaria) and *Plasmodium malariae* (quartan malaria). Clinical features are periodic attacks of shivering followed by headache, vomiting, fever and profuse sweating.

**malformation** (*mal-faw-mā-shon*). Deformity.

**Malgaigne's bulgings** (*mal-gāns bul-jings*). Bulging of the lower abdominal musculature when there is poor muscular tone. It is considered to be a sign of predisposition to inguinal hernia.

**malignant** (*ma-lig'-nant*). Virulent, fatal. A *malignant tumour* or *growth* is one which if not totally removed will spread and cause similar growths in other parts of the body until the patient dies, *e.g.* carcinoma, sarcoma.

**malignant exophthalmos** (*ma-lig-nant ek-sof-thal-mos*). Exophthalmos occurring in the absence of any marked evidence of hyperthyroidism. Proptosis is extreme and there is progressive oedema and swelling of the lids and later ulceration of the cornea, diplopia and blindness.

**malignant hypertension** (*ma-lig-nant hī-per-ten-shon*). Hypertension associated with papilloedema and evidence of renal failure.

**malignant pustule** (*ma-lig-nant pus'-tūl*). Anthrax contracted from cattle, causing gangrenous carbuncle.

**malingering** (*ma-ling'-ger-ing*). Shamming sickness.

**malleolus** (*mal-le'-ō-lus*). The projection of the ankle-bone. The inner malleolus is at the lower extremity of the tibia, the outer one at the lower extremity of the fibula.

**mallet finger.** Deformed finger with flexion of distal phalanx.

**malleus** (*ma-lē-us*). A hammer-shaped bone of the middle ear. *See* EAR.

**malnutrition** (*mal-nū-trī'-shon*). A state of undernourishment.

**Malpighian corpuscle** (*mal-pi-gi-an kor-pusl*). Mesh of capillaries which act as a filtering coil for blood passing through the kidneys.

**malpresentation** (*mal-pre-zen-tā'-shon*). Any presentation, other than the vertex, of the fetus at birth.

**malrotation of gut.** Abnormality of development in which the intestine becomes fixed to the mesentery in an abnormal way. This makes the gut liable to volvulus.

**maltase** (*mawl-tāz'*). An enzyme of the succus entericus which converts maltose into glucose.

**maltose** (*mawl-tōz*). A disaccharide composed of two molecules of glucose.

**malunion** (*ma-lū-ni-on*). Faulty union of divided tissues, as of the fragments of a broken bone.

**mammae** (*mam'-mē*). The breasts, or milk-supplying glands.

**mammaplasty** (*ma-ma-pla'-sti*). Plastic surgery on the breasts such as that done to reduce the size of very heavy breasts.

**mammary** (*ma'-ma-ri*). Relating to the breasts.

**mammilla** (*ma-mi'-la*). The nipple.

**mammography** (*ma-mo'-gra-fi*). A technique to demonstrate tissue changes in the breast: xeroradiography frequently used for this technique.

**Manchester repair.** A type of gynaecological operation for uterovaginal prolapse.

**mandible** (*man'-di-bl*). The lower jaw.

**mania** (*mā-ni-a*). Pathological combination of elation and energy. The patient is uncontrollably excited.

**manic depressive psychosis** (*sī-kō-sis*). A mental illness when intense excitement alternates with depression.

**manipulation** (*ma-ni-pū-lā'-shon*). Handling, rubbing and working with the hands to procure some healing result. Also forced movements of joints to re-establish a normal range of movement.

**mannerism** (*ma'-ne-rizm*). Habitual expression or actions of an individual which are characteristic of him. Under stress they may become exaggerated.

**manoeuvre** (*ma-noo'-ver*). Special movement by the hand or with an instrument.

**manometer** (*ma-no'-me-ter*). An instrument for measuring the pressure of gases and liquids.

**Mantoux test** (*man-too*). Test of the body's reaction to antigenic material prepared from tubercle bacilli. This material called tuberculin is injected intradermally in serial dilutions (1·0 TU; 10·0 TU; 100 TU in 0·1 ml isotonic saline). A localized inflammatory reaction within 48 hours signifies a positive response.

**manual** (*ma-nū-al*) (adjective). Done by hand.

**manubrium sterni** (*ma-nū-bri-um ster-nē*). The uppermost part of the sternum.

**manus** (*ma-nus*). Latin for hand.

**MAOI.** Mono-amine oxidase inhibitor. A drug used in some types of depression. Hypertensive crises can occur if the patient eats certain foods including cheese.

**marasmus** (*ma-ras'-mus*). Progressive emaciation.

**marble bone disease.** Familial osteosclerosis. *See* ALBERS-SCHÖNBERG'S DISEASE.

**Marfan's syndrome.** Syndrome due to abnormal development characterized by spider digits, *see* ARACHNODACTYLY, hypertonus, high-arched palate, dislocation of lenses and various cardiac anomalies, particularly atrial septal defect and coarctation of the aorta.

**marihuana.** *See* CANNABIS.

**Marion's disease** (*ma-ri-ons di-sēz*). Contracture of the bladder neck, giving rise to difficulty in passing urine.

**marrow** (*ma'-rō*). The soft substance which fills the medullary canal of a long bone and the small spaces in cancellous bone. The red cells of the blood are formed in the bone marrow.

**marrow puncture** (*ma-rō pung-cher*). Investigative procedure involving the aspiration of marrow cells, usually by puncturing the sternum with a needle.

**marsupialization** (*mar-sū-pi-a-lī-zā'-shon*). Old method of treating mesenteric cysts by opening the cavity on to the external abdominal wall, thus making a sort of kangaroo pouch.

**masochism** (*ma'-zo-kism*). Self-torture from which a sexual pleasure may be derived.

**massage** (*ma-sahj*). Manipulation and rubbing of body designed to promote blood flow.

**masseter** (*ma-se-ter*). Powerful muscle which lifts the mandible, thus closing the jaws.

**mast cells.** Cells found in the blood and the tissues which store histamine which is released when the cells are damaged. They are distinguishable by their content of basophilic granules. In the blood these cells are known as basophils.

**mastalgia** (*mas-tal'-ji-a*). Breast pains.

**mastectomy** (*mas-tek-to-mi*). Surgical removal of the breast. *Radical m*. The breast is removed together with the lymph glands of the axilla and the pectoral muscle.

**mastication** (*mas-ti-kā-shon*). Chewing.

**mastitis** (*mas-tī'-tis*). Inflammation of the breast.

**mastodynia** (*mas-tō-di-ni-a*). Pain in the breasts often in the premenstrual phase.

**mastoid** (*mas'-toyd*). Literally, breastlike. The *mastoid process* is the projecting portion of the temporal bone behind the ear; it contains numerous air spaces including the *mastoid antrum*.

**mastoidectomy** (*mas-toy-dek'-to-mi*). Excision of the inflamed cells.

**mastoiditis** (*mas-toy-dī-tis*). Inflammation of the mastoid cells.

**masturbation** (*mas-ter-bā'-shon*). Manipulation of the genitalia to produce sexual excitement.

**materia medica** (*ma-tār-i-a me-di-ka*). Branch of medical study dealing with the nature and use of drugs, *i.e.* pharmacology and therapeutics.

**matrix** (*mā-triks*). Continuous medium in which structures are embedded.

**matter.** Any substance. Pus is sometimes referred to as matter. *Grey m*. The nerve cells or non-medullated nerve fibres. *White m*. Medullated nerve fibres which are enveloped by a white sheath.

**maturation** (*ma-tū-rā-shon*). Ripening; the process of becoming fully developed.

**maxilla** (*mak-si-la'*). The upper jaw-bone.

**maxillary** (*mak-si-la-ri*). Pertaining to the maxilla.

**MCD.** Abbreviation for mean cell diameter.

**MCHC.** Abbreviation for mean cell haemoglobin concentration.

**MCV.** Abbreviation for mean cell volume.

**mean** (*mēn*). The average.

**measles** (*mē-zels*). Morbilli. An infectious disease common in children. Incubation period 10 to 12 days. Early symptoms are those of a cold, sore throat, cough and rise in temperature, Koplik's spots. The rash appears on the fourth day, about the neck and behind the ears, gradually spreading to the rest of the body and extremities. Recovery occurs about the seventh or ninth day. Most infectious period is before the rash appears. *German measles*, rubella.

**meatus** (*mē-ā'-tus*). An opening into a passage.

**mechanics of labour** (*me-ka-niks*). The series of forces which act upon the fetus while it is being driven through the birth canal, with the resistance to those forces, and the resulting effects of both upon the attitude and movements of the fetus.

**Meckel's cartilage** (*me-kels kar-ti-lāj*). Part of the articular surface of the jaw.

**Meckel's diverticulum** (*me-kels dī-ver-ti-kū-lum*). A small blind protrusion occasionally found in the lower portion of the ileum.

**meconium** (*me-kō-ni-um*). A

black, sticky substance voided from the bowels of an infant during the first day or two after its birth.

**medial** (*mē-di-al*). On the inside, *cf.* lateral (on the outside); towards the median line.

**median** (*mē-di-an*). In the middle. *M. line*, an imaginary longitudinal line dividing the body down the centre. *M. nerve*, one of the nerves of the arm.

**mediastinum** (*mē-di-as-tī'-num*). The space in the chest between the two lungs. It contains the heart, glands and important vessels.

**medical jurisprudence** (*jū-ris-prū-dens*). Medicine as it is connected with the law; for instance, in cases of suicide or murder.

**medicament** (*me-di-ka-ment*). Any medicinal drug or application.

**medication** (*me-di-kā'-shon*). A medicine given to a patient. *Pre-operative m.* One given before an operation as a basal anaesthetic.

**medicinal** (*me-di'-si-nal*). Pertaining to the science of medicine or to a drug.

**medicine** (*me'-di-sin*). (1) The treatment of disease. (2) A drug used to prevent or treat disease.

**medico-chirurgical** (*me-di-kō-shi-rer-ji-kal*). Relating to both medicine and surgery.

**Mediterranean anaemia** (*me-di-tār-ā-ne-an a-nē-mi-a*). Also known as Cooley's anaemia, *see* THALASSAEMIA. A recessively inherited abnormality in which the marrow continues to manufacture fetal haemoglobin.

**medium** (*mē-di-um*). Material to nourish cultures of tissues, cells and micro-organisms.

**medulla** (*me-du-la*). Latin for marrow.

**medulla oblongata** (*me-du-la ob-lon-ga'-ta*). The lowest part of the brain where it passes through the foramen magnum and becomes the spinal cord. It contains the vital centres which govern circulation and respiration. *See* BRAIN.

**medullary** (*me-du-la-ri*). Relating to the marrow.

**medullated nerve fibre** (*me-du-lā-ted nerv fī-ber*). Nerve fibre surrounded by a sheath of myelin.

**medulloblastoma** (*me-du-lō-bla-stō'-ma*). Malignant tumour, from embryonic cells of neuro-epithelial origin, occurring in the cerebellum.

**megacephaly** (*me-ga-ke'-fa-li*). An abnormally large head.

**megacolon** (*me-ga-kō'-lon*). Enlargement and dilatation

of the colon. *Congenital m.*
Hirschsprung's disease.

**megakaryocytes** (*me-ga-ka-ri-ō-sīts*). Large bone marrow
cells which produce the blood
platelets.

**megaloblast** (*me-ga-lō-blarst*).
Large, nucleated primitive
red blood cell. They occur in
the peripheral blood when
there is a defect of red blood
cell maturation in the bone
marrow, as for example in
vitamin $B_{12}$ deficiency.

**megalomania** (*me-go-lō-mā'-ni-a*). Insanity with delusional ideas of personal
greatness.

**Meibomian glands** (*mī-bō-mi-an glans*). Sebaceous glands
of the eyelids. *M. cyst*, Chala-
zion.

**Meig's syndrome** (*mīgs sin'-drōm*). Fibroma of the ovary
associated with pleural
exudate.

**meiosis** (*mī-ō-sis*). Successive
divisions of diploid cell to
yield haploid gametes. The
gametes (spermatozoa, ova)
must have their chromosome
number reduced by half in
order to compensate for the
doubling which occurs by fertilization. The stages in
meiosis are represented in
the accompanying figure, *cf.*
mitosis, p. 228.

**melaena** (*me-lē-na*). Black tar-
like stools, due to the pres-

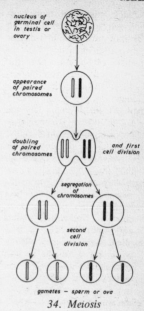

34. *Meiosis*

ence of blood which has
undergone changes in the
alimentary tract. The blood is
often from a gastric or
duodenal ulcer.

**melancholia** (*me-lan-kō-li-a*). A
state of profound depression
in which there is often a slowing down of all mental and
physical functions, feelings of
guilt and self-denigration.
Suicide is a possibility.

**melanin** (*me-la-nin*). Black

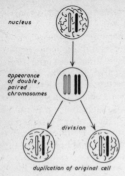

nucleus

appearance
of double,
paired
chromosomes

division

duplication of original cell

35. Mitosis

pigment formed by the
polymerization of quinonoid
molecules. It is widely distributed in nature and is the
skin pigment of man.

**melanoma** (*me-la-nō-ma*). A
tumour composed of
melanocytes, the cells which
are responsible for the production of melanin.

**melanosis** (*me-la-nō-sis*). Black
spots in the tissues.

**melanotic** (*me-la-no-tik*).
Black.

**membrane** (*mem-brān*). A thin
lining.

**membrane bone.** Bone arising
from dermal connective tissues as opposed to bone
arising from cartilage.

**menarche** (*me-nar-kā*). The
age at which menstruation
begins.

**Mendel's laws** (*men-dels lors*).
Two laws of inheritance
promulgated by Mendel. The
first states that allelomorphs
segregate, *see* MEIOSIS; and
the second that independent
assortment of alleles occur.
The second law is subject to
the genes being situated on
separate chromosomes since
it depends on the independent behaviour of chromo-
some pairs during meiosis.
When two or more genes are
located on the same chromosome the alleles are said to be
linked.

**Ménière's disease** (*mā-nē-ārs*).
Giddiness resulting from disease of the internal ear or the
equilibrating mechanism of
the brain.

**meningeal** (*me-nin-jē-al*). Pertaining to the meninges.

**meninges** (*me-nin'-jēz*). The
membranes surrounding and
covering the brain and spinal
cord. They are, from without:
the dura mater, the arachnoid, the pia mater.

**meningioma** (*me-nin-jē-ō-ma*).
Tumour derived from the
meninges.

**meningism** (*me-nin-jism*). Syndrome characterized by
symptoms and signs of
meningitis but occurring in
the absence of any causative
organism. Probably a non-
specific inflammatory reac-

tion of the meninges to circulating toxins or some other trauma.

**meningitis** (*me-nin-jī-tis*). Inflammation of the meninges due to infection by organisms. Acute bacterial or viral meningitis is characterized by fever, headache, vomiting, backache and development of a stiff neck. Stupor, coma and convulsions may follow. A more insidious onset is sometimes seen in tuberculous meningitis. There may be a rash in meningococcal meningitis in infants.

**meningocele** (*me-nin-jō-sēl*). Protrusion of meninges from a bony defect usually in the spine, *e.g.* spina bifida.

**meningococcus** (*me-nin-jō-ko-kus*). A micro-organism, the cause of cerebrospinal fever.

**meningo-encephalocele** (*me-nin-jō-en-ke-fa-lō-sēl*). A meningocele containing nerve tissue may be classed as meningoencephalocele if it contains brain, or *mening-omyelocele* if it contains spinal cord.

**meniscectomy** (*me-ni-sek-to-mi*). Removal of a semilunar cartilage from the knee joint.

**meniscus** (*me-nis-kus*). (1) A semilunar cartilage. (2) A lens. (3) The crescent-like surface of a liquid in a narrow tube.

**menopause** (*me-nō-pawz*). Cessation of menstruation. Ovulation stops and reproductive life ends. It usually occurs between 40 and 50 years of age and is associated with alterations in hormonal balance which sometimes produce troublesome symptoms such as hot flushes, etc.

**menorrhagia** (*me-no-rā-ji-a*). Excessive menstrual bleeding.

**menses** (*men-sēz*). The menstrual flow.

**menstruation** (*men-stroo-ā-shon*). Monthly discharge of uterine mucosa with resultant bleeding which occurs in the absence of pregnancy in sexually mature females.

**mental** (*men'-tal*) (1) Pertaining to the mind (2) Pertaining to the chin.

**mental defective.** See IDIOCY and classification thereunder.

**mento-anterior** (*men-tō-an-tā-ri-or*). A type of face presentation.

**mento-posterior** (*men-tō-pos-tā-ri-or*). See FACE PRESENTATION.

**meralgia paraesthetica** (*me-ral-ji-a par-ēs-the-ti-ka*). Compression of the lateral cutaneous nerve of the thigh in the groin giving rise to pain and sensory disturbances in the outer aspects of the thigh.

**mesarteritis** (*mes-ar-ter-ī'-tis*). Inflammation of the middle coat of an artery.

**mesencephalon** (*mes-en-ke-fa-lon*). The midbrain.

**mesenchyme** (*me-sen-kīm*). Embryonic connective tissue which forms bone, cartilage, connective tissue and blood, etc.

**mesenteric** (*mes-en-te-rik*). Pertaining to the mesentery.

**mesentery** (*me-sen-te-ri*). A large fold of the peritoneum to which the small intestines are attached.

**mesmerism** (*mez'-mer-izm*). Hypnosis.

**meso-appendix** (*me-sō-a-pen-diks*). The mesentery of the appendix vermiformis.

**mesocolon** (*me-sō-kō-lon*). The fold of the peritoneum attached to the colon.

**mesoderm** (*me-sō-derm*). Germ layer of cells which have migrated from the surface of the developing embryo during gastrulation and which is situated between the ectoderm and the endoderm. The mesoderm gives rise to muscle, blood and connective tissues, etc.

**mesometrium** (*me-sō-mē-tri-um*). The broad ligaments which attach the uterus to the sides of the pelvis.

**mesonephroma** (*mē'-zō-ne-frō'-ma*). Malignant tumour of ovary, whose structure resembles that of renal glomeruli and tubules.

**mesosalpinx** (*me-sō-sal-pinks*). The part of the broad ligament which lies immediately below the Fallopian tubes.

**mesothelium** (*me-sō-thē-li-um*). General term applied to the epithelium lining serous cavities.

**mesovarium** (*me-sō-vār-i-um*). A short peritoneal fold connecting the ovary to the posterior layer of the broad ligament.

**metabolic** (*me-ta-bo-lik*). Pertaining to metabolism.

**metabolic disorders.** Disorders in which there is interference with the normal processing of substances by the body. This includes a very extensive list of conditions including diabetes mellitus, renal failure, hepatic failure, etc. These disorders may be congenital or acquired.

**metabolism** (*me-ta-bo-lism*). Chemical process taking place in living cells which may be divided into constructive or building-up processes (anabolism), and destructive or breaking-down processes (catabolism).

**metabolism, inborn errors of.** Disorders due to an inherited defect in metabolism such as albinism, phenylketonuria, Wilson's disease and mucoviscidosis, etc.

**metacarpals** (*me-ta-kar-pals*). The five bones of the hand joining the fingers to the wrist.

**metacarpophalangeal** (*me-ta-kar-pō-fa-lan-jē-al*). Relating to the metacarpus and phalanges.

**metamorphosis** (*me-ta-mor-fō'-sis*). Transformation.

**metaphase** (*me-ta-fāz*). *See* MITOSIS.

**metaphysis** (*me-ta'-fi-sis*). Part between the shaft, diaphysis, and the end, epiphysis, of the long bones.

**metaplasia** (*me-ta-plā-si-a*). Term applied to the apparent transformation of adult tissues.

**metastasis** (*me-tas'-ta-sis*). Transfer or spreading of a disease from one organ to another which is remote. A malignant growth spreads in this way.

**metatarsalgia** (*met'-a-tar-sal'-ji-a*). Pain in the fore part of the foot.

**metatarsals** (*me-ta-tar-sals*). The five bones of the foot between the tarsus and toes.

**meteorism** (*mē-tē-o-rism*). Distension of the intestines by gas.

**methaemoglobin** (*met-hē-mō-glō-bin*). Haemoglobin which has been altered so that the iron which it contains is in the oxidized state ($Fe^{+++}$). In this state the haemoglobin cannot take up oxygen. The abnormal haemoglobin may be excreted in the urine (methaemoglobinuria).

**methionine** (*me-thē-ō-nin*). A sulphur-containing essential amino-acid. It acts as a donor of methyl ($-CH_3$) groups in reactions known as trans-methylations.

**metra** (*me'-tra*). The womb.

**metre** (*mē'-ter*). A measure of length, containing 100 cm, or 1,000 mm, and equal to 39·370 in.

**metric system** (*me-trik sis-tem*). System of weights and measures employing the metre and the gram as standard units which are multiplied or divided by powers of ten.

**metritis** (*me-trī-tis*). Inflammation of the womb.

**metrocolpocele** (*met-rō-kol'-pō-sēl*). Protrusion of the uterus into the vagina, the wall of the vagina being pushed in advance.

**metropathia haemorrhagica** (*me-trō-pa-thi-a hē-mō-ra'-ji-ka*). Excessive menstrual bleeding due to excess of oestrin and associated with follicular ovarian cysts.

**metroptosis** (*met-rop-tō'-sis*).
Prolapse of the womb.

**metrorrhagia** (*me-tro-rā'-ji-a*).
Bleeding from the uterus,
other than at the menstrual
period. It should always be
investigated as it is usually
due to some pathological
condition.

**microbe** (*mī-krōb*). Micro-
organism. *See* BACTERIA,
VIRUS.

**microbiology** (*mī'-krō-bī-o'-
lo-ji*). Study of micro-
organisms.

**microcephalic** (*mī-krō-ke-fa-
lik*). Having an abnormally
small head.

**micrococci** (*mī-krō-ko-kē*).
Small cocci. *See* BACTERIA.

**microcyte** (*mī-krō-sīt*). A small
red blood cell.

**microcythaemia** (*mī-krō-sī-
tē-mi-a*). Anaemia in which
the red blood cells are
diminished in size as in
iron-deficiency anaemia.
It is usually termed *microcy-
tic anaemia*.

**microglia** (*mī-krō-glē-a*). Certain type of nervous supporting tissue.

**micrognathia** (*mī-krō-na-thi-a*).
Abnormally small jaw due to
defective development of the
mandible. Occasionally it is
associated with congenital
laryngeal stridor due to lack
of tone in the aryteno-
epiglottic folds.

**microgram** (*mī-krō-gram*). µg.
One millionth part of a gram.

**micrometer** (*mī-kro'-me-ter*).
Instrument for measuring
very small distances.

**micrometre** (*mī-kro-mē-ter*).
µm. A millionth part of a
metre.

**micro-organism** (*mī-krō-or-
ga-nism*). Any microscopic
plant or animal.

**microphthalmos** (*mī-krof-
thal'mos*). Abnormal small-
ness of the eyes.

**microscope** (*mī-kro-scōp*). An
instrument which magnifies
minute objects invisible to
the naked eye.

**microsomes** (*mī-krō-sōmes*).
These are the broken-up
fragments of intracellular
membranes, *see* CELL. When
a tissue is homogenized and
the resultant material separated by density gradient
centrifugation a$_t$ number of
fractions can be isolated, *e.g.*
the fraction containing
mitochondria, the fraction
containing lysosomes, etc.
One of these fractions contains remnants of membranes
and is called the microsomal
fraction.

**microsporon** (*mī-krō-spo-ron*).
Genus of fungi some species
of which are parasitic to man.
They are able to digest keratin and thus live in the hair
and on the skin surface.

**microtome** (*mī-krŏ-tōm*). An instrument for cutting fine sections for microscopic examination.

**micturiton** (*mik-tū-rish'-on*). The act of passing urine.

**midbrain** (*mid-brān*). Small part of the brain between the forebrain and hindbrain.

**midriff** (*mid'-rif*). The diaphragm.

**midwife** (*mid'-wīf*). A woman who is trained to conduct confinements.

**midwifery** (*mid'-wif-ri*). The art and science of the conduct of pregnancy, labour and the puerperium.

**migraine** (*mē-grān'*). Paroxysmal attacks of headache, usually with nausea and often preceded by disorders of vision. Migraine is usually unilateral.

**Mikulicz's disease** (*mi-kū-liks di-sēz*). A syndrome consisting of the following triad: symmetrical enlargement both of the salivary glands, and the lacrimal glands with narrowing of the palpebral fissures. Also parchment-like dryness of the mouth. The cause is unknown.

**miliaria** (*mi-li-ār-i-a*). Prickly heat. Due to obstruction to the ducts of the sweat glands.

**miliary** (*mi-li-a-ri*). Like millet seed. Thus *miliary tuberculosis* is an acute form of infection in which the tissues are studded with small tubercles so as to resemble a mass of millet seeds.

**milium** (*mi-li-um*). Small white lumps in the skin. Frequently on the eyelids.

**milk.** The secretion of mammary glands. The average composition is:

| Protein: | Human Milk % | Cow's Milk % |
|---|---|---|
| Lactalbumin | 1·4 }2 | 0·75 }4 |
| Casein | 0·6 | 3·25 |
| Fat | 4·0 | 4·0 |
| Carbohydrate | 6·0 | 4·0 |
| Salt | 0·2 | 0·7 |
| Water | 87·8 | 87·3 |

Human milk is neutral or slightly alkaline. Cow's milk is usually slightly acid by the time it reaches the consumer. Specific gravity 1·026 to 1·036.

**milk teeth.** Primary dentition. *See* TEETH.

**Miller-Abbott tube.** A double-bore rubber tube which is passed via the mouth into the duodenum so that intestinal suction can be applied in obstruction of the upper intestinal tract.

**milliampère** (*mil-i-ahm-pār*). One thousandth part of an ampère.

**millicurie** (*mi-li-kū-ri*). Unit of

radioactivity, one thousandth of a curie (mCi).

**milligram** (*mil'-i-gram*). One thousandth part of a gram.

**millilitre** (*mil-i-lē-tr*). One thousandth part of a litre. Abbr. ml. It is almost equivalent to a cc.

**millimetre** (*mil-i-mē-tr*). One thousandth part of a metre.

**Millin's prostatectomy** (*mil-lins pro-sta-tek-to-mi*). In this operation the bladder is not incised but the prostate gland is enucleated from around the neck of the bladder. Also called retro-pubic prostatectomy.

**Milroy's disease.** Lymphangiectasis of the lymphatics of a limb. A pathological dilatation of the lymphatic vessels usually as a result of defective development.

**miner's anaemia.** *See* ANKYLOSTOMA DUODENALE.

**miner's nystagmus** (*mī-ners nis-tag-mus*). Nystagmus due to insufficient light striking the retina. The eye compensates by moving so that the maximum number of rods, (*see diagram of* EYE), are exposed to the light, a process akin to the method of seeing faint stars by not looking directly at them since the macula lutea has more cones and fewer rods than the retina. Cones are less sensitive to light than rods but are essential for colour vision. Miner's nystagmus occurs in partial blindness due to disease of the eye.

**miosis** (*mī-ō-sis*). *See* MEIOSIS.

**miscarriage** (*mis-ka'-rāj*). *See* ABORTION.

**misce** (*mis'-kā*). A direction on a prescription.

**missed abortion** (*ab-or'-shon*). *See* ABORTION.

**mitochondria** (*mī-tō-kon-dri-a*). Small membranous bodies which occur in the cell cytoplasm. They have a complex internal structure of folded membranes and harbour a great number of enzymes, particularly those connected with oxidative metabolism and the production of energy.

**mitosis** (*mī-tō-sis*). The usual process of nuclear division which occurs when a cell divides, *cf.* meiosis. Before division the cell reduplicates its chromosomes by synthesizing DNA chains complementary to those contained in the cell, *see* DEOXYRIBONUCLEIC ACID. This process takes place during the so-called *interphase*. The phases of nuclear division are *prophase*, *metaphase*, *anaphase* and *telophase*. *See also* Figs., pp. 227 and 228.

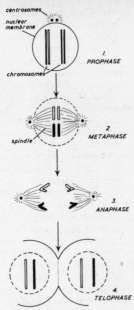

centrosomes

nuclear membrane

chromosomes

*1. PROPHASE*

spindle

*2. METAPHASE*

*3. ANAPHASE*

*4. TELOPHASE*

36. *Stages of mitosis*

**mitral valve** (*mī-tral valv*). Valve of the heart between the left atrium and the left ventricle. Disease of this valve may give rise to *mitral stenosis* when there is narrowing of the orifice of the valve or *mitral regurgitation* or *incompetence* when the valve fails to close properly.

**mittelschmerz** (*mi-tel-shmärz*) Pain occurring at the time of ovulation which may be associated with a slight loss of blood vaginally.

**MNS blood group system.** Groups are characterized by possession of one or both antigens M and N. In English population 28 per cent possess M, 22 per cent N, 50 per cent M and N. 55 per cent have antigen S, usually in association with M.

**modiolus** (*mō-di-ō'-lus*). Central axis of the cochlea.

**molality** (*mō-la'-li-ti*). Solution strength expressed as the number of moles of solute to 1 kg of solvent.

**molar teeth** (*mō-lar tēth*). The grinding teeth. *See* DENTAL FORMULA.

**molarity** (*mō-la'-ri-ti*). Solution strength expressed as the number of moles of solute dissolved per litre of solution.

**mole** (*mōl*). (1) Hairy, pigmented raised area of skin. (2) In obstetric practice, a tumour composed of coagulated blood, fetal membranes and the embryo; due to haemorrhage into a gestation sac, and followed sooner or later by abortion. *Carneous* or *fleshy m.* When mole is retained in utero for some time, the fluid part of the blood-clot becomes absorbed, leaving solid fleshy masses, in the midst of which traces of the embryo may or may not be found. *Hydatidiform or vesicular m.* Degeneration of the chorion in the early weeks of pregnancy, resulting in the death of the embryo and the conversion of the chorionic villi into beadlike cysts or vesicles which may attain the size of a grape. Two prominent symptoms are: (*a*) undue enlargement of the uterus for the period of amenorrhoea, (*b*) a watery pink discharge which may contain vesicles. No fetal parts are felt and no fetal heart heard, and the uterus feels softer than in a normal pregnancy. As soon as diagnosed the uterus should be emptied. The villi may become malignant, and invade the wall of the uterus. It is then known as *chorion epithelioma*. (3) The molecular weight of a substance in grams.

**molecule** (*mol'-e-kūl*). A combination of atoms forming a definite substance. Thus one atom of sodium with one atom of chlorine forms one molecule of sodium chloride.

**molluscum contagiosum** (*mo-lus-kum kon-ta-ji-ō-sum*). A virus disease affecting the skin.

**Mönckeberg's arteriosclerosis** (*mern-ke-bergs ar-tā-ri-ō-skle-rō'-sis*). Sclerosis of the medium and small arteries with extensive degeneration of the middle muscle lining, with atrophy and calcareous deposits in the muscle cells.

**mongolism** (*mon'-go-lism*). Down's syndrome. Due to chromosomal abnormalities occurring during meiosis. A chromosome pair fails to separate (non-disjunction) with the result that the child has a chromosome too many, *i.e.* 47 instead of 46. The syndrome is characterized by slanting eyes, short head, hypotonia and mental deficiency. Another variety of mongolism may be inherited and is due to translocation of a chromosome.

**Monilia** (*mo-ni-li-a*). See THRUSH.

**monitoring** (*mo'-ni-tor-ing*). Automatic recording of physiological functions, *e.g.* pulse, blood pressure.

**mono-amine oxidase inhibitors** (*mo-nō-ā'-mēn ok'-si-dāz in-hi'-bi-terz*). Drugs stimulating nervous system by inhibiting mono-amine oxidases and causing pressor amines to accumulate in brain tissue. If foods containing these (*e.g.* cheese, yeast extract) are taken concurrently, reaction may be severe or even fatal.

**monocular** (*mo-nok'-ū-lar*). Relating to one eye only.

**monocytes** (*mo-nō-sīts*). Largest white cells found in the blood. They are macrophages of the reticuloendothelial system.

**monocytosis** (*mo-nō-sī-tō-sis*). Term employed when moncytes comprise more than 8 per cent of the total white cell count.

**monograph** (*mon'-ō-graf*). Book on one subject only.

**monomania** (*mon-ō-mā'-ni-a*). A neurosis when the patient has fixed ideas on one particular subject.

**mononeuritis multiplex** (*mo-nō-nū-rī-tis mul-ti-pleks*). Rare form of peripheral neuritis in which there is selective involvement of isolated nerves.

**mononuclear** (*mo-nō-nū-klē-a*). With one nucleus.

**monoplegia** (*mon-ō-plē'-ji-a*). Paralysis of one limb.

**monorchid, monorchis** (*mon-or'-kid*). Having only one testicle.

**monosaccharides** (*mo-nō-sa-ka-rīds*). Simplest sugars, *e.g.* glucose.

**Monro's foramen** (*mun-rōz fo-rā-men*). Interventricular foramen. The communication between the two lateral ventricles and the third ventricle of the brain.

**mons veneris** (*monz ven'-e-ris*). The eminence just over the os pubis in women.

**Montgomery's follicles** (*munt-gum'-er-ēz fol'-ikls*). Small prominences about the nipple, which become more evident during pregnancy and lactation. *See also* AREOLA.

**Mooren's ulcer** (*moo-renz ul-ser*). Basal cell carcinoma affecting the cornea.

**morbid** (*mor'-bid*). Diseased, disordered, pathological.

**morbilli** (*mor-bi-lē*). Measles.

**morbus** (*mor'-bus*). Latin for disease.

**Morgagni, hydatids of** (*maw-ga-nyi, hi-da-tids*). Small translucent cysts arising from the embryonic pronephros which occur attached by pedicles to the fimbriated end of the Fallopian tubes.

**morgue** (*mawg*). A public mortuary.

**moribund** (*mo'-ri-bund*). In a dying state.

**morning sickness.** *See* VOMITING OF PREGNANCY.

**morphine** (*maw-fēn*). An alkaloid obtained from opium, used as a sedative or anodyne.

**morphoea** (*maw-fē-a*). Scleroderma affecting the skin only. Patches of atrophic, depigmented skin overlie connective tissue which has lost its elasticity.

**morphology** (*mor-fo-lo-ji*). The study of shape and structure of living organisms.

**mortality** (*maw-ta'-li-ti*). Death rate. The annual death rate in this country is the number of registered deaths × 1,000 divided by the mid-year population. The *infant m. rate* is the number of deaths of infants under 1 year × 1,000 divided by the number of registered live births. The *maternal m. rate* is the number of deaths of women ascribed to pregnancy or childbearing × 1,000 divided by the number of registered live and still-births.

**mortuary** (*mor'-tū-a-ri*). A place where dead bodies are kept.

**morula** (*mo'-rū-la*). Early stage in development of fertilized ovum.

**mosaic** (*mo-zā-ik*). In genetics a term applied to individuals made up of cells of different genetic constitution.

**motile** (*mō'-tīl*). Able to move independently.

**motions** (*mō'-shons*). The evacuations of the bowels. *See* FAECES.

**motor end-plate** (*mō-ter*). An accumulation of nuclei and cytoplasm of muscle fibres at the termination of motor nerves.

**motor nerves.** Nerves carrying motor neuron fibres. Motor neurons carry impulses from the central nervous system to the effector organ, *cf.* sensory nerves.

**motor neurone disease.** Disease of unknown cause characterized by the degeneration of the anterior horn cells of the spinal cord, the motor nuclei of the cranial nerves and corticospinal tracts.

**motor root.** The ventral root of the spinal cord, *cf.* dorsal root.

**mould** (*mōld*). See FUNGI.

**moulding** (*mōl'-ding*). The alteration in shape of the infant's head produced by the pressure it is subjected to whilst being driven through the birth canal.

**mountain sickness** (*mown-tān sik-nes*). Disorder resulting from lack of oxygen at high altitudes.

**movements** (fetal) (*moov-mentz*). See QUICKENING.

**moving beam radiotherapy.** Technique employed to increase the dose incident on the target tissue while reducing the skin dose by rotating the beam in an arc with its centre in the target.

**mucilage** (*mū'-si-lāj*). Aqueous solutions of gums or starch.

**mucin** (*mūsin*). Term loosely used for mucopolysaccharide and protein compounds (mucoprotein).

**mucocele** (*mū'-kō-sēl*). A cyst distended with mucus, as of the gall bladder or lacrimal sac.

**mucoid** (*mū'-koyd*). Resembling mucus.

**mucolytic** (*mū-kō-li'-tik*). Substance which reduces the viscosity of mucus.

**mucopurulent** (*mū-kō-pu-roo-lent*). With mucus and pus.

**mucosa** (*mū-kō'-za*). A mucous membrane.

**mucous membrane** (*mū-kus mem-brān*). A surface which secretes mucus. The lining of the alimentary canal, air passages, and urinogenital organs: merges into true skin at the various orifices of these canals.

**mucous polypus** (*mū-kus po-li-pus*). A small outgrowth from the mucous surface of the cervix uteri or of the nose.

**mucoviscidosis** (*mū-ko-vis-ki-dō-sis*). Fibrocystic disease of the pancreas. A recessively inherited disorder of salt secretion in which there is an inability of secreting glands to reabsorb sodium. As a result the mucous secretions are extremely viscous and obstruction of the ducts of glands results with consequent dilatation, stasis, infection and fibrosis. The extent of the involvement by the disease is variable but usually affects the pancreas and lungs.

**mucus** (*mū-kus*). Viscous fluid containing muco-protein, *see* MUCIN. It is secreted by special mucus-producing cells in mucous epithelia.

**multigravida** (*mul-ti-gra'-vi-da*). Pregnant woman who has previously had two or more pregnancies.

**multilocular** (*mul-ti-lo-kū-la*). Having many locules.

**multipara** (*mul-tip'-a-ra*). A woman who has had more than one child.

**multiple myeloma** (*mul-ti-pl mī-e-lō-ma*). Neoplasm of plasma cells which infiltrate and replace the bone marrow. Characteristic features are anaemia, bone pains and large quantities of circulating globulins of an abnormal type which may be excreted in the urine. *See* BENCE JONES PROTEIN.

**multiple pregnancy** (*mul-ti-pl preg'-nan-si*). Twins, triplets, or any larger number of fetuses gestated together by one mother.

**multiple sclerosis.** *See* DISSEMINATED SCLEROSIS.

**mumps.** Acute virus-mediated parotitis. Occasionally the

testes or ovaries ,may be involved.

**murmur** (*mer-mer*). Abnormal sound on auscultation of heart. *See* HEART SOUNDS.

**Murphy's sign** (*mer-fis sīn*). If continuous pressure is exerted over an inflamed gall bladder while the patient takes a deep breath, it causes him to 'catch' the breath just before the zenith of inspiration.

**muscae volitantes** (*mus-kē vo-li-tan'-tēs*). Spots or filaments which float in the vitreous humour of the eye and which are visible to the patient.

**muscle** (*mus'-sl*). Specialized tissue composed of highly contractile cells. There are three varieties of muscle in the body: (1) Striated, voluntary muscle. (2) Smooth, involuntary, and (3) Cardiac muscle. *M. atrophy, peroneal.* Charcot-Marie-Tooth disease. An inherited condition in which there is degeneration of the anterior horn cells of the peroneal nerves. *M. dystrophy.* A group of conditions also known as myopathies in which there is degeneration of groups of muscles without apparent nerve involvement.

**musculospiral nerve** (*mus-kū-lō-spī-ral nerv*). A nerve of the arm.

**mutant** (*mū-tant*). A gene which has undergone a mutation, or an individual possessing characteristics due to such a gene.

**mutation** (*mū-tā-shon*). Relatively permanent alteration in the coding of part of the chromosomal deoxyribonucleic acid. These alterations are infrequent and occur at random but their frequency can be greatly increased by radiation. Mutations occurring in gametes, *i.e.* spermatozoa or ova, or their precursors are important since they may produce an inherited change in the characteristics of the individual developing from them, *see* MUTANT. Mutations in a body cell (somatic mutations) are transmitted to the clone of cells to which it gives rise.

**mute** (*mūt*). Without the power of speech. Dumb.

**myalgia** (*mī-al-ji-a*). Pain in the muscles.

**myalgia, epidemic** (*mī-al-ji-a e-pi-de-mik*). Bornholm disease. Characterized by sudden onset of fever and intercostal or diaphragmatic pain. It is thought to be caused by a virus.

**myasthenia** (*mī-as-thē-ni-a*). Debility of the muscles.

**myasthenia gravis** (*mī-as-thē-*

*ni-a gra'-vis*). Disorder characterized by abnormal fatigue of striated muscle (*see* MUSCLE), with rapid recovery after rest. The cause is not known but appears to be some form of biochemical disturbance affecting the transmission of the impulse from the nerve-ending to the motor end-plate. A striking improvement in muscle power follows the administration of neostigmine. Occasionally myasthenia gravis is associated with hyperplasia of the thymus.

**myatonia** (*mī-a-tō'-ni-a*). Lack of muscle tone.

**mycelium** (*mī-sē-li-um*). The filaments of fungus forming an interwoven mass.

**mycetoma** (*mī-se-tō'-ma*). Also known as Madura foot. A tropical disease due to infection with a vegetable parasite akin to that of actinomycosis. The part affected, most commonly the foot, becomes the seat of chronic inflammatory swelling with formation of ulcers and sinuses.

**Mycobacterium** (*mī-kō-bak-tā-rē-um*). A genus of bacteria. *M. leprae* causes leprosy and *M. tuberculosis*, tuberculosis.

**mycosis** (*mī-kō-sis*). Disease caused by a fungus.

**mydriasis** (*mid-rī'-a-sis*). Increase in the size of the pupil of the eye.

**mydriatics** (*mi-dri-a-tiks*). Drugs which dilate the pupil of the eye, *e.g.* atropine, homatropine.

**myelin** (*mī-e-lin*). Phospholipid–protein complex which invests the larger nerve fibres. It is produced by Schwann cells which appear to wrap coils of their cell membrane round the fibres. The coils condense to form myelin.

**myelitis** (*mī-e-lī'-tis*). Inflammation of the spinal cord.

**myelocele** (*mī-e-lō-sēl*). *See* MENINGO-MYELOCELE.

**myelocyte** (*mī-e'-lō-sīt*). Bone marrow cell.

**myelogram** (*mī-e-lō-gram*). Radiograph of the spinal cord.

**myeloid** (*mī'-e-loyd*). Like marrow. *M. tissue*. Tissue giving rise to the cellular elements of the blood, *viz.* red cells, white cells and platelets.

**myeloma** (*mī-e-lō-ma*). Neoplasm of plasma cells, *see* PLASMA.

**myelomatosis** (*mī-e-lō-ma-tō'-sis*). Multiple myeloma.

**myelopathy** (*mī-e-lo-pa-thi*). Any neurological disorder arising from disease of the spinal cord.

**myelosclerosis** (*mī-e-lō-skle-rō'-sis*). Replacement of bone marrow by fibrous tissue.

**myocardial** (*mī-ō-kar'-di-al*). Pertaining to the muscle of the heart.

**myocarditis** (*mī-ō-kar-dī'-tis*). Inflammation of the myocardium.

**myocardium** (*mī-ō-kar'-di-um*). The heart muscle.

**myofibrils** (*mī-ō-fīb'-rilz*). Thread-like structures bound together to form muscle fibres, probably essential contractile elements of muscle.

**myogenic** (*mī-ō-je'-nik*). Originating from muscular tissue.

**myoglobin** (*mī-ō-glō-bin*). A specialized haemoglobin found in muscle which has slightly different dissociation characteristics from that in the blood so that oxygen is transferred from the blood to the muscle.

**myoma** (*mī-ō'-ma*). Any tumour composed of muscular tissue.

**myomectomy** (*mī-ō-mek'-to-mi*). Removal of a myoma; usually referring to a fibroid from the uterus.

**myometrium** (*mī-ō-mēt'-ri-um*). Uterine muscle.

**myopathy** (*mi-o-pa-thi*). Any primary disease of muscle.

**myope** (*mī-ōp*). A shortsighted person. *Myopic*, pertaining to shortsightedness.

**myopia** (*mī-ō-pi-a*). Short-sightedness; corrected by wearing a biconcave lens.

**myosarcoma** (*mī-ō-sar-kō'-ma*). A malignant tumour of muscle.

**myosin** (*mī-ō-sin*). Muscle-protein, part of the actomyosin complex.

**myosis** (*mī-ō'-sis*). Contraction of the pupil of the eye.

**myositis** (*mī-ō-sī'-tis*). Inflammation of a muscle. *M. ossificans*. May follow stretching of an injured muscle. Its fibres and haematoma are replaced by cancellous bone. The condition can be prevented by resting the injured muscle.

**myotics** (*mī-o-tiks*). Drugs which cause the pupil to contract, *e.g.* eserine.

**myotomy** (*mī-o-to-mi*). Cutting through a muscle.

**myotonia** (*mī-ō-tō-ni-a*). Tonic muscular spasm. *M. atrophica* or *dystrophica*. A hereditary disorder characterized by wasting of the muscles of the face, neck and limbs associated with cataract, frontal baldness in men and gonadal atrophy. *M. congenita*. Thomsen's disease. A dominantly inherited disorder in which the only symptom is the slow relaxation of muscles after contraction which makes it difficult, for example, for the patient to relax his grasp.

**myringa** (*mi-rin-ga*). The tympanic membrane of the ear.

**myringitis** (*mi-rin-jī-tis*). Inflammation of the tympanic membrane of the ear.

**myringotomy** (*mi-rin-go-to-mi*). Incision of the tympanic membrane of the ear, performed when the presence of pus is suspected in the middle ear.

**myxoedema** (*mik-se-dē-ma*). Syndrome due to hypothyroidism and characterized by dry atrophic skin, swelling of the limbs and face and retardation both physical and mental. The metabolic rate is diminished and the patient dislikes the cold intensely. There is usually loss of hair in the frontal and pubic regions and the outer third of the eyebrows.

**myxoma** (*mik-sō-ma*). Tumour of connective tissue containing mucoid material.

**myxosarcoma** (*mik-sō-sar-kō'-ma*). A malignant myxoma.

# N

**Naboth's follicles** (*nah'-bōts fo'-li-kels*). Small cystic bodies resulting from infection of Naboth's glands.

**Naboth's glands.** Small glandular bodies situated in the neck of the uterus.

**NAD.** Nothing abnormal diagnosed.

**Naegele's obliquity** (*nā'-gēl-e*). Tilting of the fetal head towards one or other shoulder as it enters the brim of the pelvis; by this attitude a slightly smaller transverse diameter of the head is presented to the brim.

**naevus** (*nē-vus*). Latin for mole. Usually applied to *cellular n.*, a small skin lesion resulting from the proliferation of naevus cells which are thought to be related to melanocytes, *see* MELANOMA. Naevus is also a general term for congenital skin lesions, *i.e.* birth marks, resulting from abnormalities in the development of superficial blood vessels, lymphatics, etc.

**nail** (*nāl*). Horny plate found at the tip of finger or toe.

**nape.** Back of the neck.

**napkin rash.** Rash in the napkin area due to irritation of the skin by ammonia produced by bacteria which ferment the urea in the urine.

**narcissism** (*nar-si'-sizm*). An abnormal love of oneself: named after Narcissus, who fell in love with his own reflection.

**narco-analysis** (*nar-ko-a-na'-li-sis*). Psycho-analysis practised with the patient in a state of basal narcosis. Founded on the principle that the unconscious (subconscious) thoughts are less likely to be suppressed if the patient is rendered drowsy.

**narcolepsy** (*nar-ko'-lep'-si*). A condition characterized by sudden attacks of sleep occurring repeatedly during the day.

**narcosis** (*nar-kō'-sis*). A state of unconsciousness produced by the use of narcotics.

**narcotic** (*nar-ko'-tik*). A drug which produces unconsciousness, *e.g.* paraldehyde, the barbiturates.

**nares** (*na'-rēz*). The nostrils.

**nasal** (*nā'-sal*). Relating to the nose.

**nascent** (*nās'-sent*). At the moment of birth.

**nasogastric tube** (*na'-zō-gas-trik tūb*). Tube passing through the nose to the stomach.

**nasolacrimal** (*nā-zō-la'-kri-mal*). Relating to the nose and lacrimal apparatus.

**nasopharyngeal** (*nā'sō-far-in-je'-al*). Pertaining to the nasopharynx.

**nasopharynx** (*nā'-zō-fa'-rinks*). The space between the posterior nares, the base of the skull, the soft palate, the upper end of the oesophagus, and the epiglottis.

**nates** (*nā'-tēz*). The buttocks.

**natural childbirth.** A school of opinion concerning childbirth which advocates the minimum of medical interference with the process of delivery. Childbirth is considered to be a normal physiological process and training in relaxation is given during pregnancy.

**nausea** (*naw'-sē-a*). A feeling of sickness.

**navel** (*nā'-vel*). The umbilicus, the point of connection of the umbilical cord.

**navicular** (*na-vi-kū-la*). The boat-shaped tarsal bone.

**nebula** (*ne'-bū-la*). A cloud or mist. Term applied to filmy corneal opacities.

**nebulizer** (*ne'-bū-li-zer*). *See* ATOMIZER.

**neck** (*nek*). Narrow part near the end of an organ. *Derbyshire n.* Goitre. *Wry n.* torticollis.

**necrobiosis** (*ne-krō-bī-ō'-sis*). Death of tissue. *Red n.* A type of degeneration occurring in a fibroid of the uterus if pregnancy takes place. After labour, the fibroid can recover its vitality.

**necropsy** (*ne-crop'-si*). Examination of a body after death.

**necrosis** (*ne-krō'-sis*). Death of tissue.

**necrotic** (*ne-kro'-tik*). Relating to necrosis.

**needle-holder.** Spring-loaded forceps for holding surgical needles.

**needling.** Perforation with a needle especially in cataract. *See* DISCISSION.

**negativism** (*ne'-ga-ti-vizm*). A state of mind in which the ideas and behaviour of an individual are in opposition to those of the majority and contrary to suggestion.

**Neisseria** (*nī-se-ri-a*). Genus of diplococci. *N. gonorrhoeae* causes gonorrhoea; *N. meningitidis* causes epidemic cerebrospinal meningitis.

**Nelaton's line** (*ne-la-tons*). Line from the anterior superior iliac spine to the tuberosity of the ischium.

**nematodes** (*ne-ma-tōds*). Worms including round-worms, threadworms and eelworms. Some of these are parasitic to man, *e.g.* hookworm.

**neoarthrosis** (*nē-ō-ar-thrō-sis*). A new joint.

**neocortex** (*nē'-ō-kor'-teks*). Cerebral cortex excluding hippocampal formation and piriform area.

**neonatal** (*nē-ō-nā-tal*). Relating to the first four weeks of life.

**neonate** (*nē'-ō-nāt*). Newborn infant in the first month of life.

**neoplasm** (*nē-ōplasm*). A tumour. An abnormal local multiplication of some type of cell. A neoplasm may be either *benign* if it shows no tendency to spread, or *malignant* if the growing cells infiltrate surrounding tissues and invade other parts of the body.

**nephrectomy** (*ne-frek-to-mi*). Removal of kidney.

**nephritis** (*ne-frī'-tis*). Inflammation of the kidney. The term nephritis is used to describe a large number of widely differing conditions affecting the kidney largely because of the unsatisfactory nature of most classifications of renal disease. The classification given here should be taken only as an explanatory guide: (1) *Localized renal inflammation*. (*a*) *Pyelonephritis*. Infection arising usually from the urinary tract and characterized by the presence of pus and pathogenic organisms in the urine. One or both kidneys may be involved. (*b*) *Focal nephritis*. Usually a stage in a renal infection (often chronic) characterized by haematuria. The infection is blood-borne, *e.g.* bacterial endocarditis. (2) *Diffuse, non-suppurative, bilateral renal disease* is responsible for three broad renal syndromes: (*a*) *Acute nephritis* characterized by facial oedema, oliguria, haematuria, proteinuria and hypertension. The most common cause of this syndrome is acute glomerular nephritis (*Type I nephritis*). (*b*) *Nephrotic syndrome*. (*c*) *Chronic renal failure*. The end result of a great number of widely different diseases affecting the kidneys.

**nephro** (*ne-frō*). Pertaining to the kidney.

**nephroblastoma** (*ne-frō-blastō'-ma*). Wilms's tumour. A neoplasm of the kidney which occurs in children.

**nephrocalcinosis** (*ne-frō-kalsi-nō'-sis*). A complication of hyperparathyroidism in which calcium becomes deposited in the renal tubules.

**nephrocapsulectomy** (*nef'-rōkap-sū-lek'-to-mi*). Operation to remove the kidney capsule.

**nephrolithiasis** (*ne-frō-li-thī-a-sis*). Stone in the kidney.

**nephrolithotomy** (*ne-frō-litho'-to-mi*). Removal of a stone from the interior of the kidney.

**nephroma** (*ne-frō'-ma*). Tumour of the kidney.

**nephron** (*ne-fron*). The basic unit of the kidney. Each kidney contains about a million nephrons but not all of these are working at any one time. Each nephron consists of a filtering mechanism (the glomerulus) and a long tubule which is specialized in various regions to reabsorb substances from the urine which pass through it. The modified filtrate of the blood plasma which is thus produced is collected in the renal pelvis and leaves the kidney in the ureter.

**nephropexy** (*ne-frō-pek'-si*). Stitching a movable kidney into a firm position.

**nephroptosis** (*nef'-rop-tō-sis*). Downward displacement of the kidney.

**nephrosis** (*ne-frō'-sis*). A term originally introduced to describe a group of patients with nephrotic syndrome in whom the lesion was thought to be in the tubules. Since then it has undergone several changes of meaning. In present usage it is applied to cases of nephrotic syndrome in which there is no obvious renal lesion and which respond well to steroid treatment.

**nephrostomy** (*ne-fros'-to-mi*). Surgical opening into the kidney to drain it.

**nephrotic syndrome** (*nef-ro-tik sin'-drōm*). A syndrome characterized by proteinuria, hypoproteinaemia and oedema. There are many causes of this condition including subacute glomerular nephritis (*Type II nephritis*), diabetic nephropathy, amyloid disease, systemic lupus erythematosus, poisons, *e.g.* mercury, thrombosis of the renal veins and nephrosis.

**nephrotomy** (*nef-ro-to-mi*). Cutting into the kidney.

**nephro-ureterectomy** (*nef'-rō-ū-rē'-te-rek-to-mi*). Excision of kidney and ureter.

**nerve** (*nerv*). A bundle of fibres, conveying the impulses of movement and sensation to and from the organs. *See* MOTOR NERVES, SENSORY NERVES, VASOMOTOR.

**nerve root.** Each spinal nerve arises from the spinal cord by two roots. The dorsal root carries the sensory fibres and the ventral root the motor fibres.

**nervous** (*ner-vus*). Pertaining to the nerves.

**nervous system.** *See* CENTRAL NERVOUS SYSTEM.

**n. et m., nmque.** *Nocte et mane*, *nocte maneque*, night and morning.

**nettle rash.** Urticaria.

**Neufeld reaction** (*noy'-feld rē-ak'-shon*). Capsular swelling of pneumococci visible microscopically if suspension of live organisms is mixed with serum homologous for the type. Used to identify serological types of pneumococci.

**neural** (*nū-ral*). Relating to nerves.

**neuralgia** (*nū-ral'-ji-a*). Pain in the distribution of a nerve, *e.g. trigeminal neuralgia*. Severe pain in the distribution of the trigeminal nerve (*see* CRANIAL NERVES 5). *Sciatica* is neuralgia of the sciatic nerve distribution. The cause may be irritation of the nerve by some bony structure or a tumour but frequently the cause cannot be ascertained. For intractable pain interruption of the sensory fibres of the nerve is often helpful.

**neurapraxia** (*nū-rā-prak'-si-a*). There is a temporary block to nerve conduction as after giving a local anaesthetic.

**neurasthenia** (*nū-ras-thē-ni-a*). Nervous exhaustion.

**neurectomy** (*nū-rek-to-mi*). Excision of part of a nerve.

**neurilemma** (*nu-ri-le-ma*). The sheath of a nerve fibre.

**neurinoma** (*nū-ri-nō-ma*). Tumour of neurilemma.

**neuritis** (*nū-rī-tis*). Inflammation of a nerve.

**neuroblast** (*nū-rō-blast*). Embryonic nerve cell.

**neuroblastoma** (*nū-rō-blas-tō-ma*). Malignant growth of sympathetic nerve ganglia, esp. adrenal medulla. Strictly a tumour of neuroblasts.

**neurodermatitis** (*nū-rō-der-ma-tī-tis*). *See* LICHENIFICATION.

**neuroepithelium** (*nū-rō-e-pi-thē-li-um*). Specialized nerve epithelium, *e.g.* the retina, which consists of nerve endings, rod and cone-shaped cells of the optic nerve.

**neurofibroma** (*nū-rō-fī-brō-ma*). Tumour arising from connective tissue surrounding peripheral nerves.

**neurofibromatosis** (*nū-rō-fī-brō-ma-tō'-sis*). Von Recklinghausen's disease. Generalized distribution within the body of neurofibromas.

**neuroglia** (*nū-rog-li-a*). Connective tissue cells of the central nervous system are collectively known as *glia*. Neuroglia are cells with long fibrous processes which are derived from embryonic nervous tissue and are closely related to Schwann cells. Their exact supportive function is not known. *Microglia* are similar to macrophages.

**neuroleptic** (*nū-ro-lep'-tik*). Drug affecting nervous system.

**neurologist** (*nū-ro-lo-jist*). Physician who specializes in neurology.

**neurology** (*nū-ro'-lo-jī*). Study of diseases of the nervous system.

**neuroma** (*nū-rō'-ma*). A tumour composed of nerve tissue.

**neuromuscular junction** (*nū-rō-mus-kū-la junk-shon*). The junction between a motor nerve and the effector muscle. *See* MOTOR ENDPLATE.

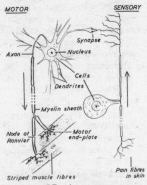

37. A neuron

**neuron** (*nū-ron*). Nerve cell which conducts the nerve impulses. It consists of a cell body from which extend collecting branches (dendrites) and a long process (axon) along which the impulse passes to the effector organ or to other nerves. Such a typical arrangement is shown in the diagram, although, of course, nerve cells take on differing shapes according to their connectivity. Connections between nerves, and between nerves and effector organs are through synapses.

**neuropathic** (*nū-ro-pa'-thik*). Relating to neuropathy.

**neuropathy** (*nu-ro'-pa-thi*). A disorder affecting the structure and function of the nervous system, esp. applied to the peripheral nervous system.

**neuroplasty** (*nū-ro-plas'-ti*). Operative repair of a nerve.

**neurorrhaphy** (*nū-ro'-ra-fi*). Operation to suture a severed nerve.

**neurosis** (*nū-rō-sis*). A disorder of mental function whereby patients are abnormally emotionally vulnerable but retain appreciation of external reality, *cf.* psychosis. Neuroses include behaviour disorders such as hysterical and obsessive compulsive reactions and disturbances of 'affect', as, for example, in anxiety states.

**neurosurgery** (*nū-rō'-ser-je-ri*). Surgery of peripheral and central nervous system.

**neurosyphilis** (*nū-rō-si'-fi-lis*).

Involvement of the central nervous system by syphilis.

**neurotic** (*nū-ro-tik*). Relating to a neurosis.

**neurotmesis** (*nū-rō-tmē-sis*). The nerve trunk is severed and there can be no useful recovery without surgery.

**neurotomy** (*nū-ro-to-mi*). Division of a nerve.

**neurotripsy** (*nū-ro-trip'-si*). Crushing a nerve.

**neutral** (*nū'-tral*). Neither acid nor alkaline.

**neutropaenia** (*nū-trō-pē-ni-a*). Insufficiency of neutrophil polymorphonuclear leucocytes in the blood.

**neutrophil** (*nū-trō-fil*). Predilection for neutral dyes, *i.e.* not acidophil or basophil. A term used to describe the majority of polymorphonuclear leucocytes which do not demonstrate any characteristically staining granules in their cytoplasm, *cf.* basophil, eosinophil.

**Newcastle disease** (*nū-kah-sel di-sēz*). Highly infectious virus fowl disease, causing acute conjunctivitis in humans.

**nicotine poisoning.** Result of overindulgence in smoking. Cardinal features are the paralysis of autonomic ganglia and constriction of the coronary arteries.

**nicotinic acid** (*ni-ko-ti-nik*

*a-sid*). Pellagra-preventing factor of vitamin B complex.

**nictitation** (*nik-ti-tā-shon*). Involuntary blinking of the eyelids.

**nidation** (*ni-dā-shon*). Implantation.

**Niemann-Pick's disease** (*nē-man-piks*). A lipoid storage disease in which lecithin is deposited. An inherited defect of phospholipid metabolism which leads to widespread deposition of lecithin in the tissues. It is associated with mental retardation.

**night blindness** (*nīt blīnd-nes*). Inability to see in the dark, also called *nyctalopia*. Usually the result of vitamin A deficiency.

**night sweats** (*nīt swets*). Profuse sweating at night characteristic of tuberculosis.

**nigrescent** (*ni-gre-sent*). Growing black.

**nigrites** (*ni-gri-ti-ēs*). Blackness. *N. linguae*, a condition in which the filiform papillae of the tongue are hypertrophied and darkly pigmented.

**nipple** (*ni-pel*). Small eminence in the centre of each breast. *N. shields*. Coverings of glass or india-rubber put on the nipples to protect them when they are sore.

**Nissl's granules** (*ni-sels gra-*

*nūls*). Cytoplasmic organelles visible in the cell body of neurons.

**nit.** The egg of the louse.

**nitrogen** (*ni'-tro-jen*). A colourless inert gas, forming 78 per cent of the atmosphere and acting as a diluent. Nitrogenous foods, *see* PROTEIN. *N. mustard*. Cell-destroying drug, used in the treatment of certain malignant tumours and especially Hodgkin's disease.

**nitrous oxide** (*nīi-trus ok-sīd*). Laughing gas; an anaesthetic.

**nocturia** (*nok-tū-ri-a*). Passing urine at night.

**nocturnal** (*nok-ter-nal*). At night. *N. enuresis*. Bed wetting during sleep.

**nodding spasm.** *See* SPASMUS NUTANS.

**node** (*nōd*). A swelling. *Atrioventricular n.* At the base of the interatrial septum from which impulses pass down the Bundle of His. *Heberden's ns*. Deformity of the terminal joints in the fingers in osteo-arthritis. *Sinuatrial n.* The pace-maker of the heart, found at the opening of the superior vena cava into the right atrium. *N. of Ranvier*. The constriction in the neurilemma of a nerve fibre.

**nodule** (*no-dūl*). A little knob.

**non compos mentis.** Not sound of mind.

**non-viable** (*non-vī-abl*). Unable to survive, especially as to a child of less than 28 weeks' gestation.

**noradrenaline** (*no-ra-dre-na-lin*). Hormone of the adrenal medulla. Raises blood pressure by a general vasoconstriction. Given in shock, etc.

**normal** (*nor-mal*). The average or usual form.

**normoblasts** (*nor-mō-blasts*). Immature nucleated red cells present in bone marrow.

**normocyte** (*nor-mō-sit*). A normally sized erythrocyte.

**nose** (*nōz*). The organ of smell and used for warming, filtering and moistening the air breathed in.

**nosology** (*nō-zo'-lo-ji*). Classification of disease.

**nostalgia** (*nos-tal-ji-a*). Homesickness or yearning for the past.

**nostrils** (*nos-trils*). The anterior apertures of the nose.

**notch.** Indentation.

**notifiable** (*nō-ti-fī-abl*). A term applied to certain cases of disease and other occurrences which must be made known to the Area Medical Officer *e.g.* smallpox, tuberculosis, typhoid fever, dysentery, food poisoning, acute poliomyelitis, diphtheria, measles, whooping cough, etc.

**noxious** (*nok'-shus*). Harmful.

**NPN.** Non-protein nitrogen.

**nucha** (*nu-ker*). The nape, or back of the neck.

**Nuck** (*nuk*). *See* CANAL OF.

**nucleated** (*nū-klē-ā-ted*). With a nucleus.

**nucleic acid** (*nū-kle-ik a-sid*). Long chain of nucleotides. Two major types are found: *deoxyribonucleic acid* (*DNA*) and *ribo-nucleic acid* (*RNA*). DNA is formed from nucleotides the components of which are deoxyribose, phosphoric acid and the four bases adenine, guanine, thymine, cytosine (symbolized A, G, T, C). The chromosomes are composed of a double helix of DNA in which the bases are paired A–T and G–C. The coding of genetic information is considered to occur as triplet combinations of those bases. RNA is composed of ribose, phosphoric acid and the bases adenine, guanine, cytosine and uracil (A, G, C, U). There are several types of RNA: *messenger* RNA which is formed as a chain complementary to DNA and which takes the message to the sites of protein synthesis. *Transfer RNA* transports selected amino-acids to the ribosomes. Other types of RNA also exist.

**nucleolus** (*nū-klē-ō-lus*). A small dense body containing RNA which is situated in the nucleus, *see* CELL. It disappears during mitosis and is thought to represent a condensation of some chromosomal material. Its function continues to remain obscure.

**nucleoprotein** (*nū-kle-ō-prō-tēn*). Compound of nucleic acid and protein, *e.g.* the ribosomes.

**nucleotide** (*nū-klē-ō-tīd*). Compound formed from a pentose sugar, phosphoric acid and a nitrogen-containing base.

**nucleus** (*nū-klē-us*) (pl. **nuclei**). (1) Of cell: the spherical body containing the chromosomes. *See also* CELL, etc. (2) of brain: demarcated mass of cell bodies, *e.g.* basal nuclei.

**nucleus pulposus** (*nū-klē-us pul-pō-sus*). A pulpy mass in the centre of the intervertebral disc.

**nullipara** (*nu-li-pa-ra*). A woman who has never had a child.

**nummulated** (*nu-mū-lā-ted*) or **nummular** (*nu-mū-la*). Coin-shaped.

**nutation** (*nū-tā-shon*). Involuntary nodding of the head.

**nutrient** (*nū-tri-ent*). Nourishing. *N. foramen*, opening in a bone for the nourishing vessels.

**nutrition** (*nū-tri-shon*). Science of feeding.

**nyctalopia** (*nik-ta-lō-pi-a*). See NIGHT BLINDNESS.

**nyctophobia** (*nik-to-fō-bi-a*). Abnormal fear of darkness.

**nymphomania** (*nim-fō-mā-ni-a*). Excessive sexual desire in females.

**nystagmus** (*nis-tag-mus*). Involuntary oscillations of the eyeball; sometimes congenital; sometimes a symptom of brain disease, ocular affection, or lesion in the internal ear.

## O

**obesity** (*o-bē-si-ti*). Excessive fatness.

**objective** (*ob-jek'-tiv*). (1) The object glass of a microscope. (2) Pertaining to things lying external to one's self.

**oblique diameters of pelvis** (*ob-lēk dī-a-me-ters*). See DIAMETERS.

**oblique muscles** (*ob-lēk mu-sels*). (1) Two external muscles of the eyeball, an upper and a lower. (2) Two large muscles of the abdominal wall, an internal and an external.

**obsession** (*ob-se'-shon*). An idea of which the patient cannot rid himself. Minor obsessions are common in perfectly healthy people; but long-standing ones are especially frequent in the insane.

**obsessional neurosis** (*ob-se'-shon-al nū-rō-sis*). A mental illness in which the patient's mind gets taken up with forbidden thoughts and in which he has to engage in many rituals to try and free himself from these thoughts.

**obsolete** (*ob-sō-lēt*). No longer used.

**obstetric** (*ob-ste-trik*). Pertaining to the practice of midwifery.

**obstetrician** (*ob-ste-tri-shon*). Doctor who practises obstetrics.

**obturator** (*ob-tū-rātor*). That which stops up a hole or cavity. The obturator of a sigmoidoscope for example, is the blunt-ended rod which fills up the end of the instrument when it is introduced into the rectum, and thus prevents any scratching of the mucous membrane. The *o. foramen* is a hole on each side of the pelvis, closed by the powerful *o. ligament*. The *o. muscles* are two muscles on each side in the same region, and there are also *o. vessels* and *nerves*.

**obtusion** (*ob-tū'-zhon*). A blunting, as of sensitiveness.

**occipital** (*ok-si'-pi-tal*). Relating to the back of the head.

**occipito-anterior** (*ok-si-pi-tō-an-tār-i-or*), **occipito-posterior.** The two kinds of vertex presentation, according to the back of the head (occiput) being directed forwards or backwards.

**occiput** (*ok'-si-put*). The back of the head or skull.

**occlusion** (*ok-klū'-zhon*). Closure.

**occlusive therapy** (*o-kloo'-siv the'-ra-pi*). Application of ointments under impervious dressing.

**occult blood** (*o'-kult blud*). Not visible to naked eye. Term used to describe blood passed in faeces in such small amounts that no dark colour is present. This blood can only be demonstrated by the occult blood test.

**Occultest.** Tablets containing reagents for the demonstration of occult blood.

**occupational disease** (*o-kū-pā'-sho-nal di-sēz*). Illness induced by the patient's occupation.

**occupational therapy.** Any occupation given to a patient to help in his recovery, both mentally and physically.

**ocular** (*o'-kū-la*). Relating to the eye.

**oculist** (*o'-kū-list*). An eye specialist.

**oculogyric** (*o'-kū-lō-jī'-rik*). Rolling eyes.

**oculomotor nerves** (*o-kū-lō-mō'-tor*). The third pair of cranial nerves which help to move the eyeball.

**Oddi, sphincter of** (*o'di sfink-ter ov*). Muscular sphincter at the opening of the common bile duct into the duodenum.

**odontalgia** (*ō-don-tal'-ji-a*). Toothache.

**odontoid** (*o-don'-toyd*). Tooth-like. *O. process.* Peg-like projection of second cervical vertebra.

**odontolith** (*o-don'-to-lith*). Calcareous matter deposited on teeth; tartar.

**odontology** (*ō-don-to'-lo-ji*). Dentistry.

**odontoma** (*o-don-tō'-ma*). Tumour arising from a tooth or a developing tooth.

**oedema** (*e-dē'-ma*). Abnormal amount of fluid in the tissues causing a puffy swelling. The fluid tends to collect in the dependent parts, *e.g.* oedema of the ankles.

**Oedipus complex** (*ē'-di-pus*). A persistence of the normal love of a boy for his mother so that it rivals that of his father. Named after Oedipus who, according to Greek mythology, unknowingly married his mother.

**oesophageal** (*ē-so'-fa-je-al*). Pertaining to the oeso-

phagus. *O. atresia.* A congenital closure of the oesophagus needing urgent operative treatment. *O. varices.* Varicose veins in the lower part of the oesophagus resulting from hypertension in the hepatic portal system which occurs in cirrhosis of the liver.

**oesophagectasis** (*ē-so-fa-jek'-ta-sis*). Dilatation of a stricture in the oesophagus.

**oesophagectomy** (*ē-so-fa-jek-to-mi*). Resection of the oesophagus.

**oesophagitis** (*ē-so-fa-jī-tis*). Inflammation of the oesophagus, esp. *reflex o.*, due to hiatus hernia when stomach acid regurgitates into the lower part of the oesophagus causing damage and inflammation of the wall.

**oesophagoscope** (*ē-so'-fa-go-skōp*). An instrument for viewing the interior of the oesophagus.

**oesophagoscopy** (*ē-so'-af-go'-sko-pi*). Study of the oesophagus by means of the oesophagoscope.

**oesophagostomy** (*ē-so'-fa-gos-to-mi*). An artificial opening is made into the oesophagus.

**oesophagotomy** (*ē-so'-fa-go'-to-mi*). Cutting into the oesophagus.

**oesophagus** (*ē-so'-fa-gus*). The

canal which runs from the pharynx into the stomach.

**oestrogen** (*ēs-tro-gen*) or **oestrogenic substance** or **hormone.** Any substance usually a steroid, capable of producing genital tract changes characteristic of the follicular phase of the menstrual cycle: an oestrogen, probably oestradiol, is secreted by the ovaries. Oestrogens are also produced by the placenta during pregnancy and by the adrenal cortex. The female secondary sexual characteristics are under the influence of oestrogens. Oestrogens may be used to control menopausal symptoms and combined with progestogens are used in the contraceptive pill.

**ohm** (*ōm*). Unit of electrical resistance.

**ointment.** A soft application to promote healing, usually consisting of a base impregnated with some drug.

**olecranon** (*ō-le'-kra-non*). The bone composing the point of the elbow. The extreme upper end of the ulna, the inner of the two bones of the forearm.

**olfactory** (*ol-fak'-to-ri*). Relating to the sense of smell.

**oligaemia** (*o-le-gē'-mi-a*). Lack of blood.

**oligo-** (*o-li'-gō*). Prefix meaning deficiency.

**oligodendroglia** (*o-li-gō-den-drō-gli-a*). Glial cells, *see* NEUROGLIA, with few dendrites or processes. Probably equivalent to microglia.

**oligohydramnios** (*o-li-go-hī-dram'-ni-os*). Deficiency of amniotic fluid.

**oligomenorrhoea** (*o-li-gō-me-nor-rē-a*). Sparse menstrual flow.

**oligospermia** (*o-li-gō-sper-mi-a*). Abnormally small numbers of spermatozoa in the semen.

**oligotrophia** (*o-li-gō-trō'-fi-a*). Lack of nourishment.

**oliguria** (*o-li-gū'-ri-a*). A diminution in the amount of urine secreted.

**olivary body** (*o-li-va-ri bo-di*). An oval mass of grey matter behind the anterior pyramid of the medulla oblongata.

**omentocele** (*ō-men-tō-sēl*). Hernial sac containing omentum.

**omentopexy** (*ō-men-to-pek-si*). Fixation of the omentum.

**omentum** (*ō-men-tum*). A fold of the peritoneum. The *greater o.* is suspended from the greater curvature of the stomach and hangs in front of the gut. The *lesser o.* passes from the lesser curvature of the stomach to the transverse fissure of the liver.

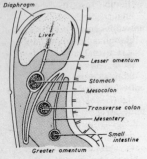

Diaphragm
Liver
Lesser omentum
Stomach
Mesocolon
Transverse colon
Mesentery
Small intestine
Greater omentum

38. The omentum

**omphalitis** (*om-fa-lī'-tis*). Inflammation of the umbilicus.

**omphalocele** (*om'-fa-lō-sēl*). An umbilical hernia.

**omphaloproptosis** (*om'-fa-lō-prop-tō'-sis*). Umbilical protrusion.

**onychia** (*ō-ni'-ki-a*). Inflammation of the matrix of a nail.

**onychocryptosis** (*o-ni-kō-krip-tō-sis*). Ingrowing nail.

**onychogryphosis** (*o-ni-kō-gri-fō-sis*). Bizarre overgrowth of the nails, often the nail of the big toe.

**onychomycosis** (*o-ni-kō-mī-kō'-sīs*). Infection of the nails by fungi.

**oocyte** (*o'-ō-sīt*). An ovum before it has left the Graafian follicle.

**oogenesis** (*o-o-je'-ne-sis*). The production of ova in the ovary.

**oophorectomy** (*o-o-fo-rek-to-mi*). Removal of an ovary. Also called ovariectomy.

**oophoritis** (*o-o-fo-rī-tis*). Inflammation of an ovary.

**oophoron** (*o-of'-o-ron*). That portion of the ovary which produces the ova; or the ovary itself.

**oophorosalpingectomy** (*o-o'-fo-ro-sal-pin-jek-to-mi*). Removal of the ovary and its associated Fallopian tube.

**opacity** (*ō-pa'-si-ti*). Want of transparency, cloudiness.

**opaque** (*ō-pāk*). Not transparent.

**opening snap.** Adventitious heart sound which often precedes the mid-diastolic murmur of mitral stenosis.

**ophthalmia** (*of-thal'-mi-a*). Inflammation of the eye. The term is applied especially to severe inflammations of the conjunctiva. There is an acute infectious form which occurs in epidemics, especially in schools and military camps.

**ophthalmia neonatorum** (*of-thal-mi-a nē-o-nah-tor-um*). Severe inflammation of the eyes in the newly born, due to gonorrhoeal or septic infection of the conjunctiva during the passage of the head through the vagina.

**ophthalmic** (*of-thal'-mik*). Pertaining to the eye.

**ophthalmitis** (*of-thal-mī'-tis*). Inflammation of the eye.

**ophthalmologist** (*of-thal-mo-lo-jist*). A surgeon specializing in diseases of the eye.

**ophthalmology** (*of-thal-mo'-lo-ji*). The study of diseases of the eye.

**ophthalmoplegia** (*of-thal-mo-plē-jī-a*). Paralysis of the muscles of the eye.

**ophthalmoscope** (*of-thal'-mo-skōp*). A small instrument, fitted with a lens, used to examine the interior of the eye.

**ophthalmotonometer** (*of-thal'-mō-tō-no-me-ter*). Instrument to measure the intraocular tension of the eye.

**opiate** (*ō'-pē-āt*). An opium preparation. A hypnotic.

**opisthotonos** (*o-pis-tho'-tō-nos*). Backward retraction of the head and lower limbs with arched back; seen in severe cases of tetanus, meningitis and in strychnine poisoning.

**opium** (*ō'-pi-um*). A preparation of poppy juice, much used to induce sleep and to allay pain. It contains the alkaloids, morphine, codeine, papaverine and narcotine. Can cause addiction.

**opponens** (*op-pō'-nens*). Opposing. Applied to muscles, *e.g.* *o. pollicis* which brings the thumb towards the little finger.

**opsonins** (*op-so'-nins*). Class of globulins found in the blood serum that are said to prepare the bacteria for phagocytosis.

**optic** (*op'-tik*). Relating to the sight.

**optic atrophy** (*op-tik a-tro-fi*). Degeneration of the optic nerve.

**optic chiasm** (*op-tik ki-as-m*). The crossing of the fibres of the optic tract, *see* CHIASM.

**optic disc** (*op'-tik disk*). The point where the optic nerve enters the eye. This point is insensitive to light and is known as the blind spot.

**optic neuritis** (*op-tik nū-rī-tis*). Inflammation of the optic nerve.

**optician** (*op-ti'-shon*). One who is trained to test eyes, make and dispense prescriptions for lenses and fit contact lenses.

**optics** (*op'tiks*). The study of the properties of light.

**optimum** (*op-ti'-mum*). The best possible conditions for a particular function.

**optometry** (*op-to'-me-tri*). Measurement of visual powers.

**oral** (*aw'-ral*). Pertaining to the mouth.

**orbicularis** (*or-bi-ku-lā-ris*). A name given to a muscle which encircles an orifice, *e.g. o. oris*, around the mouth.

**orbit** (*aw'-bit*). The bony cavity in the skull which holds the eye.

**orbital** (*aw-biptal*). Pertaining to the orbit.

**orchidectomy** (*aw-ki'-dek'-to-mi*). Removal of one or both testicles. Castration.

**orchidopexy** (*or-ki'-dō-pek-si*). The bringing down of an imperfectly descended testicle into the scrotum and fixing it there by sutures.

**orchiepididymitis** (*aw-ki-e'-pi-di-di-mī-tis*). Inflammation of the testis and epididymus.

**orchis** (*aw'-kis*). Testicle.

**orchitis** (*aw-kī'-tis*). Inflammation of the testicles.

**organ** (*aw-gan*). A part of the body constructed to exercise a special function.

**organic** (*aw-ga'-nik*). Relating to the organs; thus, organic disease of the heart means that the structure itself is affected *O. chemistry.* Chemistry relating to the carbon compounds.

**organism** (*aw'-ga-nism*). A living cell or cells.

**organophosphorus** (*aw-gan'-ō-fos'-for-us*). Type of insecticides which act mainly as cholinesterase inhibitors producing toxic effects in man, often delayed for several hours after contact.

**orgasm** (*aw'-gazm*). The crisis of sexual excitement.

**Oriental sore** (*o-ri-en-tal saw*). Delhi boil.

**orientation** (*o-ri-en-tā'-shon*). The location of one's position and attitude in relation to surrounding objects.

**orifice** (*o'-ri-fis*). An opening.

**ornithosis** (*aw-ni-thō'-sis*). Repiratory disease of birds, transmissible to man.

**orogenital syndrome** (*o-rō-je-ni-tal*). Syndrome of severe riboflavine deficiency characterized by stomatitis, cheilitis, glossitis and an eczematous eruption round the genitalia.

**oropharynx** (*o-rō-fa-rinks*). Posterior part of the pharynx below the soft palate and above the hyoid bone.

**orphan viruses** (*aw-fan vī-ruses*). *See* ADENOVIRUS.

**orthodontics** (*or-tho-don-tiks*). The correction of irregular placing of the teeth often undertaken for cosmetic reasons.

**orthopaedics** (*or-thō-pē'-diks*). The medical speciality concerned with all aspects of the bony skeleton including development, disease and damage.

**orthopnoea** (*or-thop'-nē-a*). Breathlessness, the patient gaining relief only in an upright position.

**orthoptics** (*or-thop'-tiks*). Term applied to correcting defective vision in a squint by exercises, etc.

**orthostatic.** Pertaining to or caused by standing upright.

**os** (*os*). (1) Bone. (2) Mouth or opening, *e.g. external os*, of cervix, etc.

**os calcis** (*os kal-sis*). The bone of the heel.

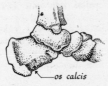

*39. The os calcis (calcaneum)*

**oscheal** (*os'-kē-al*). Pertaining to the scrotum.

**oscillation** (*os-si-lā'-shon*). A swinging movement.

**Osgood Schlatter's disease** (*osgood shla-ter*). Osteochondritis of unknown cause affecting the tibial tuberosity.

**Osler's disease** (*o'-zler*). Polycythaemia.

**Osler's nodes** (*o'-zlerz nōdz*). Small tender inflamed areas in the skin due to small emboli; occurs in bacterial endocarditis.

**osmol** (*oz'-mōl*). Unit for measuring ability of dissolved substances to cause osmosis and osmotic pressure; is equal to one gram molecule (or mole) of non-diffusible and non-ionizable dissolved substance.

**osmolality** (*oz'-mō-la'-li-ti*). Degree of osmotic activity shown by solution or mixture, expressed in osmols or milliosmols (mosmols).

**osmosis** (*oz-mō'-sis*). When a solution of a substance is separated from the solvent by a *semi-permeable* membrane impermeable to the solute, solvent passes through the membrane. If aqueous solutions are separated by such a membrane, the water will move in such a way as to equilibrate the strength of the solutions. This process is known as osmosis.

**osmotic fragility test** (*oz-mo-tik fra-ji-li-ti*). Method of determining the fragility of red blood cells.

**osmotic pressure** (*oz-mo-tik pre-sher*). Pressure required to prevent the passage of water by osmosis. The osmotic pressure depends on the number of solute molecules in solution.

**osseous** (*os'-se-us*). Like bone, bony.

**ossicle** (*os'-si-kel*). *Lit.*, a small bone. Name applied to the tiny bones of the middle ear. *See* EAR.

**ossification** (*os-si-fi-kā'-shon*). Hardening into bone.

**osteitis** (*os'-tē-ī'-tis*). Inflammation of bone. *O. fibrosa*, a disease of bone caused by an adenoma of the parathyroid glands. As the result of excessive secretion calcium is absorbed from the bones into the blood.

**osteitis deformans.** *See* PAGET'S DISEASE.

**osteoarthritis** (*os-tē-o-ar-thrī-tis*) or **osteoarthrosis** (*os-tē-ō-ar-thrō-sis*). Disorder due to excessive wear and tear to joint surfaces. Affecting chiefly weight-bearing joints, late in life, and resulting in pain, especially at night, deficient movement, and deformity.

**osteoarthropathy** (*os-tē-ō-ar-thro'-pa-thi*). Damage or disease affecting the bones and joints.

**osteoarthrotomy** (*os'-tē-ō-ar-thro'-to-mi*). Excision of joint and neighbouring bone.

**osteoblasts** (*os'-tē-ō-blasts*). Cells producing the intercellular bone matrix in the same way as fibroblasts may be considered to manufacture connective tissue matrix.

**osteochondritis** (*os'-tē-ō-kon-drī'-tis*). Combined inflammation of bone and cartilage. *O. deformans juvenilis.* A form occurring in children in which the head of the femur is affected. Perthes' disease. *O. dissecans.* Separation of loose bodies from the joint surface.

**osteochondroma** (*os-tē-ō-kon-drō'-ma*). Benign tumour derived from bone and cartilage.

**osteoclastoma** (*os-tē-ō-klas-tō-ma*). Tumour of osteoclasts.

**osteoclasts** (*os-tē-ō-klasts*). Multinucleated cells which break down the calcified bone matrix. Remodelling of bone by the combined activity of osteoclasts and osteoblasts occurs continuously during bone growth.

**osteocyte** (*os-tē-ō-sīt*). Osteoblasts which have become incorporated into bone.

**osteogenesis** (*os'-tē-ō-je'-ne-sis*). Formation of a bone. *O. imperfecta.* Abnormally fragile bones.

**osteogenic sarcoma** (*os-tē-ō-je-nik sar-kō-ma*). Sarcoma derived from osteoblasts.

**osteolytic** (*os-tē-ō-li-tik*). Bone destroying.

**osteoma** (*os-tē-ō'-ma*). A bony tumour.

**osteomalacia** (*os-tē-ō-ma-lā'-ki-a*). Softening of bones in adults.

**osteomyelitis** (*os-tē-ō-m-ī-lī'-tis*). Inflammation of bone including the marrow, the bone around it and the cartilage covering the end of the bone.

**osteopath** (*os-tē-ō-path*). One who practises osteopathy.

**osteopathy** (*os-tē-o'-pa-thē*). The study and treatment of disease based on the belief of maladjustments in the joints of the body as a cause of disease. The majority of osteopaths are not medically qualified.

**osteopetrosis** (*os-tē-ō-pe-trō'-sis*). *See* MARBLE BONE DISEASE.

**osteophony** (*os-tē-o'-fo-ni*). Conduction of sound by bone.

**osteophyte** (*os'-tē-ō-fīt*). A bony outgrowth or nodosity; occurs in osteoarthritis.

**osteoplastic** (*os-tē-ō-plas-tik*). Pertaining to the repair of bones.

**osteoporosis** (*os-tē-ō-po-rō'-sis*). Fragility of bones due to reabsorption of calcium.

**osteosarcoma** (*os-tē-ō-sar-kō'-ma*). A malignant tumour growing from a bone.

**osteosclerosis** (*os-tē-ō-skle-rō'-sis*). Increase in bone density.

**osteotome** (*os'-ti-o-tōm*). A surgical instrument resembling a chisel and used for cutting through bones. The instrument is bevelled on both sides.

**osteotomy** (*os-tē-o'-to-mi*). Operation of cutting through a bone.

**ostium** (*os'-ti-um*). An opening. The orifice of any tubular passage.

**otalgia** (*ō-tal'-ji-a*). Ear-ache.

**otitis externa** (*ō-tī'-tis ex-ter-na*). Inflammation of the skin of the external ear. Sometimes a form of eczema. In children can be caused by a foreign body in the external ear.

**otitis interna** (*o-tī'-tis in-ter-na*). Inflammation of the inner ear affecting the organs of balance.

**otitis media** (*mē-di-a*). Inflammation of the middle ear.

**otologist** (*ō-to-lo-jist*). Ear specialist.

**otology** (*ō-to'-lo-ji*). Study of diseases of the ear.

**otorrhoea** (*ō-tor-rē'-a*). A purulent discharge from the ear.

**otosclerosis** (*ō-tō-skle-rō'-sis*). A chronic, progressive thickening of the structures of the internal ear leading to deafness.

**otoscope** (*ō'-to-skōp*). Auriscope.

**ounce** (*owns*). In fluid measure, about two tablespoonfuls; in apothecaries' weight, 8 drachms.

**outlet of pelvis** (*owt'-let*). The space bounded by the lower edges of the pubes, ischium, sacrum and coccyx and by the sacrosciatic ligaments.

**ovarian cyst** (ō-va'-rē-an sist). Cyst of the ovary; may be developmental or associated with ovarian tumour.

**ovarian follicle** (ō-va'-rē-an folli-kl). See FOLLICLE.

**ovarian tumour** (tū-mer). A growth in the ovary which can be benign or malignant.

**ovariectomy** (ō-vā-rē-ek-to-mi). Oophorectomy. Surgical removal of ovary.

**ovaries** (ō'-va-rēz). Two small oval bodies situated on either side of the uterus; the female organs in which the ova are formed. They are also endocrine glands.

**ovariotomy** (ō-vā-rī-ō'-to-mi). The operation of cutting into an ovary.

**ovaritis** (ō-va-rī-tis). See OOPHORITIS.

**ovary.** See OVARIES.

**overcompensation** (ō-ver-com-pen-sā-shon). (1) Homeostasis is achieved by the body compensating for changes brought about in various circumstances. When the compensatory mechanism too far outweighs the change which it opposes, overcompensation is said to have taken place. (2) In psychiatry applies to exaggerated compensatory

behaviour, e.g. extreme aggressiveness in response to a feeling of inadequacy.

**overdosage** (ō-ver-dō-sij). Excessive concentration of a drug in the blood. This may be an accumulation from repeated doses or from too high a dose. May also be caused by the body's inability to excrete or break down the drug.

**overextension** (o-ver-eks-ten'-shon). Extension beyond the normal, e.g. of a joint or muscle.

**oviduct** (o'-vi-dukt). The Fallopian tube between the ovary and the womb, conveying the ova. See OVARIES.

**ovulation** (o-vū-lā'-shon). The development and discharge of ova from the ovary.

**ovum** (ō'-vum). The egg cell produced in the female ovary.

**oxaluria** (ok-sa-lu'-ri-a). Presence of oxalic acid crystals in the urine.

**oxidation** (ok-si-dā'-shon). Process involving the loss of electrons from the oxidized substance.

**oxycephaly** (ok-si-ke-fa-li). Abnormal development of the skull with resultant egg-shaped appearance.

**oxygen** (ok'-si-jen). Gas forming 20 per cent of the atmosphere. Essential for human life. *O. administration*. By (1) nasal catheters at approximately 2 litres per minute. This will raise the alveolar oxygen to approximately 30 per cent. (2) *O. tent*. Rate of flov depends upon amount of disturbance for nursing care. With average care, the alveolar oxygen can be kept at 45 per cent. (3) Masks. There are various types available: some allow different concentrations of oxygen dependent upon the oxygen flow to the mask; some allow humidification to be provided. Oxygen may be used in high concentrations following open heart surgery.

**oxygen debt** (*ok-si-jen det*). If the metabolic requirement for oxygen exceeds the supply, the metabolic processes are carried on under partially anaerobic conditions until at a later time the 'oxygen debt' is repaid.

**oxygenation** (*ok-si-je-nā-shon*). To saturate with oxygen.

**oxyhaemoglobin** (*ok-si-hē-mo-glō-bin*). Oxygenated haemoglobin.

**oxyntic** (*ok-sin-tik*). Term applied to cells secreting hydrochloric acid in the stomach.

**oxytocin** (*ok-si-tō'-sin*). Polypeptide hormone secreted by the posterior lobe of the pituitary which produces a strong contraction of uterine muscle.

**oxyuriasis** (*ok'-si-ū-rī-a-sis*). Infection with oxyuris vermicularis.

**oxyuris vermicularis** (*ok'-si-ū-ris ver-mi-kū-lā'-ris*). Threadworm found in the rectum and large intestine, especially in children.

**ozone** (*ō'-zōn*). $O_3$. An oxidizing agent sometimes used as a disinfectant.

## P

**Pacchioni's bodies** (*pa-ki-ō-nis*). Villi from the arachnoid membrane. A path for draining cerebrospinal fluid into the venous sinuses.

**Paccini's corpuscles** (*pa-chē-nis kor'-pu-sels*). Specialized sensory receptors which register pressure and to some extent vibration. They are situated in the deeper connective tissues of the skin and consist of nerve-endings surrounded by concentric lamallae of fibrous tissue.

**pacemaker** (*pās-mā-ker*). *See* AURICULO – VENTRICULAR BUNDLE. *P. artificial*. Electrical appliance which can be fitted surgically to act as the initiator of the cardiac impulse if the sinuatrial node does not function normally.

**pachy-.** A prefix denoting thickness.

**pachydermia** (*pa-ki-der'-mi-a*). Thickening of the skin.

**pachymeningitis** (*pa-ki-me-nin-ji'-tis*). Inflammation of the dura mater, with thickening of the membrane.

**pack.** Moistened material applied to the patient.

**paediatrician** (*pē-dē-a-tri-shon*). Specialist in diseases of children.

**paediatrics** (*pē-dē-a-triks*). Study of diseases of children.

**Paget's disease.** (1) Of bone, *Osteitis deformans*, is a disorder of unknown cause which usually affects a number of bones to greater or lesser extent. Clinically the features are pain, tendency to pathological fractures and hyperdynamic circulation. (2) Of nipple. Eczema of the nipple associated with underlying duct carcinoma of the breast.

**pain** (*pān*). Specific form of unpleasant, sensory experience, usually aroused by incipient or actual damage to cells or tissue.

**palate** (*pa'-lāt*). The roof of the mouth.

**palatoplegia** (*pa'-la-to-plē'-ji-a*). Paralysis of soft palate.

**palliative** (*pa'-li-a-tiv*). A medicine which relieves but does not cure.

**pallidectomy** (*pal-li-dek-to-mi*). Operation used in Parkinson's disease to decrease the activity part of the lentiform nucleus in the base of the brain.

**pallidotomy** (*pa'-li'-do'-to-mi*). Operation performed to relieve tremor in Parkinson's disease. Fibres from the cerebral cortex are severed.

**pallor** (*pa'-lor*). Paleness.

**palm** (*pahm*). The hollow or flexor surface of the hand.

**palmar** (*pal'-mar*). Pertaining to the palm of the hand.

**palpation** (*pal-pā-shon*). Examination by the hand.

**palpebra** (*pal-pe'-bra*). The eyelid.

**palpitation** (*pal-pi-ta'-shon*). Rapid beating of the heart, producing consciousness of the heart's action.

**palsy** (*pawl'-zē*). Paralysis. *See* ERB'S PARALYSIS.

**pan.** A prefix signifying all, total.

**panacea** (*pa-na-sē'-a*). A medicine which is claimed or advertised to cure all diseases.

**panarthritis** (*pan-ahr-thrī'-tis*). Generalized inflammation of joints.

**pancarditis** (*pan-kar-dī-tis*). Generalized inflammation of the heart.

**Pancoast's tumour.** Tumour occurring at the apex of the

lung involving the lower part of the brachial plexus producing Horner's syndrome and pain, weakness and wasting down the arm.

**pancreas** (*pan'-krē-as*). Sweetbread. A gland situated in the mesentery in relation to the duodenum and crossing the mid-line of the body. It secretes an alkaline mixture of digestive enzymes through the pancreatic duct into the duodenum when stimulated by the hormone *secretin*. Contains groups of cells which secrete insulin into the blood. *See* ISLETS OF LANGERHANS.

**pancreatectomy** (*pan-krē-a-tek'-to-mi*). Excision of pancreas.

**pancreatin** (*pan-krē-a-tin*). Extract of pancreatic glands used in the treatment of mucoviscidosis.

**pancreatitis** (*pan'-kre-a-tī'-tis*). Inflammation of the pancreas.

**pandemic** (*pan-de'-mik*). A widely spread epidemic..

**panhypopituitarism** (*pan-hī-pō-pi-tū-i-ta-rism*). Simmond's disease. Deficient secretion of all the anterior pituitary hormones with secondary reduction in production of hormones by the thyroid and adrenal cortex.

**pannus** (*pan'-nus*). Vascularization of the cornea; in joints

the replacement of cartilage by granulation tissue.

**panophthalmia** or **panophthalmitis** (*pan-of-thal-mī'-tis*). Generalized inflammation of the eyeball.

**panotitis** (*pa-no-tī-tis*). Inflammation of the middle and internal ear.

**Papanicolaou stain** (*pa-pa-ni-kō-law*). Stain frequently employed for the examination of vaginal and cervical smears. *See* CERVICAL SMEAR.

**papilla** (*pa-pil'-la*)(pl. **papillae**). (1) A small nipple-shaped eminence. (2) The optic disc. *Circumvallate papillae.* These are found at the root of the tongue. *Filiform papillae.* The common *p.* of the tongue and found at its tip. *Fungiform papillae* are the broad *p.* of the tongue.

**papillitis** (*pa-pi-lī-tis*). Inflammation of the optic disc.

**papilloedema** (*pa-pi-le-dē'-ma*). Oedema of the optic nerve.

**papilloma** (*pa-pil-lō'-ma*). Benign neoplasm of epithelial cells.

**papovaviruses** (*pa-pō'-va-vī'-ru-sez*). Group of viruses associated with induction of papillomata and polyoma in rabbits and in warts in man.

**papule** (*pa'-pūl*). A small solid pimple.

**para-aminobenzoic acid** (*pa-ra-a-mī'-nō-ben-zo-ik as-id*).

A bacterial growth factor antagonized by the sulphanilamides.

**para-aortic** (*pa-ra-ā-or'-tik*). Near the aorta.

**paracentesis** (*pa-ra-sen-tē'-sis*). Withdrawing fluid from body cavity. *See* ASPIRATION.

**paracusis** (*pa-ra-kū-sis*). Disordered hearing.

**paraesthesia** (*pa-res-thē'-zi-a*). Disordered sensation, such as tingling and pins and needles.

**para-influenza** (*pa'-ra-in-flū-en'-za*). Used of viruses suspected of causing common cold. They included Sendai, haemadsorption 1 and 2, and croup-associated viruses.

**paralysis** (*pa-ra'-li-sis*). Loss of nervous function, usually *motor*, but may be applied to sensory paralysis. In motor paralysis the loss of nerve function results in the inability to stimulate contraction of muscles. This does not necessarily mean that the muscles become *flaccid* since this follows only the paralysis of lower motor neurones. Upper motor neurone paralysis causes *spastic* paralysis. *P. agitans. See* PARKINSON'S DISEASE.

**paralytic ileus** (*pa-ra-li-tik ī-lē-us*). Intestinal obstruction due to paralysis of muscles of peristalsis.

**paramedian** (*pa-ra-mē'-di-an*). Close to the middle.

**parametritis** (*pa-ra-me-trī-tis*). Inflammation of the parametrium. Also called *pelvic cellulitis.*

**parametrium** (*pa-ra-mē-tri-um*). The connective tissue around the uterus, chiefly found round large vessels and between the layers of the broad ligament.

**paramnesia** (*par-am-nē'-si-a*). False memory; usually memory of events which did not occur in the connection related.

**paranoia** (*pa-ra-noy'-a*). Feelings of persecution; may be due to reality or in some psychiatric illness be delusional.

**paranoid** (*pa-ra-noyd*). Relating to paranoia.

**paraphimosis** (*pa-ra-fī-mō'-sis*). Retraction of the prepuce behind the glans penis with inability to restore it to the natural position.

**paraplegia** (*pa-ra-plē-ji-a*). Paralysis of both lower limbs.

**pararectal** (*pa-ra-rek'-tal*). Around the rectum.

**parasite** (*pa-ra-sīt*). Any living thing which lives on or in another organism.

**parasiticide** (*pa-ra-sī-ti-sīd*). Substance lethal to parasites.

**parasympathetic system** (*pa-ra-sim-pa-the-tik sis-tem*).

Part of the autonomic nervous system.

**parathormone** (*pa-ra-thor'-mōn*). The hormone of the parathyroid glands.

**parathyroid** (*pa-ra-thī'-royd*). Small endocrine glands which control calcium and phosphate metabolism. They are usually four in number and they are situated in the vicinity of the thyroid gland.

**paratyphoid** (*pa-ra-tī-foyd*). An infectious disease resembling typhoid fever and caused by an organism not identical with but closely allied to the bacillus of typhoid. *See* ENTERIC.

**paravertebral** (*pa-ra-ver'-tebral*). To one side of the spinal column.

**parenchyma** (*pa-ren'-kī-ma*). The functional part of an organ.

**parenteral treatment** (*pa-rente-ral'*). Therapy by drugs given by routes other than the alimentary tract.

**paresis** (*pa-rē-sis*). A partial paralysis.

**parietal** (*pa-rī'-e-tal*). The two bones which form the crown and sides of the cranium. *See* FONTANELLE.

**parietes** (*pa-rī-e-tēz*). The walls of any cavity of the body.

**parity** (*pa'-ri-ti*). The number of children a woman has borne.

**Parkinson's disease** (*par'-kin-sonz*). Degeneration affecting the basal ganglia of the brain especially affecting the substantia nigra and the surrounding tissues. It is characterized by a combination in varying degrees of muscular *rigidity* and a *tremor* which is temporarily abolished by the voluntary movement of the part affected.

**paronychia** (*pa-ro-ni'-ki-a*). Whitlow; inflammation and abscess at the end of a finger near the nail.

**parosmia** (*pa-ros-mi-a*). Perverted sense of smell.

**parotid** (*pa-ro'-tid*). Near the ear; applied to a salivary gland under the ear.

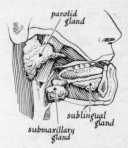

*parotid gland*

*sublingual gland*

*submaxillary gland*

40. *The salivary glands*

**parotitis** (*pa-ro-tī'-tis*). Inflammation of the parotid gland. (1) Mumps. (2) Spread of infection from a septic mouth.

PAR  268

**parovarium** (*pa-ro-vā'-ri-um*). A vestigal structure in the broad ligament of the uterus which occasionally gives origin to small cysts in this region.

**paroxysm** (*pa'-rok-sizm*). A sudden temporary attack.

**paroxysmal nocturnal dyspnoea** (*pa-rok-sis-mal nok-ter-nal dis-nē-a*). Attacks of breathlessness occurring at night due to accumulation of fluid in the lungs resulting from left ventricular failure.

**paroxysmal nocturnal haemoglobinuria** (*hē-mō-glo'-bi'-nū-ri-a*). Marchiafava-Micheli syndrome. The passage of haemoglobin in the urine occurring at night. The cause is not known.

**paroxysmal tachycardia** (*ta'-ki-kār-di-a*). Is due to the regular and rapid discharge of impulses from an ectopic focus in the atrial walls of the heart. The focus thus replaces the sinuatrial node as the cardiac pacemaker and drives the heart at a rate of about 180 beats per minute (normal about 80). Attacks may last anything from a minute to several days.

**parrot disease.** Psittacosis.

**parthenogenesis** (*par-the-nō-ge'-ne-sis*). Development of an ovum into a new individual without being fertilized.

**parturient** (*par-tū'-ri-ent*). In the condition of giving or being just about to give birth to a child. The *P. canal* is the passage traversed by the fetus during birth, from the brim of the pelvis to vulva.

**parturition** (*par-tū-ri'-shun*). The act of giving birth to a child.

**Paschen bodies** (*pash-en*). Minute bodies containing the virus of smallpox.

**passive.** Submissive. Not active or spontaneous. *P. immunity. See* IMMUNITY. *P. movements* are performed on a patient's joints by a physiotherapist to increase the mobility, prevent contractures and to improve the circulation.

**Pasteurella** (*pahs-ter-e'-la*). Plague bacteria.

**pasteurization** (*pas'-tū-rī-zā'-shon*). Method of sterilization of fluids introduced by Pasteur which involves heating for 30 minutes at 70°C.

**patella** (*pa-tel'-la*). The knee-cap. A sesamoid bone in front of the knee joint.

**patellar bursae** (*ber'sē*). The bursae around the patella. Inflammation of the prepatellar bursa used to be called housemaid's knee, as it occurs after much kneeling.

**patellectomy** (*pa-tel-lek-to-mi*).

Operation to excise the patella.

**patent** (*pā'-tent*). Open.

**patent ductus arteriosus** (*pā-tent duk-tus ah-tār-i-ō-sus*). Failure of the ductus arteriosus to close at birth.

**patent foramen ovale** (*fo-ra-men ō-vā-le*). Failure of closure of the foramen ovale.

**pathogenesis** (*pa-thō-je'-ne-sis*). The origin and progress of disease.

**pathogenic** (*path-ō-je-nik*). Capable of causing disease.

**pathognomonic** (*pa-tho-nō-mon'-ik*). Characteristic of, or peculiar to, a particular disease.

**pathological** (*pa-tho-lo'-ji-kal*). Relating to pathology. Morbid, abnormal.

**pathology** (*pa-tho'lo-ji*). The study of disease, particularly regarding the changes in the tissues resulting from disease.

**pathophobia** (*pa-thō-fō-bi-a*). Neurotic fear of disease.

**patulous** (*pa'-tū-lus*). Open wide.

**Paul's tube.** Transparent drainage tube.

**Paul-Bunnell test** (*pawl-boo-nel*). A serological test for glandular fever (infective mononucleosis).

**PD.** Papillary distance.

**peau d'orange** (*pō-do-ranj'*). Orange-skin appearance of skin overlying carcinoma of the breast which is caused by obstruction to superficial lymphatics.

**pectin** (*pek'-tin*). A polysaccharide found in fruit.

**pectoral** (*pek'-to-ral*). Relating to the chest. *P. muscles* are on the anterior surface of chest.

**pectus** (*pek'-tus*). The thorax, chest.

**pediatrics** (*pē'-di-a'-triks*). See PAEDIATRICS.

**pedicle** (*pe-di-kl*). The stalk of a collection of tissue which contains the supply of vessels and nerves.

**pediculosis** (*pe-di-kū-lō'-sis*). Infestation with lice.

**pediculus** (*pe-di'-kū-lus*). The louse, a parasite infesting the hair and skin. *P. capitis* infests the head; *P. corporis*, the body and clothing; *P. pubis*, the pubic hair. These three varieties are different in shape and size.

**pedunculated** (*pe-dung'-kū-lā-ted*). Possessing a pedicle.

**Pel-Ebstein's fever** (*pel-eb-stīns*). A regularly remitting fever which sometimes occurs in Hodgkin's disease.

**pellagra** (*pel-la'-gra*). Syndrome caused by deficiency of nicotinic acid characterized by dementia, diarrhoea and dermatitis.

**pellet** (*pel'-et*). Small pill.

**pellicle** (*pel'-li-kl*). A thin skin or membrane.

**pelvic** (*pel'-vik*). Relating to the pelvis. *P. cellulitis. See* PARAMETRITIS. *P. exenteration.* Operative removal of organ from pelvis.

**pelvimetry** (*pel-vi'-me-tri*). Measurement of internal diameters of pelvis.

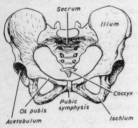

41. The pelvis

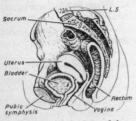

42. Sagittal section of the female pelvis

**pelvis** (*pel'-vis*). The bony cavity composed of the hips and the lower bones of the spine and holding the bowels, bladder and organs of generation.

**pemphigus** (*pem'-fi-gus*). Disease characterized by the formation of large blisters on the skin and mucous membranes. *P. neonatorum* is a misnomer. It is an acute staphylococcal impetigo occurring in newborn infants.

**pendulous** (*pen'-dū-lus*). Hanging down.

**penetration** (*pe-ne-trā'-shon*). Entering into.

**penicillin** (*pe-ni-si-lin*). First of the antibiotic agents to be used in therapy. It is a substance synthesized by the *Penicillium* mould.

**penis** (*pē'-nis*). The male organ of coition containing the urethra.

**pentagastrin test meal** (*pen'-ta-gas-trin test mēl*). Test of responsiveness of gastric mucosa to stimulation by the hormone pentagastrin.

**pentose** (*pen-tōz*). Monosaccharide sugar with five carbon atoms, *e.g.* ribose, deoxyribose.

**pentosuria** (*pen-tō-sū-ri-a*). Renal defect in which there is failure to reabsorb pentoses from the urine with the result that the urine contains sugar.

**pepsin** (*pep'-sin*). An enzyme which breaks down proteins in acid solution to form peptides (*a peptidase*). It is secreted in the stomach with hydrochloric acid.

**peptic** (*pep'-tik*). Pertaining to digestion. *P. ulcer*, a gastric, duodenal or gastrojejunal ulcer.

**peptic ulcer diet.** Diet used in the treatment of peptic ulcer. Formerly a bland one but now more varied.

**peptide** (*pep-tīd*). Compound of two or more amino-acids. The peptide link, which is split by peptidases, *see* PEPSIN, is formed between the amino group of one amino-acid and the carboxyl group of the next. When many are joined together they form so-called *polypeptides*. Polypeptides join together to form protein.

**peptonized food** (*pep'-tō-nīzed*). A partially predigested food. As a rule, milk, beef-tea, or other simple fluid food is chosen. May be prescribed for acute gastritis.

**perception** (*per-sep-shon*). An awareness. Receiving impressions through the senses.

**percolation** (*per-ko-lā'-shon*). The passage of a liquid through a solid but porous substance. Liquid extracts are made in this way. The drug is coarsely powdered, packed into a cylindrical vessel and the solvent trickles slowly through.

**percussion** (*per-ku'-shon*). Striking upon the body, the sound heard being helpful in diagnosis. The note emitted is resonant or dull according to the condition of the organ underneath.

**perforation** (*per-fo-rā'-shon*). A hole in an organ caused by disease or injury. The act of perforating.

**peri-.** Prefix signifying around, near, about.

**perianal** (*pe-ri-ā'-nal*). Around the anus.

**periarteritis** (*pe-ri-ar-te-rī'-tis*). Inflammation of the outer coat of an artery. *P. nodosa*. A disease of unknown cause which is characterized by the production of multiple nodules in the connective tissues surrounding the smaller arteries. The symptoms and signs associated with this disorder depend on the distribution of the lesions.

**periarthritis** (*pe-ri-ar-thrī-tis*). Inflammation of the tissues round a joint.

**pericardial** (*pe-ri-kar-di-al*). Pertaining to the pericardium. *P. adhesions*. Fibrosis of the pericardium which may follow pericarditis in which the two layers of the pericardium become stuck together.

**pericardiotomy** (*pe-ri-kar-di-*

*o-to-mi*). An opening made into the pericardium.

**pericarditis** (*pe-ri-kar-dī'-tis*). Inflammation of the pericardium.

**pericardium** (*pe-ri-kar'-di-um*). Membranes which surround the heart leaving a potential space and thus enabling changes in shape and volume of the heart to take place.

**perichondritis** (*per-i-kon-drī'-tis*). Inflammation of perichondrium.

**perichondrium** (*per-i-kon'-dri-um*). The membranous covering of a cartilage.

**pericolitis** (*pe-ri-ko-lī'-tis*). Inflammation round the colon.

**pericolpitis** (*per-i-kol-pī'-tis*). Also called paracolpitis. Inflammation of the structures around the vagina.

**pericranium** (*per-i-krā'-ni-um*). The membrane covering the bones of the skull.

**perilymph** (*pe-ri-limf*). Clear fluid in the osseous labyrinth of the ear.

**perimeter** (*pe-ri'-me-ter*). The outside or circumference, often applied to the width of visual fields.

**perimetritis** (*pe-ri-me-trī'-tis*). Inflammation of the peritoneum covering the uterus.

**perinatal** (*pe'-ri-nā'-tal*). The period of time before, during and after childbirth.

**perineal** (*pe-ri-nē-al*). Pertaining to the perineum. *P. body*. Wedge-shaped muscular body which forms the focus of the pelvic floor.

**perineorrhaphy** (*pe-ri-nē-o-ra-fi*). Operative repair of perineal tear.

**perinephric** (*pe-ri-nef-rik*). Round about the kidney. *P. abscess*, a collection of pus in the tissues round the kidney.

**perineum** (*pe-ri-nē-um*). The region of the pelvic floor anterior to the anus.

**perineurium** (*pe-rī-nū-ri-um*). A sheath investing a bundle of nerve fibres.

**periodic syndrome** (*pe-ri-o-dik sin'-drōm*). Cyclical vomiting attacks of unknown cause which may occur in children. Often associated with headache, fever and abdominal pain.

**periosteal** (*pe-ri-os-te-al*). Pertaining to periosteum. *P. sarcoma*, sarcoma growing from periosteum.

**periosteum** (*pe-ri-os-tē-um*). The membrane covering a bone.

**periostitis** (*pe-ri-os-tī'-tis*). Inflammation of the periosteum.

**peripheral** (*pe-ri-fe-ral*). Relating to the circumference or outer surface. *P. neuritis*.

Inflammation of the peripheral nerves.

**periproctitis** (*pe-ri-prok-tū-tis*). Inflammation of tissue around rectum or anus.

**perisalpingitis** (*pe-ri-sal-pin-jī'-tis*). Inflammation of peritoneum covering the uterine tube.

**perisplenitis** (*pe-ri-sple-nī-tis*). Inflammation of the connective tissues surrounding the spleen.

**peristalsis** (*pe-ri-stal'-sis*). The contractions and movements of the alimentary tract forcing on the contents.

**peritomy** (*pe-ri-to-mi*). Incision of the conjunctiva near the margin of the cornea for the cure of pannus.

**peritoneal** (*pe-ri-tō-nē-al*). Pertaining to peritoneum.

**peritoneum** (*pe-ri-tō-nē-um*). The membrane or sac which surrounds the intestines and most other abdominal viscera, and which also lines the abdominal cavity. It secretes a serous fluid which reduces friction.

**peritonitis** (*pe-ri-tō-nī-tis*). Inflammation of the peritoneum.

**peritonsillar abscess** (*pe-ri-ton-si-la ab-ses*). Abscess in the pharynx near the tonsils. *See also* QUINSY.

**periurethral** (*pe-ri-ū-rē-thral*). Around the urethra.

**permanent teeth.** Teeth of the second dentition.

**permeable** (*per-mē-abl*). Capable of being penetrated.

**pernicious** (*per-ni-shus*). Tending to a fatal issue. *P. anaemia.* Anaemia resulting from cyanocobalamin (vitamin $B_{12}$) deficiency. *P. vomiting. See* VOMITING OF PREGNANCY.

**pernio** (*per'-ni-ō*). Chilblains.

**perniosis** (*per-ni-ō-sis*). Chilblains.

**peroneal** (*pe-rō-nē-al*). Pertaining to the fibula.

**peroral** (*per-aw'-ral*). Through the mouth.

**perseveration** (*per-se-ve-rā-shon*). A recurring idea, feeling or way of action from which the patient finds it difficult to escape.

**persistent ductus arteriosus.** *See* PATENT DUCTUS ARTERIOSUS.

**personality** (*per-so-na-li-ti*). Individual characteristics of behaviour.

**perspiration** (*per-spi-rā-shon*). Sweat.

**Perthe's disease.** Pseudocoxalgia. Osteochondritis affecting the head of the femur. Usually occurs in boys before their teens.

**pertussis** (*per-tus'-sis*). Whooping cough. A disease of childhood characterized by a cough with a typical 'whoop' on inspiration. Caused by haemophilus pertussis.

**perversion** (*per-ver-shon*). Turned away from the normal course *e.g. sexual perversion*, aberrations of normal sexual behaviour.

**pes** (*pāz*). Foot. *Pes cavus*. Exaggerated longitudinal arch of foot. *Pes planus*. Flat foot. Loss of longitudinal arch.

**pessary** (*pes'-sa-ri*). (1) A device placed in vagina to remedy malpositions of uterus or vaginal prolapse. (2) A medicated vaginal suppository.

**pestilence** (*pes'-ti-lens*). Epidemic disease.

**petechiae** (*pe-tē'-chi-ē*). Small red spots on the skin formed by effusion of blood.

**petit mal** (*pe-ti mal*). See EPILEPSY.

**Petri dish** (*pe-tri*). A small flat glass dish used in bacteriological laboratories.

**pétrissage** (*pā'-tris-sahj*). A type of kneading massage.

**petrous** (*pe-trus*). Stony; a term given to a hard part of the temporal bone.

**Peyer's patches** (*pā-yers pa-ches*). Collections of lymphoid tissue associated with the small intestine.

**pH.** Expression of the hydrogen ion concentration of a solution. $pH = -$ logarithm $(H^+)$ where $(H^+)$ represents the hydrogen ion concentration. The scale ranges from 0 to 14. Between 0 and 7 is *acid* and between 7 and 14 is *alkaline*; 7 is neutral.

**phaeochromocyte** (*fē'-ō-krō-mō-sīt*). One of two cell-types present in the adrenal medulla and in the sympathetic ganglion.

**phaeochromocytoma** (*fē-ō-krō-mō-sī-to-ma*). Adrenal medullary tumour which secretes adrenaline and noradrenaline, causing episodes of raised blood pressure.

**phage typing** (*fāj tī-ping*). Method of identifying bacteria which depends on their sensitivity to lysis by bacteriophage viruses.

**phagocytes** (*fa-gō-sīts*). The polymorphonuclear white cells of the blood, so called from their property of being able to ingest and destroy micro-organisms which may be circulating in the blood or attacking the tissues.

**phagocytosis** (*fa-gō-sī-tō-sis*). Process of ingestion of material by cells such as phagocytes and macrophages. Most cells are considered to be capable of phagocytosis at least to some extent. In an attempt to distinguish this type of ingestion from the defensive, *e.g.* anti-bacterial, ingestion of the phagocytes and macrophages, the term *pinocytosis* has been introduced. The mechanism is similar but the average size of ingested particles is smaller.

**phalanges** (*fa-lan-jes*). The small bones of the fingers and toes.

**phallus** (*fa-lus*). The penis.

**phantom limb** (*fan-tom lim*). Sensation often experienced by patient, after an amputation, that the limb is still there.

**pharmaceutical** (*far-ma-sū-ti-kal*). Pertaining to drugs.

**pharmacogenetics** (*far'-ma-kō-je-ne'-tiks*). Study of genetically determined variations in response to, and metabolism of, drugs.

**pharmacology** (*far-ma-ko'-lo-ji*). The study of drug action.

**Pharmacopoeia** (*far-ma-kō-pē-a*). An authorized handbook of drugs. *British P.* has a legal status.

**pharmacy** (*far-ma-si*). The science of preparing and mixing medicines or drugs. The place where drugs are dispensed.

**pharyngeal** (*fa-rin-jē-al*). Pertaining to the pharynx. *P. pouch*. Diverticulum in the wall of the pharynx which

may form between the two portions of the inferior constrictor muscle of the pharynx.

**pharyngectomy** (*fa-rin-jek'-to-mi*). Excision of part of the pharynx.

**pharyngismus** (*fa-rin-jis-mus*). Spasm of the pharynx.

**pharyngitis** (*far-in-jī''-tis*). Inflammation of the pharynx.

**pharyngotympanic tube** (*fa-rin-gō-tim-pa-nik tūb*). Eustachian tube, running from the pharynx to the middle ear.

**pharynx** (*făr-inks*). The musculo-membranous sac at the back of the mouth leading to the oesophagus and to the larynx.

**phase-contrast microscopy** (*fāz-kon-trahst mī-kros'-ko-pi*). Microscopic examination of living unstained biological material using two light-beams, one retarded by $\frac{1}{4}$ wavelength in relation to the other. Their difference in intensity causes the object to stand out.

**phenol** (*fē-nol*). Substance consisting of benzene nucleus to which hydroxyl groups are attached. In pharmacology applies especially to carbolic acid, $C_6H_5OH$, used in liquid form as dental analgesic, in aqueous form as antiseptic, in other solutions as a sclerosing agent for haemorrhoids, intrathecal injection for intractable pain. It is poisonous, and sufficient can be absorbed through intact skin to be fatal.

**phenotype** (*fē'-no-tīp*). Property shown by an individual, due to the expression of characters of his genotype.

**phenylalanine** (*fe-nil-al-a-nin*). Essential amino-acid.

**phenylketonuria** (*fe-nīl-kē-tō-nū-ri-a*). Genetically determined error of metabolism in which there is an inability of the liver to convert phenylalanine to tyrosine. Instead phenylalanine is broken down to phenyl-pyruvic acid which is excreted in the urine. There is associated mental deficiency. Screening is done for this and other inborn errors of metabolism by the Guthrie test soon after birth.

**phimosis** (*fī-mō-sis*). Contraction of the orifice of the prepuce; usually treated by the operation of circumcision.

**phlebectomy** (*fle-bek-to-mi*). Excision of a vein.

**phlebitis**(*fle-bī'-tis*). Inflammation of the veins.

**phlebolith** (*fle-bō-lith*). Calcified venous thrombus.

**phlebothrombosis** (*fle-bo-throm-bō'-sis*). Thrombosis in veins, particularly the veins of the legs, due to prolonged haemostasis.

**Phlebotomus** (*fle-bo'-to-mus*). Genus of disease-carrying flies.

**phlebotomy** (*fle-bo-to-mi*). Bleeding a patient by opening a vein. Venesection.

**phlegm** (*flem*). Thick mucoid expectoration.

**phlegmasia** (*fleg-mā-si-a*). Inflammation. *P. alba dolens*, white leg; a form of phlebitis occurring sometimes after labour. The leg becomes swollen, white and tense, and is very painful.

**phlyctenule** (*flik-te-nūl*). Red pimples on surface of eye. *Phlyctenular conjunctivitis*, a form of disease when phlyctenules appear on the conjunctiva, each becoming the centre of a small inflamed patch. They then rupture, forming a small ulcer which readily heals. *Phlyctenular keratitis*, when cornea is similarly affected.

**phobia** (*fō-bi-a*). Fear of sufficient intensity to affect the life of the patient, *e.g.* cancerophobia, claustrophobia.

**phonation** (*fō-nā-shon*). The utterance of vocal sounds.

**phonetic** (*fo-ne-tik*). Relating to the voice.

**phonocardiogram** (*fō-nō-kar-di-ō-gram*). Instrument recording heart sounds.

**phonocardiograph** (*fō-nō-kah'-di-ō-grahf*). Instrument recording heart sounds.

**phosphate** (*fos-fāt*). Salt of phosphoric acid.

**phosphaturia** (*fos-fa-tū-ri-a*). Excess of phosphates in the urine.

**phospholipid** (*fos-fō-li-pid*). A lipid containing phosphates, *e.g.* lecithin. Phospholipids are particularly useful in living systems for forming membranes. Since they have

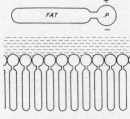

*43. Phospholipids*

a long lipid 'body' with a small charged 'head', the molecules arrange themselves in parallel rows.

**phosphonecrosis** (*fos-fō-ne-krō-sis*). Necrosis of the jaw, caused by inhaling phosphorus; occurs in certain trades, such as match-making, but is rare.

**photobiology** (*fō-tō-bi-o'-lo-ji*). The study of the effect of light on life.

**photochemistry** (*fō-tō-kem'-is-tri*). The study of the effect of light on chemical reactions.

**photophobia** (*fō-to-fō-bi-a*). Intolerance of light.

**photosensitization** (*fō-to-sen-si-tī-zā-shon*). Tendency of tissues to react abnormally to light, usually as the result of the presence in tissues of certain chemicals which magnify the damaging effect of the incident radiation.

**phrenic** (*fre-nik*). Relating to the diaphragm.

**phrenicotomy** (*fren-i-ko'-to-mi*). Division of the phrenic nerve.

**phrenoplegia** (*fre-nō-plē-ji-a*). Paralysis of the diaphragm.

**phrynoderma** (*fri-nō-der-ma*). Follicular keratosis as occurs, for example, in vitamin A deficiency.

**Phthirus pubis** (*thī-rus pū-bis*). The pubic louse.

**phthisis** (*fthi-sis*). Tuberculosis affecting the lungs.

**physic** (*fi-sik*). (1) The art of medicine. (2) Any medicinal preparation.

**physician** (*fi-si'-shon*). Qualified medical practitioner.

**physicist** (*fi-si-sist*). An expert in the science of physics.

**physics.** The science which deals with the forces and forms of nature.

**physiological saline** (*fi-si-ō-lo-ji-kal sā-līn*). A solution, 0·9 per cent, of sodium chloride in water.

**physiology** (*fi-si-o-lo-ji*). The study of processes occurring in living systems.

**physiotherapy** (*fi-zi-ō-the-ra-pi*). Therapy by physical means, *i.e.* heat, light, electricity, massage, etc.

**physique** (*fi-zēk*). The form and constitution of the body.

**phytic acid** (*fī-tik a'-sid*). Substance which prevents absorption of calcium from the gut. Found in wholemeal flour but partially destroyed if yeast is used in preparation of bread.

**pia mater** (*pē-a mā-ter*). The fine membrane surrounding the brain and spinal cord.

**pica** (*pē-ka*). A desire to eat substances unsuitable for food. Occurs most commonly in small children who are emotionally upset.

**Pick's disease** (*piks di-sēz*). (1) Disorder affecting serous membranes resulting in effusions in the peritoneum, pericardium and pleura. The cause is unknown. (2) Presenile dementia due to cerebral atrophy.

**pigment** (*pig-ment*). Coloured material, *e.g.* haemoglobin, melanin.

**piles** (*pīls*). Enlarged veins about the anus; haemorrhoids.

**pilonidal** (*pī-lō-nē-dal*). Containing hair as in some cysts.

**pilonidal sinus** (*pī-lō-nē-dal sī-nus*). Sinus leading from encysted hairs usually in the sacral region.

**pilosis** (*pī-lō-sis*). Abnormal growth of hair.

**pilula** (*pi-lū-la*). A pill; abbreviation, *pil.*

**pineal body** (*pi-nē-al bo-di*). The so-called 'third eye'. Develops from outgrowths of the forebrain, part of which forms an eye-like structure in the lamprey. In man it is a gland-like structure whose function is entirely unknown.

**pinguecula** (*ping-gwe-kū-la*). Small yellow patch of connective tissue on conjunctiva occurring in old age.

**pink disease.** No longer seen. It was a disease of infants caused by mercury in teething powders.

**pink eye** (*pink ī*). Infectious conjunctivitis.

**pinna** (*pin-na*). The outspread part of the ear.

**pinocytosis** (*pi-nō-sī-tō-sis*). Particles are surrounded by cell membrane and are included in the cytoplasm. *See* PHAGOCYTOSIS.

**pint** (*pīnt*). Twenty fluid ounces.

**pipette** (*pi-pet*). A small graduated glass tube for taking up liquids.

**pisiform** (*pē-si-fawm*). Pea-shaped; applied to a bone of the wrist.

**pitting.** Pits are formed in the skin on pressure, as in oedema.

**pituitary gland** ((*pi-tū-i-ta-ri*). Endocrine gland in the base of the skull. There are two lobes separated by a cleft. The *anterior lobe* secretes thyrotrophic hormone (TSH), corticotrophic hormone (ACTH), gonadotrophic hormones (FSH, LH), growth hormone (GH) and prolactin. The *posterior lobe* secretes anti-diuretic hormone (ADH) and oxytocin.

**pityriasis rosea** (*pi-ti-rī-a-sis rō-sē-a*). Skin disease characterized by scaly, erythematous macular eruption. Thought to be caused by a virus related to the measles virus.

**placebo** (*pla-sē-bō*). Medicine made of inert material and flavouring which may be used as a control during trials on an active drug or as a token to satisfy a patient's need for help.

**placenta** (*pla-sen-ta*). The after-birth; a circular flesh-like tissue through which the mother's blood nourishes the fetus; it is expelled from the womb after the birth of the child. *P. praevia.* The placenta attached partially or totally to the lower uterine segment thus endangering the normal delivery of a baby.

**placental barrier** (*pla-sen'-tal ba'-ri-er*). Layer of placental epithelium separating maternal from fetal blood.

**plagiocephaly** (*pla-ji-ō-ke-fa-li*). Type of craniostenosis in which there is unilateral involvement of a coronal or lambdoid suture thus producing an asymmetrical head.

**plague** (*plāg*). An acute epidemic infectious disease caused by *Pasteurella pestis* derived from infected rats and transmitted to man by fleas.

**plantar** (*plan-ta*). Relating to the sole of the foot. *P. response.* Reflex movement of toes when the sole of the foot is stroked.

**plasma** (*plas'-ma*). The liquid in which the cells of the blood are suspended. *P. proteins.* These are *fibrinogen*, *albumin* and *globulins*.

**plasmodium** (*plas-mō-di-um*). *See* MALARIA.

**plaster** (*plas-ter*). (1) Adhesive tape used to secure dressings, etc. (2) Plaster of Paris. Material used to immobilize part of the body.

**plastic surgery.** Restoration of tissue to its normal shape and appearance by operative means.

**platelets** (*plāt-lets*). Blood cells concerned with the clotting of blood.

**platybasia** (*pla-ti-bā-si-a*). Flattening of the base of the skull.

**Platyhelminthes** (*pla-ty-hel-min-thes*). Flat worms.

**pleomorphism** (*plē-ō-maw'-fizm*). Having several different forms.

**plethora** (*ple-tho-ra*). Fullness; an excess of blood.

**pleura** (*plū-ra*). A thin membrane which covers each lung and lines the inner surface of the thoracic cavity.

**pleural rub** (*plū-ral rub*). A grating feeling and sound produced by friction between the layers of the pleura.

**pleurisy** (*plū'-ri-si*). Inflammation of the pleura.

**pleurodynia** (*plū-rō-di-ni-a*). Pain in the side, usually intercostal myalgia. *See* BORNHOLM DISEASE.

**plexor** (*plek'-sor*). Small hammer used in testing deep reflexes, etc.

**plexus** (*plek-sus*). A network of vessels or nerves.

**plica** (*plē-ka*). A fold.

**plicate** (*pli'-kāt*). Folded.

**plombage** (*plom'-bahj*). Filling a cavity with an inert substance.

**plumbism** (*plum-bizm*). Lead-poisoning.

**Plummer-Vinson syndrome** (*plu-mer-vin-son sin-drōm*). Also known as Kelly-Patterson syndrome. Glossitis and dysphagia due to iron deficiency.

**PMB** Abbreviation for post-menopausal bleeding.

**pneumatocele** (*nū-ma'-tō-sēl*). A swelling containing air or gas.

**pneumaturia** (*nū-maptū-ri-a*). Diagnostic feature of vesico-intestinal fistula. Air is passed per urethra.

**pneumococcal** (*nū-mō-ko-kal*). Pertaining to the pneumococcus.

**pneumococcus** (*nū-mō-ko-kus*). A microbe which causes pneumonia. *See* BACTERIA.

**pneumoconiosis** (*nū-mō-kō-ni-ō-sis*). Fibrosis of the lungs caused by working in an atmosphere contaminated with irritant dusts. *See* SILICOSIS, BAGASSOSIS and BYSSINOSIS.

**pneumomycosis** (*nū-mō-mī-kō-sis*). Fungus disease of the lungs.

**pneumonectomy** (*nū-mo-nek-to-mi*). Surgical removal of a lung.

**pneumonia** (*nū-mō'-ni-a*). An

infective disease characterized by inflammation of the lungs. In double pneumonia, both lungs are diseased. *Hypostatic p.* is caused by lack of movement in a debilitated patient. May occur after operation or in the aged. *Lobar p.*, affecting one or more lobes of the lung. *Lobular p.*, see BRONCHO-PNEUMONIA.

**pneumonitis** (*nū-mō-nī'-tis*). Inflammation of the lung.

**pneumoperitoneum** (*nū-mō-pe-ri-to-nē'-um*). Air in the peritoneal cavity.

**pneumothorax** (*nū-mō-tho'-raks*). Air in the pleural space. *Spontaneous p.* Due to rupture of one of the air passages which may lead to a rise in pressure inside the chest (*tension p.*) and difficulty in breathing. *Artificial p.* Air is introduced into the chest through a needle or incision.

**pock** (*pok*). A pustule or the scar left by it.

**podalic version** (*pod-al'-ik ver-shon*). A turning round of the fetus in utero, so that the breech presents in delivery.

**poikilocytosis** (*poy-ki-lō-si-to-sis*). Variation in the form of the red blood cells.

**poison** (*poy'-son*). A substance deleterious to the body if absorbed in toxic concentra-tions. The term is usually reserved for substances which are toxic in low concentrations, *e.g.* cyanide.

**polar body** (*pō-la bo'-di*). Two small cells formed after mitotic division of the primary oocyte.

**polio** (*pō'-li-o*). Prefix denoting grey. Journalese abbreviation of poliomyelitis.

**polioencephalitis** (*pō'-li-ō-en-ke-fa-lī-tis*). Inflammation of the grey matter of the brain.

**poliomyelitis** (*pō-li-ō-mī-e-lī'-tis*). Acute virus-mediated infection causing degeneration of the anterior horn cells of the spinal cord and consequent paralysis of the appropriate muscles.

**Politzer's bag** (*po-lit-zers*). An india-rubber bag with long tube and nozzle. Used for inflating the middle ear through the nose and Eustachian tube.

**pollution** (*pō-lū'-shon*). The act of rendering impure.

**poly-** (*po-li*). A prefix denoting much or many.

**polyarteritis nodosa** (*po-li-ar-te-rī-tis no-dō-sa*). See PERIARTERITIS NODOSA.

**polyarthritis** (*po-li-ar-thrī'-tis*). Inflammation of many joints.

**Polya's operation** (*pol-yus o-pe-rā-shon*). Operation for duodenal ulcer in which the stump of the stomach is anastomosed to the side of the jejunum.

**polychondritis** (*po'-li-kon-drī'-tis*). Inflammation of cartilaginous tissues at several sites in the body.

**polychromasia** (*po-li-krō-mā-si-a*). Term given to staining characteristics of young red blood cells.

**polycystic** (*po-li-sis-tik*). Composed of many cysts.

**polycythaemia** (*po-li-sī-tē-mi-a*). (1) *Primary p.* An increased number of red cells. (2) *Secondary p.* Increase in the number of red blood cells in the blood due to stimulation of the bone marrow, *e.g.* by anoxia at high altitudes or due to respiratory disease.

**polydactyly** (*po-li-dak-ti-li*). The presence of supernumerary fingers or toes.

**polydipsia** (*po-li-dip'-si-a*). Abnormal thirst.

**polyglandular** (*po-li-glan-dū-la*). Pertaining to several glands.

**polyhedral** (*po-li-hē-dral*). Having many surfaces.

**polymazia** (*po-li-mā-zi-a*). Accessory breasts.

**polymenorrhoea** (*po-li-me-no-rē-a*). Frequent menstruation.

**polymorphonuclear** (*po-li-maw-fō-nū-klē-a*). Having nuclei of various shapes.

Name given to the most numerous form of white blood cell, of which there are normally about 70 per cent of total. These are the chief phagocytes, and therefore they are increased in number in the presence of most bacteria.

**polymyositis** (*po-li-mī-ō-sī-tis*). Weakness and wasting of muscles due to inflammation of unknown aetiology.

**polyneuritis** (*po-li-nū-rī-tis*). Multiple neuritis. *Syn.* peripheral neuritis.

**polyopia** (*po-li-ō-pi-a*). Seeing multiple images of the same object.

**polypeptide** (*po-li-pep-tīd*). See PEPTIDE.

**polypoid** (*po-li-poyd*). Like a polypus.

**polyposis intestini** (*po-li-pō-sis in-tes-ti-ni*). Familial adenomatous polyposis of the colon. An inherited disorder. Distinguish from *Peutz-Jehger's intestinal polyposis* in which there is characteristic circumoral pigmentation.

**polypus** (*po-li-pus*). A small tumour occurring in the ear, nose, uterus or rectum.

**polysaccharides** (*po-li-sa-ka-rīds*). A group of carbohydrates which contain more than two molecules of simple carbohydrates combined with each other, *e.g.* starch, glycogen.

**polyuria** (*po-li-ū-ri-a*). Excessive production of urine.

**polyvalent** (*po-li-vā-lent*). As applied to sera, meaning those which are active against many different strains of the same micro-organisms.

**pompholyx** (*pom-fō-liks*). A vesicular eruption occurring on the palms and soles. Probably a form of eczema.

**pons.** Part of the brain stem between the medulla oblongata and the thalamus.

**pontine** (*pon-tēn*). Pertaining to the pons.

**POP.** Persistent occipito-posterior presentation of fetus.

**popliteal** (*pop-li-tē-al*). Pertaining to the popliteal space, the area behind the knee.

**pore** (*paw*). A small space.

**porphyria** (*paw-fi-ri-a*). General term used to describe a variety of syndromes due to an excess of porphyrins in the blood and tissues.

**porphyrins** (*paw-fi-rins*). Pyrrole derivatives produced in the metabolism of haemoglobin.

**portal hypertension** (*paw-tal hī-per-ten-shon*). Hypertension in the hepatic portal system usually resulting from cirrhosis of the liver.

**portal vein** (*paw-tal vān*). A vein carrying blood between capillary networks, usually *hepatic portal vein.*

**position** (*po-si-shon*). Attitude or posture.

**positive pressure ventilation** (*po'-zi-tiv pre'sher-ven-ti-lā'-shon*). Artificial respiration by blowing air into the lungs.

**posological** (*pō-sō-lo-ji-kal*). Pertaining to dosage.

**posset** (*po'-set*). In infant feeding, to regurgitate a feed.

**post.** Behind or after.

**postclimacteric** (*pōst-klī-mak-te-rik*). After the menopause.

**postdiphtheritic paralysis** (*pōst-dif-the-ri-tik pa-ra-li-sis*). Paralysis as a result of the diphtheria toxin acting on the nervous system. These may be palatal, ocular, cardiac, pharyngeal, laryngeal and respiratory paralysis.

**postencephalitis** (*pōst-en-kef-a-lī'-tis*). Condition which may remain after encephalitis.

**posterior chamber of eye** (*post-ār-i-or chām-ber*). Small space lying behind the iris and containing aqueous humour.

**posterior nerve root.** Dorsal nerve root. *See* NERVE ROOT.

**postganglionic** (*pōst-gang-gli-o'-nik*). Behind or after a ganglion.

**postgastrectomy syndrome** (*pōst-gas-trek-to-mi sin'-drōm*). A number of syndromes may follow gastrectomy including dumping syndrome hypoglycaemic attacks and malnutrition.

**posthumous** (*pos-tū-mus*). After death.

**postmaturity** (*pōst-ma-tū-ri-ti*). Birth of an infant considered to have matured beyond the normal fetal stage. More than one of the following criteria should be satisfied: pregnancy exceeding 290 days; fetal length exceeding 54 cm; fetal weight exceeding 4 kg (about 8¾ lb). The skin is often dry and scaling, the nails may have grown beyond the ends of the fingers and toes and the liquor may be stained with meconium.

**post mortem** (*pōst maw-tem*). After death. Usually *post mortem examination*. See NECROPSY.

**post-natal** (*pōst-nā-tal*). Following birth.

**postoperative** (*pōst-op-er-a-tiv*). After operation.

**post-partum** (*pōst-par'-tum*). After labour. *Post-partum haemorrhage* is excessive vaginal bleeding occurring either immediately after the birth of the baby (primary), or within a few days (secondary).

**postprandial** (*pōst-pran'-di-al*). After meals.

**postural** (*pos-tū-ral*). Pertaining to posture, *e.g. postural drainage*, position adopted to facilitate expectoration of material in lung diseases.

**post-vaccinial** (*pōst-vak-si-ni-al*). Occurring after vaccination.

**potential** (*pō-ten-shal*). (1) Capability; *e.g. potential space*, a space which is capable of forming. (2) *Electrical potential*, the tendency of electrons to flow in a specified direction, measured in volts.

**Pott's disease.** Tuberculosis of the spine.

**Pott's fracture** (*frak-tūr*). Fracture-dislocation of the ankle in which the fibula and the medial malleolus are fractured with lateral displacement of the foot.

**pouch of Douglas** (*powch*). See DOUGLAS'S POUCH.

**pouch, pharyngeal** (*fa-rin-jē-al*). See PHARYNGEAL POUCH.

**pouch, postprostatic** (*powch pōst-pro-sta-tik*). Diverticulum of the bladder which sometimes develops behind a hypertrophied middle lobe of the prostate.

**pouch, urethral** (*ū-rē-thral*). Diverticulum of the male urethra.

**poultices** (*pōl-ti-sis*). Hot moist

material applied as an external counter-irritant.

**Poupart's ligament** (*poo-pahts*). The ligament of the groin, stretching between the anterior superior spine of the ilium and the os pubis.

**poxviruses** (*poks'-vī'-ru-sez*). Group of large DNA viruses associated with vaccinia, variola and allied animal diseases.

**p.p.m.** Parts per million.

**p.r.** Per rectum. Examination made with one finger in the rectum, by which information can be obtained of the condition of the rectum and adjacent structures.

**preauricular sinus** (*prē-aw-ri-kū-la sī-nus*). Opening at the root of the tragus of the ear due to imperfect fusion of the processes which form the ear.

**precancerous** (*prē-kan-se-rus*). A state before a cancer has arisen but which may become cancerous.

**precipitate labour** (*pre-si-pi-tāt lā-ber*). Labour which is concluded in a time very much shorter than the average.

**precipitation** (*pre-si-pi-tā-shon*). The process of separating solids from the liquids which hold them in solution, by the application of heat or cold, or the addition of chemicals.

**precipitins** (*pre-si-pi-tins*). Antibodies.

**precocious puberty** (*pre-kō-shus pū-ber-ti*). Two groups are recognized. (*a*) Those in which true sexual maturity is reached at an early age and in which ovulation or spermatogenesis commences, and (*b*) those in which there are advanced secondary sex changes but no spermatogenesis or ovulation occur.

**precordium** (*prē-caw-di-um*). The area of the chest over the heart.

**precursor** (*prē-ker-ser*). Forerunner.

**predigestion** (*prē-di-jes-chon*). Breakdown of foodstuffs before ingestion.

**predisposed** (*prē-dis-pōsd*). Susceptible.

**pre-eclampsia** (*prē-ek-lamp-si-a*). State before eclampsia develops and when it can still be prevented. There is proteinuria, raised blood pressure and swelling of the ankles.

**prefrontal** (*prē-fron-tal*). Lying in the anterior part of the frontal lobe of the brain. *P. leucotomy. See* LEUCOTOMY.

**pregnancy** (*preg-nan-si*). The state of being with child. Usual period 280 days. *See also* ECTOPIC GESTATION.

**premature labour** (*pre-ma-tūr lā-ber*). Labour at or before 36 weeks of gestation and resulting in birth of a premature baby, *i.e.* one weighing 5½ lb or less.

**premedication** (*prē-me-di-kā-shon*). Drug given as a narcotic before a general anaesthetic.

**premenstrual** (*prē-men-stroo-al*). Before menstruation. *P. tension syndrome*. Syndrome consisting of tension, anxiety, aches, depression and often accident-proneness which occurs for a few days before menstrual period in some women. It is thought to be hormonal in origin.

**premolar** (*prē-mō-la*). The two bicuspid teeth in each jaw which lie between the canine and the molars. *See* TEETH.

**premonitory** (*prē-mo-ni-to-ri*). Giving warning beforehand.

**prenatal** (*prē-nā-tal*). Prior to birth, during the period of pregnancy.

**prepuce** (*pre-poos'*). Loose skin covering the glans penis: foreskin.

**presbyopia** (*pres-bi-ō-pi-a*). Long-sightedness due to inability to make the lens of the eye convex by contraction of the ciliary muscles, *i.e.* failure of adaptation of the lens.

**prescription** (*pres-krip-shon*). A formula written by the physician to the dispenser. Consists of the heading, usually the symbol R̸ meaning 'take', the names and quantities of the ingredients, the directions to the dispenser, the directions to the patient, the date and the signature.

**presentation** (*pres-sen-tā'-shon*). The part of the fetus which first engages or tends to engage in the pelvis is said *to present*, and the description of this part is the presentation.

**presenting symptom** (*prē-sen-ting simp'-tom*). The symptom of a disease which causes the patient to seek medical advice.

**pressor** (*pre-sor*). Substance causing rise in blood pressure, *e.g. P. amines* are substances such as noradrenaline and adrenaline which constrict the blood vessels and cause an elevation of the blood pressure.

**pressure areas** (*pre-sher ā-rē-us*). Parts of the body where the bone is near the skin surface and where a pressure sore is likely to occur if there is prolonged pressure owing to diminished blood supply to these parts.

**pressure points** (*pre'-sher poynts*). Points at which

pressure may be applied to check haemorrhage.

**presytole** (*prē-sis-to-lē*). Period in the cardiac cycle before systole.

**priapism** (*prī-a-pism*). Painful erection of the penis.

**prickle cells** (*pri-kel*). Epidermal cells. So called because they have specialized areas of attachment to each other (called *desmosomes*) which allow extracellular fluid to circulate between them. In fixed microscopic preparations these regions of attachment look like tiny interlocking spines.

**prickly heat.** Miliaria papillosa.

**primary focus** (*prī-ma-ri fō-kus*). First site of infection in tuberculosis. Healing usually takes place uneventfully.

**primary lesion** (*prī-ma-ri le-jon*). Original lesion from which others may arise.

**primary sore.** Initial site of infection in syphilis.

**primigravida** (*pri'-mi-gra'-vi-da*). A woman pregnant for the first time.

**primipara** (*prī-mi-pa-ra*). A woman who has borne one child.

**primordial** (*prī-maw-di-al*). Pertaining to the beginning.

**probe** (*prōb*). A slender rod, sometimes of silver, used for exploring wounds.

**process** (*prō-ses*). A prolonga-tion or eminence of a part.

**procidentia** (*pro-si-den-shi-a*). Prolapse. A falling down.

**proctalgia** (*prōk-tal-ji-a*). Pain about the rectum.

**proctectomy** (*prok-tek-to-mi*). Excision of rectum.

**proctitis** (*prok-tī-tīs*). Inflam-mation of the rectum.

**proctocele** (*prok-tō-sēl*). Pro-lapsed rectum.

**proctoclysis** (*prok-tō-klī-sis*). Introduction into the rectum of saline solution for absorp-tion.

**proctorrhaphy** (*prok-to'-ra-fi*). Suturing of the rectum.

**proctoscope** (*prok-tō-skōp*). An instrument for viewing the interior of the rectum.

**prodromal period** (*prō-drō-mal pā-ri-od*). The period that elapses in an infectious dis-ease between the appearance of the first symptoms and the development of the rash, *e.g.* in smallpox, three days.

**progeria** (*prō-je-ri-a*). A con-dition in which premature senility is combined with infantilism.

**progesterone** (*prō-jes-te-rōn*). A steroid hormone secreted by the corpus luteum respon-sible for preparing the repro-ductive organs for pregnancy and for maintaining these changes if pregnancy occurs. A synthetic form used with oestrogen in the contraceptive pill.

**proglottis** (*pro-glo-tis*). Segment of tapeworm.

**prognosis** (*prog-nō-sis*). The considered opinion as to the course of a disease.

**progressive muscular atrophy** (*prō-gre-siv mus-kū-la a-tro-fi*). Loss of power and wasting of muscles. Degenerative changes are found in the motor cells of the brain and anterior horns of the spinal cord. *See also* MOTOR NEURONE DISEASE.

**projection** (*pro-jek-shon*). Painful thoughts, feelings and motives are relieved by transferring them on to someone else, *e.g.* blaming one's own mistake on to another person.

**prolactin** (*prō-lak-tin*). Milk-producing hormone of the anterior lobe of the pituitary.

**prolapse** (*prō-laps*). Falling forwards or downwards.

**proliferation** (*prō-li-fe-rā-shon*). Reproduction. Cell genesis.

**promontory** (*pro-mon-tō-ri*). A projecting part. An eminence.

**pronation** (*prō-nā-shon*). Downward turning of the palm of the hand.

**prone** (*prōn*). Lying with the face downward.

**propensity** (*prō-pen'-si-ti*). Inclination or tendency.

**prophylactic** (*pro-fi-lak-tik*). Tending to prevent disease.

**proprietary** (*prō-prī-e-ta-ri*). A remedy with a registered trade name.

**proprioceptor** (*prō-pri-ō-sep-tor*). Sensory end organ which detects changes in position, *e.g.* of muscles or joints or fluid in the balancing apparatus of the inner ear.

**proptosis oculi** (*prop-tō-sis o-kū-lī*). Protrusion of eyeballs.

**prostaglandins** (*pros'-ta-glan'-dinz*). Group of substances extractable from prostate gland, seminal vesicles and plasma. Role in physiology remains undetermined and properties are not fully understood, but they are powerful stimulators of smooth muscle contraction.

**prostate** (*pros-tāt*). A gland associated with the male reproductive system. Its size and secretion are under the influence of androgens. Its function is not clear but it appears to supply supportive substances to the spermatozoa in the seminal vesicles.

**prostatectomy** (*pros-ta-tek-to-mi*). Operation of removing the prostate gland. The operation may be suprapubic when the bladder is first incised, or retropubic, *see* MILLIN'S PROSTATECTOMY, or transurethral.

**prostatic** (*pros-ta-tik*). Pertaining to the prostate. *P. bar.* Form of benign prostatic enlargement.

**prostatitis** (*pros-ta-tī-tis*). Inflammation of the prostate gland.

**prosthesis** (*pros-thē-sis*). The replacement of an absent limb or organ by an artificial apparatus.

**prostration** (*pros-trā-shon*). Extreme exhaustion.

**protein** (*pro-tēn*). Very complex organic compound, made up of a large number of amino-acids, which are synthesized by living systems, *see* NUCLEIC ACIDS. There are twenty different amino-acids commonly found in proteins and these are arranged in different sequences which give the specific characteristics to the proteins.

**proteinuria** (*prō-tē-nū-ri-a*). Protein in the urine.

**proteolysis** (*prō-tē-ō-lī'-sis*). The breakdown of proteins to form polypeptides, peptides and amino-acids.

**proteolytic enzymes** (*prō-tē-ō-li-tik en-zīms*). Enzymes capable of proteolysis. Several different such

enzymes are usually required to digest protein.

**prothrombin** (*prō-throm-bin*). The precursor of thrombin. *See* BLOOD COAGULATION.

**protoplasm** (*prō-tō-plas-m*). The substance of a cell, thus excluding material which has been ingested or is to be secreted.

**prototype** (*prō-tō-tīp*). The original form from which others are copied.

**protozoa** (*prō-tō-zō-a*). A class of unicellular organisms forming the lowest division of the animal kingdom, *e.g.* amoeba.

**proud flesh** (*prowd*). Excessive granulation tissue in a wound.

**provitamin** (*prō-vi-ta-min*). A precursor of a vitamin.

**proximal** (*proksi-mal*). Nearest to the centre.

**prurigo** (*proo-rī-gō*). A skin disease marked by irritating papules.

**pruritus** (*proo-rī-tus*). Itching.

**pseudarthrosis** (*sūd-ar-thrō-sis*). A false joint.

**pseudo** (*sū-dō*). A prefix meaning false or spurious.

**pseudo-angina** (*sū-dō-an-ji-na*). A neurotic disease resembling angina pectoris.

**pseudo bulbar palsy** (*sū-dō-bul-ba pawl-si*). A form of motor neurone disease affecting the nerves arising from the brain stem.

**pseudocoxalgia** (*sū-dō-kok-sal-ji-a*). *See* PERTHE'S DISEASE.

**pseudocyesis** (*sū-dō-sī-ē-sis*). Changes mimicking pregnancy but without a fetus.

**pseudohermaphrodite** (*sū-dō-her-ma-frō-dit*). Individual in whom the secondary sexual characteristics do not correspond to the generative organs. In females this may be due to hypersecretion of androgens by the adrenal cortex. In males the condition is genetically determined and presumably due to a metabolic abnormality whereby oestrogens are produced by the adrenal cortex or by the testes. In true hermaphroditism there is ambivalence in the development of the organs of generation.

**pseudomyxoma peritonei** (*sū-dō-mik-sō-ma pe-ri-tō-nā-ē*). Condition in which rupture of ovarian cyst or mucocele of the appendix gives rise to huge jelly-filled cysts throughout the peritoneal cavity.

**pseudopodium** (*sū-dō-pō-di-um*). Temporary protrusion of cell serving as method of locomotion and phagocytosis.

**psittacosis** (*si-ta-kō-sis*). A virus disease found in parrots and other birds which is communicable to man. It manifests itself as an atypical pneumonia.

**psoas** (*sō'-as*). An important muscle attached above to the lumbar vertebrae and below to the femur. It flexes the femur on the trunk. *P. abscess. See* ABSCESS.

**psoriasis** (*so-rī-a-sis*). Abnormality of keratinization producing skin lesions consisting of raised, red, scaly areas.

**psyche** (*sī-kē*). The mind.

**psychiatric social worker** (*sī-kē-a-trik sō-shal*). One who works under a psychiatrist to rehabilitate mentally ill people.

**psychiatrist** (*si-kī-a-trist*). A physician who specializes in psychiatry.

**psychiatry** (*si-kī-a-tri*). The study and treatment of mental disorders.

**psychical** (*si-ki-kal*). Relating to the mind.

**psycho-analysis** (*sī-kō-a-na-li-sis*). A method of treatment for psychiatric conditions based on Freudian theories whereby relief is allegedly obtained by tracing neuroses to their genesis.

**psychogenic** (*sī-kō-je'-nik*). Originating in the mind.

**psychologist** (*sī-ko'-lo-jist*). One who studies psychology.

**psychology** (*sī-kō-lo-ji*). The study of behaviour patterns.

**psychoneurosis** (*sī-kō-nū-rō-sis*). *See* NEUROSIS.

**psychopath** (*sī-kō-path*). Somebody suffering from a severe personality disorder.

**psychopathology** (*si-kō-pa-tho-lo-ji*). The pathology of mental diseases.

**psychosis** (*sī-ko-sis*). An organic disorder of the mind.

**psychosomatic** (*sī-kō-sō-ma'tik*). Relating to mind and body.

**psychotherapeutics, psychotherapy** (*sī-kō-the-ra-pū-tiks, si-kō-the-ra-pi*). Treatment of the mind. A term which includes any treatment for functional nervous disorders, *e.g.* by hypnotism, suggestion, psycho-analysis, etc.

**psychotic** (*sī-ko-tik*). Relating to a psychosis.

**pterygium** (*te-ri-ji-um*). Mucous membrane growing on the conjunctiva and tending to grow on to the cornea.

**pterygoid** (*te'-ri-goyd*). Literally, wing-shaped.

**pterion** (*te-ri-on*). The point of junction of the frontal, parietal, temporal and sphenoidal bones.

**ptosis** (*tō-sis*). Drooping of the upper eyelid.

**ptyalin** (*ti-a-lin*). An enzyme found in saliva which can digest starch (amylase).

**ptyalism** (*tī-a-lism*). Excessive salivation.

**puberty** (*pū'-ber-ti*). The period of sexual development.

**pubes** (*pū-bēs*). The pubic bones.

**pubiotomy** (*pū-bi-o-to-mi*). Cutting the pubis; an operation sometimes performed to enlarge a contracted pelvis and so facilitate delivery.

**pudenda** (*pū-den-da*). The external genital organs.

**pudendal block** (*pū-den'-del blok*). Method of anaesthesia in second stage of labour by injecting pudendal nerves transvaginally.

**puerperal** (*pū-er-pe-ral*). Relating to the 6 weeks following childbirth. *P. fever.* Fever associated with sepsis of the genital tract following delivery. Elevation of temperature on about the tenth day of the puerperium may be a sign of phlebothrombosis. *P. psychosis.* Psychosis occasionally occurring after delivery probably due to hormonal alterations occurring at that time.

**puerperium** (*pū-er-pār-i-um*). The period after a confinement until the uterus is involuted.

**Pulex irritans** (*pū-leks i-ri-tans*). Common flea. *See* FLEA.

**pulmonary** (*pul-mo-na-ri*). Relating to the lungs.

**pulmonary embolism** (*pul-*

*mo-na-ri em-bo-lism*). *See*
EMBOLISM.

**pulmonary eosinophilia** (*ē-ō-si-nō-fi-li-a*). A group of conditions characterized by a varying degree of cough, constitutional disturbance, infiltration of the lungs and eosinophilia of the blood. The major causes of this syndrome are infestation by worms such as microfilaria and the larvae of *Ascaris lumbricoides* or infection by a fungus, *e.g.* aspergillus. It also occurs in periarteritis nodosa and in asthma.

**pulmonary hypertension** (*pul-mo-na-ri hī-per-ten-shon*). Increase of the pressure in the pulmonary circulation.

**pulmonary oedema** (*e-dē-ma*). Exudation of fluid into the lungs.

**pulmonary stenosis** (*ste-nō'-sis*). Narrowing of the pulmonary valve of the heart.

**pulmonary valve.** The valve at the exit of the right ventricle into the pulmonary artery.

**pulp.** The interior, fleshy part of vegetable or animal tissue.

**pulsation** (*pul-sā-shon*). Beating of the heart, or of the blood in the arteries.

**pulse.** *See* ANACROTIC.

**pulsus alternans** (*pul-sus ōl-ter-nans*). Alternate weak and strong pulse waves.

**pulsus bisferiens** (*pul-sus bis-fe-ri-ens*). Double pulse wave which occurs in patients with combined aortic stenosis and regurgitation.

**pulsus paradoxus** (*pa-ra-dok-sus*). The pulse decreases on inspiration and may disappear. It is the result of pericardial constriction.

**pulvis.** A powder.

**punctate** (*punk-tāt*). Dotted.

**puncture** (*punk-cher*). To make a hole with a sharp instrument.

**pupa** (*pū-pa*). Second stage of insect development following the larval stage.

**pupil** (*pū-pil*). The orifice in the centre of the iris.

**pupillary** (*pū-pi-la-ri*). Pertaining to the pupil.

**purgative** (*per-ja-tiv*). A medicine for causing evacuation of the bowels.

**purine** (*pū-rēn*). Organic nitrogen-containing base.

**Purkinje cells** (*per-kin'-ji selz*). Nerve cells found in the cortex of the cerebellum.

**purpura** (*per-pū-ra*). Purple-coloured spots due to haemorrhage into the tissues. There are many causes of purpura which may be roughly categorized as due to: (*a*) deficiency of clotting mechanism, *e.g.* essential thrombocytopaenia; (*b*) capillary damage; (*c*) both.

293 **PYL**

**purpura, Henoch-Schönlein**
(*per-pū-ra hĕ-nock shern-līn*). This is a syndrome also
known as anaphylactoid pur-
pura characterized by
urticaria, pain, and effusions
into the joints, intestinal
bleeding and colic and purpura. Usually occurs in children and often follows a
streptococcal throat infection.

**purulent** (*pu-roo-lent*). Pus-
like.

**pus.** Matter. Consists of dead
leucocytes in an albuminous
fluid.

**pustula maligna** (*pus-tū-là ma-
lig-na*). Anthrax.

**pustulation** (*pus-tū-lā-shon*).
The formation of pustules.

**pustule** (*pus-tūl*). A pimple containing pus.

**putrefaction** (*pū-tre-fak-shon*).
The rotting away of animal
matter. Decomposition ad-
vanced to an offensive stage.

**p.v.** Abbreviation for per vaginam. Examination of the
pelvic organs by inspection or
palpation through the vagina.

**pyaemia** (*pī-ē-mi-a*). The circulation of septic emboli in the
bloodstream causing mul-
tiple abscesses.

**pyarthrosis** (*pī-ar-thrō-sis*).
Suppuration in a joint.

**pyelitis** (*pī-e-lī-tis*). Inflammation of the kidney.

**pyelography** (*pī-e-lo-gra-fi*). To

demonstrate kidneys, ureters
and bladder following intravenous injection of contrast
medium opaque to x-rays.
*Retrograde p.* To demon-
strate kidneys and ureters
following introduction of
ureteric catheter into which
contrast medium is injected.

**pyelolithotomy** (*pī-e-lō-li-tho-
to-mi*). Operation to remove
a stone from the renal
pelvis.

**pyelonephritis** (*pī-e-lō-nef-rī-
tis*). Inflammation of the kidney and its pelvis.

**pyknic.** A body type which
tends to be thick set.

**pyknosis** (*pik-nō-sis*). Contraction of nuclear material to
form a dense mass. Often
seen preceding cellular
death.

**pylorectomy** (*pī-lo-rek-to-mi*).
Removal of the pyloric end of
the stomach.

**pyloric stenosis** (*pī-lo-rik ste-
nō-sis*). Narrowing of the
pylorus. (1) A condition
found in infants, more commonly male than female. It is
not apparently present at
birth and is usually noted
after the age of ten days. Pro-
jectile vomiting after all
feeds, constipation, wasting,
are the chief symptoms, while
on examination visible peristalsis may be present and a
hard tumour to the right of

the umbilicus may be felt. Condition is supposed to be due to muscular spasm and consequent hypertrophy of muscle surrounding the pylorus, so preventing the passage of food. The stomach is always dilated. The condition can be treated in its early stages by gastric lavage, and small and frequent feeds; but once a tumour is felt, it is best to open the abdomen and divide hypertrophied muscle (Ramstedt's operation). (2) In adults when it is usually due to a gastric ulcer, or to a neoplasm.

**pyloroplasty** (*pī-lo-rō-plas-ti*). Operation for widening a contracted pylorus.

**pylorus** (*pī'-lor'-us*). Region of the junction between the stomach and the duodenum. There is a thickening of the circular muscle at this point which acts as a sphincter allowing the passage of food out of the stomach.

**pyocolpos** (*pī-ō-kol-pos*). Pus retained in the vagina.

**pyoderma** (*pī-ō-der-ma*). Any septic skin lesion.

**pyogenic** (*pī-ō-je-nik*). Pus-producing, forming pus.

**pyometra** (*pī-ō-mē-tra*). Pus retained in the uterus.

**pyonephrosis** (*pī-ō-nef-rō-sis*). Pus in the kidney.

**pyopericardium** (*pī-ō-pe-ri-*kar-di-um*). Pus in the pericardium.

**pyopneumothorax** (*pī-ō-nū-mō-tho-raks*). Pus and air in the pleural cavity.

**pyorrhoea** (*pī-o-rē-a*). A flow of pus. Generally used as meaning the same as *P. alveolaris*, a condition in which pus oozes out from the gums around the roots of the teeth. This is also known as Rigg's disease.

**pyosalpinx** (*pī-ō-sal-pinks*). Abscess in one of the Fallopian tubes.

**pyramid** (*pi-ra-mid*). Elevation on the medulla oblongata caused by the pyramidal tract.

**pyramidal** (*pi-ra-mi-dal*). Shaped like a pyramid. *P. cells*. Cells in the cerebral cortex giving out impulses to voluntary muscles. *P. system*. Tracts in the brain and spinal cord transmitting impulses from the pyramidal cells.

**pyrexia** (*pī-rek-si-a*). Fever. Elevation of the body temperature. *Intermittent p.* Temperature is high at night but below normal in the morning. *Remittent p.* Temperature high at night, less in the morning, but never reaching normal.

**pyridoxin** (*pi-ri-dok-sin*). Formerly called vitamin $B_6$.

Required as coenzyme in cell metabolism.

**pyrosis** (*pī-rō-sis*). *See* HEART-BURN.

**pyuria** (*pī-yū-ri-a*). Pus in the urine.

## Q

**'Q' fever.** Also called Queensland fever. An acute disease resembling pneumonia and caused by *Rickettsia burneti*.

**quack** (*kwak*). One who pretends to knowledge or skill, usually medical, which he does not possess.

**quadriceps** (*kwod'-ri-seps*). Four-headed: name given to four separate muscles, covering the front of the thigh, which are all inserted into the tubercle of the tibia, and extend the knee.

**quadriplegia** (*kwo-dri-plē-ji-a*). Paralysis of both legs and arms. Also known as tetraplegia.

**quarantine** (*kwo-ran-tēn*). A period of separation of infected persons or contacts from others, and which is necessary to prevent the spread of disease.

**quartan** (*kwaw'-tan*). *See* MALARIA.

**Queckenstedt's test** (*kwe-ken-stetz*). To elicit the presence of spinal block, *e.g.* tumour. A lumbar puncture is per-formed. If the manometer shows no increase of intraspinal pressure when the jugular veins are pressed, there is spinal block.

**quickening** (*kwik'-ning*). The first perception of movement of the fetus in the womb, usually felt by the mother at the end of the fourth month.

**quiescent** (*kwē-es-sent*). Not active. Dormant.

**quinsy** (*kwin'-zē*). A peritonsillar abscess, situated immediately outside the capsule of the tonsil. *See* TONSILLITIS.

**quotient** (*kwō-shent*). Result obtained by dividing one quantity by another.

## R

**rabies** (*rā'-bēz*). A specific and fatal infective disease which chiefly affects rodents and canines; transmissible to man through the saliva by means of a bite from an infected dog. Also called HYDRO-PHOBIA.

**racemose** (*ra'-sē-mōs*). Resembling a bunch of grapes. *R. glands.* Having the cells arranged in saccules with numerous ducts leading to a main duct, *e.g.* salivary glands.

**rachis** (*ra'-kis*). The spine.

**rachitic** (*ra-ki'-tik*). Due to rickets.

**rachitis** (*ra-ki'-tis*). *See* RICKETS.

**rad.** Formerly a unit of measurement for energy absorbed by tissue exposed to x or gamma radiation. Replaced by gray (Gy).

**radial** (*rā-di-el*). Relating to radius.

**radiation** (*rā-di-ā'-shon*). Emanation of energy from a source. The energy may be in a number of different forms. The usual form is that of *photons* which according to their frequency of emission are known as radio-waves, light, x-rays, gamma rays, etc. Subatomic particles such as *electrons, neutrons, protons,* and *positrons, mesons* and many subnuclear particles may also be radiated. Most of these latter particles have such short life-spans that they scarcely travel any appreciable distance from the source and therefore they are of limited interest in biology. Helium nuclei, two protons and two neutrons, have a short track length but are sometimes used to irradiate biological material. They are a natural product of certain radioactive elements and are known as α-rays. High-energy neutrons may be produced by atomic explosions and certain special equipment. Electrons are also a natural product of radioactivity and are known as β-rays. Radiation damages living tissue. *R. sickness.* Illness resulting from overexposure to radiation.

**radical** (*ra'-di-kal*). That which goes to the root; thus radical treatment aims at an absolute cure, not palliation.

**radiculitis** (*ra-di-kū-lī-tis*). Neuritis affecting the nerve root.

**radioactive fallout** (*rā-di-ō-ak'-tiv fawl-owt*). Radioactive isotopes distributed in the atmosphere as the result of atomic explosions. It constitutes a biological hazard since isotopes may be ingested in food.

**radioactive isotopes** (*rā-di-ō-ak'-tiv ī-sō-tōps'*). Radioisotopes. Variants of elements which exhibit the same chemical properties as those elements but which have a greater number of neutrons in their nucleus, *i.e.* have a higher atomic number. For example radioactive carbon $C^{14}$ (usually written $^{14}C$) has an excess of 2 neutrons over ordinary carbon $^{12}C$. There is a tendency for $^{14}C$ to decompose giving rise to $^{12}C$. As a result of this decomposition energy is emitted, which in the case of radioactive carbon is in the form of electrons (β-rays, *see* p. 58).

**radioactivity** (*rā-di-ō-ak-ti'-vi-ti*). Spontaneous decomposition of an element with emission of energy.

**radiobiology** (*rā'-di-ō-bī-o'-lo-ji*). The study of the effects of radiation of living tissue.

**radiographer** (*rā-di-o'-gra-fer*). Person trained to take x-rays.

**radiography** (*rā-di-o'-gra-fi*). Science of examination by means of x-rays.

**radiologist** (*rā-di-o'-lo-jist*). A doctor who has made a special study of radiology.

**radiology** (*rā-di-o-lo-ji*). Study of diagnosis by means of x-rays.

**radiosensitive** (*rā'-di-ō-sen'-si-tiv*). Term applied to a structure, especially a tumour, responsive to radiotherapy.

**radiotherapy** (*rā'-di-ō-the'-ra-pi*). Treatment of disease by radiation.

**radium** (*rā'-di-um*). Natural radioactive element.

**radius** (*rā'-di-us*). The outer bone of the forearm.

**radon** (*rā-don*). Radioactive gas derived from radium. *R. seeds.* Sealed containers of radon.

**râle** (*rahl*). Slight rattling sound heard in the air passages upon auscultation.

**Ramstedt's operation** (*ram-stets*). *See* PYLORIC STENOSIS.

**ramus** (*rā-mus*). A branch, thus ramification of vessels.

**ranula** (*ra-nū-la*). Cyst of mucous gland.

**raphe** (*rā'-fē*). Fibrous junction between muscles.

**rapport** (*ra-paw'*). A good relationship between two people.

**rarefaction** (*rār-e-fak-shon*). The process of becoming less dense.

**rash.** Skin eruption.

**rat-bite fever** (*rat-bīt fē-ver*). Disease which occurs in China and Japan. It is conveyed by the bite of an infected rat. The organism is known as the *Spirillum minus.*

**Rathke's pouch** (*rath-kes powch*). Diverticulum in the roof of the developing mouth which becomes part of the pituitary gland.

**rationalization** (*ra-sho-na-lī-zā-shon*). A justification to oneself of one's action or behaviour. The explanation is based on unconscious or instinctive motives.

**raucous** (*raw-kus*). Hoarse.

**ray fungus.** The organism which causes actinomycosis.

**Raynaud's syndrome** (*rā-nōs sin'-drōm*). Syndrome characterized by intense spasm of the digital arteries producing cold, white, pulseless fingers often associated with impairment of sensation and fine movement. There are many possible causes, one of which is *Raynaud's disease* which is an idiopathic hypersensitivity of the digital vessels to cold.

**reaction** (*rē-ak-shon*). Response to stimulus.

**reagent** (*rē-ā-jent*). An agent taking part in a reaction.

**recalcitrant** (*re-kal'-si-trant*). Resistant, especially of a disease to its treatment.

**recall** (*re-kawl'*). Bring back a memory.

**receptaculum chyli** (*rē-sep-ta-kū-lum kī-lē*). The lower expanded portion of the thoracic duct.

**receptor** (*re-sep'-tor*). A sense organ which receives stimuli, *e.g.* light, sound, vibration, movement, pressure, etc. and converts this information into nerve impulses which are transmitted via the sensory nerves.

**recessive** (*re-se'-siv*). Tending to disappear. In *genetics*: a gene which tends not to be expressed unless it is present in a homozygous state, *cf. dominant.*

**recipient** (*re-si-pi-ent*). One who receives, *e.g.* recipient of blood transfusion.

**Recklinghausen's disease** (*rek-ling-how-sens*). See NEUROFIBROMA.

**recrudescence** (*re-kroo-de-sens*). Return of symptoms.

**rectal** (*rek'-tal*). Relating to the rectum.

**rectocele** (*rek'-tō-sēl*). Prolapse of posterior vaginal wall. Strictly the term applies to any herniation of the rectum.

**rectopexy** (*rek-to-pek'-si*). Surgical procedure to fix a prolapsed rectum.

**rectoscope** (*rek'-tō-skōp*). Proctoscope.

**rectosigmoidectomy** (*rek-tō-sig-moy-dek-to-mi*). Operation to excise the rectum and the sigmoid colon.

**rectovesical** (*rek-tō-ve-sī-kal*). Of the rectum and bladder.

**rectum** (*rek'-tum*). The lower part of the large intestine from the colon to the anal canal. *See* BOWEL.

**rectus** (*rek'-tus*). Straight; applied to certain muscles. *R. abdominis.* Two external abdominal muscles, one each side of the mid-line, running from pubic bone to ensiform cartilage and the fifth, sixth and seventh ribs. It is enclosed in a strong sheath. There are also four short muscles of the eye, external, internal, superior and inferior rectus. *R. femoris.* Muscle on the front of the thigh, one of the four forming the quadriceps extensor.

**recumbent** (*re-kum'-bent*). Lying down.

**recuperate** (*re-kū-pe-rāt*). To get better.

**recurrent** (*re-ku-rent*). Returning. *R. laryngeal nerve* is so-called because this branch of the vagus, *see* CRANIAL NERVES 10, comes back from below the thyroid to supply the larynx.

**red blood cell or corpuscle.** These are the blood cells which contain haemoglobin (*erythrocytes*). There are about 5,000,000 in each ml of blood and they carry nearly all the oxygen required by the body cells. Red blood cells are formed in the bone marrow, normally at a rate of about a million a second and are notable for the absence of a nucleus in the mature state. They do not divide and have a lifetime of about 120 days when they are destroyed in the spleen.

**reduction** (*re-duk-shon*). (1) Replacing to a normal position, *e.g.* after fracture, dislocation or hernia. (2) In chemistry: the addition of electrons to the reduced substance.

**referred pain.** Pain felt in the distribution of a sensory nerve supplied from the same segment as the nerve stimulated, *e.g.* pain felt in the shoulder due to irritation of the diaphragm, for both are supplied by nerves from the same spinal segments.

**reflex** (*rē'-fleks*). Simplest form of nervous behaviour whereby a stimulus produces an almost instantaneous and predictable response due to an established nerve pathway, the *reflex arc*.

**reflux** (*rē-fluks*). Flowing back, *e.g.* oesophageal *reflux* is the flow of stomach acid into the oesophagus.

**refraction** (*re-frak-shon*). The bending of light rays as they pass from one medium to another. This bending is an essential part of the process by which the image of an object is focused on the retina of the eye. Errors of refraction are caused when the eyeball is too short or too long or when the muscles which make the lens focus are weakened through disease or age; the rays of light are prevented from converging accurately on the retina. Spectacles will correct the error in most cases.

**refractory** (*re-frak-to-ri*). Stubborn; not amenable to treatment.

**refrigeration** (*re-fri-je-rā-shon*). The cooling of part of the body to reduce its metabolic requirements or to anaesthetize a part.

**regeneration** (*rē-ge-ne-rā-shon*). Renewal of damaged tissue such as regenerating nerve fibres.

**regimen** (*re-ji-men*). A rule of diet or of hygiene, or of life.

**regional ileitis.** *See* CROHN'S DISEASE.

**regression** (*re-gre-shon*). Reverting to a more primitive stage. In psychology, reverting to childlike behaviour as may be seen in severe physical illness or emotional upset.

**regurgitation** (*re-ger-ji-tā-shon*). Backward flow as occurs with defective valves, *e.g.* in the heart and veins, etc. Also applied to the reverse flow of gastric contents.

**rehabilitation** (*rē-ha-bi-li-tā'-shon*). Fitting a patient to take his place in the world again, *e.g.* rehabilitation of an amputee.

**Reiter's syndrome** (*rī-ters sin'-drōm*). Syndrome consisting of arthritis, conjunctivitis and urethritis and occasionally other manifestations, *e.g.* fever, rash, malaise, etc. The cause is not known.

**rejection** (*rē-jek'-shon*). Refusal to accept; used especially of grafted tissues and organs.

**relapse** (*re-laps*). A return of

disease after convalescence has once begun.

**relapsing fever.** Famine fever. A tropical disease caused by spirochaetes of the genus *Borrelia*.

**relaxation** (*rē-lak-sā-shon*). Reduction of muscle tone.

**remission** (*re-mi-shon*). Period when a disease subsides and shows no symptoms.

**remittent** (*re-mi-tent*). Returning at regular intervals; applied to certain fevers. *R. pyrexia. See* PYREXIA.

**renal** (*rē-nal*). Relating to the kidney.

**renal calculus** (*rē-nal kal-kū-lus*). Stone in the kidney.

**renal colic** (*rē-nal ko'-lik*). Colic of the ureter due to stone in the ureter or renal pelvis.

**renal dwarfism** (*dwaw-fism*). Dwarfism due to malfunction of the kidneys, usually due to stunting of skeletal growth due to *renal rickets. See* FANCONI SYNDROME.

**renal failure.** *Acute renal failure* presents as a sudden inability of the kidneys to produce urine. *Chronic renal failure*, *see* NEPHRITIS.

**renal threshold** (*rē-nal thresh'-hōld*). Concentration of substance in the blood at which it appears in the urine.

**renal tubular acidosis** (*rē-nal tū-bū-la a-si-dō-sis*). Defective renal tubular function in which there is a failure to secrete hydrogen ions into the urine with consequent inability to reduce the acidity of the blood in the normal way. Consequently there is excessive loss of compensatory ions with generalized metabolic disturbance.

**rennin** (*re-nin*). Enzyme secreted in the stomach of infants which clots milk by converting caseinogen to casein which precipitates as a calcium salt.

**replantation** (*rē-plahn-tā-shon*). Used especially of replacing tooth in socket.

**repression** (*re-pre-shon*). (1) In psychiatry: the shutting away of undesirable information from consciousness. (2) In genetics: the ability to prevent certain types of protein synthesis from taking place within a cell.

**resection** (*rē-sek'-shon*). A complete removal.

**resectoscope** (*rē-sek'-tō-skōp*). Instrument to view and remove pieces of tissue in transurethral prostatectomy.

**residual air** (*re-si-dū-al ār*). That remaining in the lungs after forced expiration.

**residual urine** (*ū-rin*). That left in the bladder after the organ has apparently been emptied naturally, measured by catheterization.

**resistance** (*re-sis-tans*). The degree of opposition to an action.

**resolution** (*re-so-lū-shon*). (1) A resolve. (2) Stage in an inflammation, in particular, term used in pathological description of lobar pneumonia.

**resonance** (*re-so-nans*). Increase of sound by reverberation, applied to voice sounds in auscultation.

**resorption** (*rē-sawp-shon*). Absorption of secreted matter.

**respiration** (*res-pi-rā-shon*). Breathing. Rate should be in infants 50 to the minute, in children 36, in adults 16. *Inverted r.* The pause is after inspiration instead of after expiration; noticed in babies with broncho-pneumonia.

**respirator** (*res-pi-rā-tor*). (1) Appliance worn over the mouth and nose to prevent the inhalation of poisonous gas. (2) Apparatus used to assist the muscles of respiration when paralysed, *e.g.* in poliomyelitis. There is a variety of types of these respirators.

**respiratory acidosis** (*res-pi-ra-to-ri a-si-dō-sis*). Acidosis caused by inability to excrete $CO_2$ (carbon dioxide), usually the result of chronic lung disease.

**respiratory alkalosis** (*res-pi-ra-to-ri al-ka-lō-sis*). Alkalosis due to hyperventilation with excessive loss of $CO_2$.

**respiratory distress syndrome.** Also known as the pulmonary syndrome of the newborn. Very much more common in premature babies. Rapid heart beat, grunting respiration and intercostal inspiratory recession are followed by respiratory failure.

**respiratory quotient** (*qwō-shent*). *RQ*. This is the ratio of the volumes of carbon dioxide expired and the oxygen consumed during the same time.

**restitution** (*res-ti-tū'-shon*). In obstetric practice this term means the rotation of the fetal head towards the right or left side immediately after it has completely passed the vulva; the occiput is thus turned (in a vertex presentation) towards the same side of the mother as that on which it originally entered the pelvis.

**resuscitation** (*rē-su-si-tā'-shon*). Reviving those who are apparently dead.

**retardation** (*rē-tar-dā-shon*). A slowing down of activity; backwardness.

**retching** (*ret-ching*). Ineffectual efforts to vomit.

**retention** (*rē-ten'-shon*). A holding back. Inability to void urine.

**reticular** (*re-ti'-kū-la*). Resembling a network. Applied to tissue.

**reticulocyte** (*re-ti-kū-lō-sīt*). Immature red blood cell in which nuclear remnants persist as basophilic threads in the cytoplasm.

**reticulocytosis** (*re-ti-kū-lō-sī-tō-sis*). Excessive reticulocytes found in the bloodstream.

**reticulo-endothelial system** (*re-ti-kū-lō-en-dō-thē-li-al sis-tem*). A system of phagocytic macrophages in the blood and tissues which free the body fluids of foreign particles. They can be recognized by injecting particles of India ink or certain other dyes into the body. The particles are selectively taken up by cells of the reticulo-endothelial system. *See also* MACROPHAGE, PHAGOCYTE, KUPFFER CELLS, etc.

**reticulosis** (*re-ti-kū-lō'-sis*). A group of neoplasms arising from lymphoid tissue, *e.g.* Hodgkin's disease, lymphosarcoma.

**reticulum cell sarcoma** (*re-ti-kū-lum sah-kō'-ma*). A reticulosis similar to Hodgkin's disease. It is alleged to arise from a more primitive cell than other reticuloses, a so-called stem cell known as a reticulum cell.

**retina** (*re-ti-na*). Layer lining the interior of the eye which contains the light-sensitive receptors, the *rods* and the *cones*, *see illustration*, p. 143.

**retinal** (*re-ti-nal*). Pertaining to the retina.

**retinitis** (*re-ti-nī-tis*). Inflammation of the retina.

**retinoblastoma** (*re-ti-nō-blas-tō-ma*). Tumour arising from germ cells in the retina.

**retinopathy** (*re-ti-no-pa-thi*). Pathological lesion affecting the retina, *e.g.* diabetic retinopathy, hypertensive retinopathy.

**retraction** (*re-trak'-shon*). Withdrawal or shortening. Retraction of the lower segment of the first stage of labour. There is a progressive increase in the tone of the longitudinal muscle fibres with consequent shortening of the muscles.

**retractor** (*rē-trak-ter*). Instrument used to withdraw structures obscuring the field of operation.

**retro-** (*rē-trō*). Prefix denoting backwards, behind.

**retrobulbar** (*rē-trō-bul-ba*). Behind the globe of the eye.

**retrocaecal** (*re-trō-sē-kal*). Behind the caecum.

**retroflexion** (*rē-trō-flek'-shon*). A bending back, as of the body of the uterus on the cervix.

**retrograde pyelography** (*rē-trō-grād pī-e-lo-gra-fi*). See PYELOGRAPHY.

**retrogression** (*re-trō-gre'-shon*). Retreating.

**retrolental fibroplasia** (*rē-trō-len-tal fī-brō-plā-si-a*). The posterior part of the capsule of the lens of the eye becomes fibrosed and blindness may result. Occurred in babies, usually premature, who were given too high a concentration of oxygen after birth. Condition seldom seen since this danger was recognized.

**retroperitoneal** (*rē-trō-pe-ri-to-nē-al*). Behind the posterior layer of the peritoneum.

**retropharyngeal** (*re-trō-fa-rin-jē-al*). Behind the pharynx. *R. abscess.* A collection of pus behind the wall of the pharynx and anterior to the cervical vertebrae. An acute abscess may develop from inflammation of two glands near the mid-line, a chronic one from cervical caries.

**retropubic** (*rē-trō-pū-bik*). Behind the pubis. *R. prostatectomy. See* MILLIN'S PROSTATECTOMY.

**retrospection** (*rē-trō-spek'-shon*). Looking back into the past.

**retrosternal** (*rē-trō-ster-nal*). Behind the sternum.

**retroversion** (*rē-trō-ver-shon*). A turning backwards. The uterus is normally turned considerably forwards, that is, the cervix is directed towards the lower end of the sacrum and the fundus towards the suprapubic region. Any deviation from this in the backward direction is termed retroversion. *Retroversion of the gravid uterus* may prevent the enlarging uterus from rising out of the pelvis.

**rhachitis** (*ra-kī′-tis*). Technical misnomer for rickets.

**rhagades** (*ra-ga-dēs*). A crack or fissure of skin causing pain; a term especially used of radiating scars at angle of mouth due to congenital syphilis. Now most commonly due to ill-fitting dentures or vitamin deficiencies.

**Rhesus (Rh) factor** (*rē-sus*). See BLOOD GROUPING.

**rheumatic** (*roo-ma′-tik*). Pertaining to rheumatism. *R. fever.* Acute rheumatic fever is a disorder affecting connective tissue, particularly that of the heart and the joints. The cause is considered to be an allergic reaction to toxins from haemolytic streptococcus (Lancefield group A). *R. heart disease.* Chronic rheumatic heart disease is the result of severe damage and deformation of the valves of the heart due to rheumatic fever.

**rheumatism** (*roo-ma-tism*). General non-technical term covering diverse conditions which have in common rather ill-defined pains in the muscles or joints.

**rheumatoid** (*roo-ma-toyd*). Similar to rheumatism. *R. arthritis.* A subacute or chronic form of arthritis. Gross changes occur in the joints leading to deformity and ankylosis.

**rhinitis** (*rī-nī-tis*). Inflammation of the nose.

**rhinolith** (*rī-nō-lith*). A calculus formed in the nose.

**rhinoplasty** (*rī-nō-plas′-ti*). Making a false nose.

**rhinorrhoea** (*rī-no-rē-a*). Discharge from the nose.

**rhinoscope** (*rī-no-skōp*). Nasal speculum.

**rhizotomy** (*rī-zo-to-mi*). Division of spinal nerve roots.

**rhodopsin** (*rō-dop-sin*). Visual purple contained in the retina.

**rhonchus** (*ron-kus*). A dry wheezing sound heard in the chest on auscultation. May be high pitched or sibilant; low pitched or sonorous.

**rhythm** (*rithm*). A patterned sound or movement.

**riboflavine** (*rī-bō-flā-vin*). Vitamin B$_2$. It forms part of a number of enzymes required for oxidative metabolism in cells.

**ribonuclease** (*rī-bō-nū'-klē-ās*). Enzyme which degrades RNA.

**ribonucleic acid** (*rī-bō-nū-klē-ic a-sid*). RNA. *See* NUCLEIC ACID.

**ribosomes** (*rī'-bō-sōmz*). Minute intracytoplasmic bodies composed of ribonucleic acid (RNA) and protein, present in most animal cells and plentifully in those actively growing or synthesizing secretory proteins.

**ribs.** Long lateral bones enclosing the chest. The upper seven ribs on each side join the sternum by separate cartilages, and are called true ribs, the lower five ribs being termed false ribs. Of the latter, the upper three pairs are attached to the sternum by a common cartilage on each side; while the lower two ribs on each side are not attached to the sternum at all, and are therefore called floating ribs.

**rice-water stools.** Characteristic stools of cholera.

**Richter's hernia** (*rik-ters her-ni-a*). Hernia which involves only a portion of the lumen of the intestine.

**rickets** (*ri-kets*). Deficiency of calcification of the skeleton. The most usual cause is vitamin D deficiency.

**Rickettsia** (*ri-ket-si-a*). Group of organisms which fall between bacteria and viruses in a classification based on size and properties. Typhus fever is a rickettsial disease.

**Riedel's thyroiditis** (*rē-dels thī-roy-dī-tis*). A fibrosing inflammation of the thyroid.

**Rigg's disease.** *See* PYORRHOEA.

**rigor** (*rī-gaw*). Sudden feeling of cold accompanied by shivering which raises the body temperature above normal. Due to disorder of the thermoregulatory centre of the brain caused by toxins, etc. Common in malaria.

**rigor mortis** (*rī-gaw maw-tis*). The stiffening of the body after death.

**rima** (*rē-ma*). A fissure; thus *rima glottidis*, slit between vocal cords.

**ring pessary.** Pessary in circular form.

**Ringer's solution** (*ring-ers so-lū-shon*). Physiological saline which includes sodium, potassium, calcium, magnesium and some other ions normally present in extracellular fluid.

**ringworm** (*ring-werm*). Fungus infection of keratinized structures such as hair, nails and skin. There are several species of fungus which are parasitic to man.

**Rinne's test** (*rin-nes*). A vibrating tuning-fork is placed on the mastoid process until no longer heard, then quickly put in front of the meatus; normally the vibration is still heard. The test is negative when obstruction exists in the external or middle ear.

**Ripple mattress.** Apparatus designed to reduce the incidence of pressure sores by rhythmically shifting the patient from one side to the other by pumping air into linear compartments causing the mattress to 'ripple'.

**risus sardonicus** (*rē-sus sar-do-ni-kus*). A convulsive grin, symptomatic of tetanus.

**RNA.** Ribonucleic acid.

**RNA viruses.** Viruses in which genetic material is RNA.

**ROA.** Right occipito-anterior presentation of fetus.

**rodent ulcer** (*rō-dent ul-ser*). Basal cell carcinoma of the skin. More common on parts of the skin exposed to the sun. Only spreads locally.

**rods** (*rodz*). Sensitive light receptors in the retina.

**Romberg's sign** (*rom-bergs sīn*). Inability to stand erect when the eyes are closed and the feet placed together; seen in tabes dorsalis.

**Röntgen rays** (*rernt-jen rās*). X-rays. *See* RADIATION.

**Röntgen unit** (*rernt-jen ū'-nit*). Unit of radiation defined as the quantity of radiation necessary to produce 1 electrostatic unit of charge (1 esu) in 1 ml of dry air under standard pressure and temperature conditions. This is not a satisfactory unit for estimating the biological effects of radiation and a number of alternative units have been introduced. One of these is the *röntgen equivalent man* (rem) which can be regarded as an index of risk of exposure to radiation. For λ rays, x-ray and β-rays 1 rem = absorbed energy of 100 ergs/gram tissue; for α rays and neutrons 1 rem = absorbed energy of 10 ergs/gram tissue.

**ROP.** Right occipito-posterior presentation of fetus.

**rosacea** (*rō-zā-sē-a*). Vasculomotor disturbance affecting the face with associated hyperplasia of the sebaceous glands.

**roseola** (*rō-sē-ō-la*). A rose-coloured rash.

# 307 **RUP**

**rotation** (*rō-tā-shon*). Twisting. Applied to the twisting of the head upon the shoulders of the fetus as it passes down the birth canal and follows the curves.

**rotators** (*rō-tā-ters*). Muscles which cause circular movement.

**roughage** (*ru-fāj*). Cellulose part of food which gives bulk and aids peristalsis.

**round ligaments.** Ovarian ligaments.

**roundworm.** *See* ASCARIS LUMBRICOIDES.

**Rovsing's sign** (*rov-sings sīn*). In appendicitis, pressure in the left iliac fossa will cause pain in the right iliac fossa.

**RQ.** Respiratory quotient.

**rubefacients** (*roo-be-fā-si-ents*). Mild irritants which cause redness of the skin.

**rubella** (*roo-be-la*). Also called German measles. A mild infectious disease caused by a virus. Incubation period 14–20 days, infectivity less than measles. There may be slight catarrh and fever and swelling of suboccipital glands. The rash begins on the face and spreads to the body and fades quickly. Complications are few but if a woman has the disease during the first 4 months of pregnancy, she may have a deformed child with eyes, ears and heart commonly affected. All girls and women should now be immunized against rubella at least 3 months before becoming pregnant.

**rugae** (*roo'-jē*). Wrinkles or creases.

**rugose** (*rū-jōs*). Wrinkled.

**rumination** (*rū-mi-nā-shon*). Regurgitation of feeds by infants. Analogous to chewing the cud. Can cause failure to thrive. Infant may be seen inducing a vomit with fingers at the back of the mouth.

**rupture** (*rup'-cher*). A bursting. In popular language a rupture means a hernia. In obstetric practice *rupture of the perineum* is not uncommon as a result of labour, especially in primiparae; *rupture of the uterus* is a rare event due to unrelieved obstructed labour, or more rarely still to unskilful attempts at delivery by the use of instruments; *rupture of the membranes* is the normal sequence of full dilatation of the cervix in labour, and marks the commencement of the second stage. *Rupture of a tubular extra-uterine pregnancy* may result in severe internal haemorrhage and would require immediate operation.

**Russell traction** (*rus'el trak'-shon*). A type of traction used in treatment of fractures of the femur.

**Ryle's tube** (*rīls tūb*). Narrow-bore rubber tube, slightly weighted, used for giving a test meal or aspirating the stomach.

## S

**Sabin's vaccine** (*sā-bins vak-sēn*). A vaccine against poliomyelitis which consists of an attenuated strain of virus which is taken orally, *cf.* Salk vaccine.

**sac.** A small pouch, such as a hernial sac.

**saccharin** (*sak'-a-rin*). A glucoside used as a sugar substitute, having no food value.

**Saccharomyces** (*sa-ka-rō-mī-sēs*). A group of fungi including yeasts. One is the cause of thrush.

**sacculated** (*sa-kū-lā-ted*). Bagged or pursed out.

**sacral** (*sā-kral*). Pertaining to the sacrum. Sacral analgesia, *see* CAUDAL ANALGESIA.

**sacro-iliac synchondrosis** or **joint** (*sā-krō-i-li-ak sin-kon-drō-sis*). The articulation between the sacrum and the hip-bone. Normally there is no movement at this joint. During pregnancy the joint becomes more movable and this, to a slight extent, facilitates the birth of the child.

**sacrum** (*sā-krum*). The division of the backbone, forming part of the pelvis.

**saddle-nose** (*sa-del-nōs*). A flattened bridge of the nose.

**sadism** (*sā'-dism*). A sexual perversion in which pleasure is derived from inflicting cruelty upon another.

**sagittal** (*sa'-gi-tal*). Arrowlike. *S. section.* Section made by cutting through a specimen from top to bottom so that there are equal right and left halves. *S. suture.* The suture between the parietal bones.

**St. Vitus' dance** (*sānt vī-tus dans*). Chorea.

**sal.** A salt.

**saline** (*sā-līn*). A solution of salt (NaCl). In medical practice this normally refers to 'physiological' saline.

**saliva** (*sa-lī-va*). The secretion of the salivary glands.

**salivary glands** (*sa-li-va-ri glans*). Three pairs of glands. The sublingual and submaxillary situated in the floor of the mouth; the parotid above the angle of the lower jaw. *See* PAROTID.

**salivation** (*sa-li-vā-shon*). The act of secretion of saliva.

**Salk's vaccine** (*salks vak-sēn*). A vaccine against poliomyelitis made from dead virus and given by injection. Seldom used.

**Salmonella** (*sal-mo-nel-la*). Group of Gram negative bacteria which include the typhoid bacteria and a number of others causing food-poisoning.

**salpingectomy** (*sal-pin-jek-to-mi*). Removal of one or both Fallopian tubes.

**salpingitis** (*sal-pin-jī'-tis*). Inflammation of a tube, usually applied to the Fallopian tubes.

**salpingocyesis** (*sal-pin-go-sī-ē-sis*). Tubal pregnancy.

**salpingography** (*sal-pin-go-gra'-fi*). Technique of examination of the Fallopian tubes by x-rays.

**salpingo-oophorectomy** (*sal-pin-gō-oo-fo-rek'-to-mi*). Removal of Fallopian tubes and ovaries.

**salpingostomy** (*sal-pin-gos-to-mi*). Opening artificially a Fallopian tube whose aperture has been closed by inflammation.

**salpinx** (*sal-pinks*). A tube, either Eustachian or Fallopian.

**salt** (*sawlt*). A substance resulting from the combination of an acid and a base.

**salve** (*salv*). An ointment.

**sanatorium** (*sa-na-taw-ri-um*). Any institution for convalescent patients can technically be called a sanatorium. Formerly used for the open-air treatment of tuberculosis.

**sandfly fever** (*sand-fli fē'-ver*). Tropical disease due to infection by organism transmitted by sandfly bites.

**sanguine** (*san-gwin*). (1) Full-blooded. (2) Hopeful.

**sanguinous** (*san-gwi-nus*). Blood-stained. Containing blood.

**sanitary** (*sa-ni-ta-ri*). Pertaining to health.

**sanitation** (*sa-ni-tā-shon*). The use of methods conducive to public health.

**sanity** (*sa'-ni-ti*). Being of sound mind.

**saphena varix** (*sa-fē-na vār-iks*). Saccular enlargement of the termination of the long saphenous vein often without obvious varicose veins.

**saphenous nerve** (*sa-fē-nus nerv*). Large branch of the femoral nerve.

**saphenous opening.** Just below groin near inner side of thigh where superficial saphenous vein passes deep to enter femoral vein.

**saphenous veins.** Superficial leg veins. *Long s.v.* begins on the foot and extends to the groin. *Short s.v.* joins the popliteal vein at the knee.

**sapo** (*sa-pō*). Soap. *S. mollis.* Soft soap.

**saponify** (*sa-po-ni-fī*). To make into a soap.

**saprophytes** (*sa-prō-fīts*). Organisms that exist only in dead matter.

**Sarcina** (*sah-sē-na*). A genus of Schizomycetes which form rectangular bundles as they divide; usually non-pathogenic.

**sarcoid** (*sar-coyd*). Resembling flesh.

**sarcoidosis** (*sah-coy-dō'-sis*). A syndrome resulting from what appears to be a disturbance of the immunological mechanism. It is characterized by widespread lesions of a characteristic histological appearance resembling tuberculosis. Symptoms depend on the situation of these lesions. In a proportion of cases there is an associated disturbance of calcium metabolism.

**sarcolemma** (*sah-kō-le-ma*). The membrane which covers each fibril of muscle.

**sarcology** (*sah-co-lo-ji*). Anatomy of the soft tissues as distinguished from osteology.

**sarcoma** (*sah-kō-ma*). Malignant tumour of mesodermal origin.

**Sarcoptes scabiei** (*sah-kop-tēs skā-bi-ā-ē*). The itch mite or insect causing scabies. It burrows into the skin where it lays its eggs which hatch out. The 'burrows' often terminate in a papule on the skin. The disease is treated with benzyl benzoate.

**sartorius** (*sah-to-ri-us*). The long ribbon-shaped muscle of the front of the thigh.

**saturation** (*sa-tūr-ā-shon*). The condition of holding in solution the full amount of a solid capable of being dissolved.

**scab.** An incrustation formed over a wound.

**scabies** (*skā-bēs*). *See* SARCOPTES.

**scald** (*skawld*). Burn caused by hot fluids.

**scale** (*skāl*). Aggregation of keratinized cells.

**scalenus anterior syndrome** (*skā-lē-nus an-tār-i-or sin'-drōm*). Is characterized by pain in the arm and tingling of the fingers with loss of power and muscle wasting due to compression of the lower fibres of the brachial plexus by the scalenus anterior muscle.

**scalp** (*skalp*). The skin covering the cranium.

**scalpel** (*skal'-pel*). Knife used in surgery and dissection.

**scanning speech.** Speech in which syllables tend to be separated. Usually a sign of a lesion affecting the cerebellum.

**scaphocephaly** (*skā-fō-ke-fa-li*). Deformity of skull due to premature fusion of sutures producing a long narrow head.

**scaphoid** (*skā-foyd*). Boat-shaped. The name of a bone of the carpus and of the tarsus.

**scapula** (*ska-pū-la*). The shoulder blade.

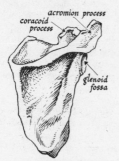

coracoid process  
acromion process  
glenoid fossa

*44. The scapula*

**scar** (*skah*). The connective fibrous tissue found after any wound has healed.

**scarification** (*ska-ri-fi-kā'-shon*). Shallow incisions just penetrating the epidermis.

**scarlatina** (*skah-la-tē-na*). Scarlet fever. The cardinal sign is a widespread erythematous rash produced by a toxin released by haemolytic streptococci which are commonly found in the throat where they give rise to an infection.

**Scarpa's triangle** (*skah-pahs trī-an-gel*). The femoral triangle bounded by Poupart's ligament, the adductor longus and sartorius.

**Scheuermann's disease** (*shoyer-mans*). Vertebral osteochondritis found in adolescents. It affects the two rings of cartilage and bone around the margin of both superior and inferior surfaces of the vertebral body. The condition does not cause general ill health.

**Schick test** (*shik*). Skin test to detect whether an individual has immunity against diphtheria. Small amounts of diphtheria toxin are used.

**schistosomiasis** (*skis-to-so-mī-a-sis*). See BILHARZIA.

**Schizomycetes** (*ski-zo-mī-sē-tēs*). Yeasts.

**schizophrenia** (*ski-zō-frē-ni-a*). The generic term used for a group of disorders characterized by a progressive loss of emotional stability, judgement and contact with reality. The cause is not yet known but there are probably genetic and biochemical components.

**Schlatter's disease** (*shla-ters*). See OSGOOD SCHLATTER'S DISEASE.

**Schlemm's canal** (*shlems*). Lymphatic channel leading to a venous plexus at the root of the ciliary body of the eye. It allows the intra-ocular fluid (aqueous humour) to drain. Failure of the canal to drain results in raised hydrostatic pressure in the anterior chamber of the eye (glaucoma).

**Schwann cell** (*schvun*). Supporting cell of the peripheral nervous system, see NEUROGLIA. The Schwann cells invest the nerves and form the myelin sheath which surrounds many of the larger fibres.

**sciatica** (*sī-a-ti-ka*). Neuralgia of the sciatic nerve, the large nerve of the thigh. It may be caused by pressure on the nerves in the spinal canal or the pelvis.

**scirrhous** (*si-rus*). Hard and fibrous in nature.

**scissor-leg deformity** (*si-ser-leg de-faw-mi-ti*). Deformity due to exaggerated tone in the adductor muscles usually resulting from cerebral damage.

**sclera** (*sklār-a*). The opaque outer coat of the eyeball, forming five-sixths of the globe of the eye, the remaining one-sixth being formed by the cornea. See EYE.

**scleritis** (*skle-rī-tis*). An inflamed sclera.

**sclerodactylia** (*skle-rō-dak-ti-li-a*). See ACROSCLEROSIS.

**scleroderma** (*skle-rō-der-ma*). Disorder of connective tissue in which there is probably increased amounts of elastic fibres laid down resulting in loss of elasticity of the connective tissues and atrophic changes in the structures which they support.

**sclerosis** (*skle-rō-sis*). Hardening. See also DISSEMINATED SCLEROSIS.

**sclerosis tuberous** (*skle-rō-sis tu-be-rus*). Epiloia. Dominantly inherited defect characterized by sebaceous adenomas in a butterfly distribution on the face, multiple gliomas of the brain, and tumours of the heart, kidney and retina.

**sclerotic** (*skle-ro-tik*). Pertaining to the sclera.

**sclerotomy** (*skle-ro-to-mi*). An operation on the sclerotic coat of the eye, for the relief of glaucoma.

**scolex** (*skō-leks*). Head of a tapeworm.

**scoliosis** (*skō-li-ō-sis*). Lateral curvature of the spine.

**scotoma** (*skō-tō-ma*). A blind spot in the field of vision.

**screening** (*skrē-ning*). Radiological examination by means of a fluorescent screen. Term used more generally for ways of detecting early disease in clinically healthy people.

**scrofuloderma** (*skro-fū-lō-der-ma*). Tuberculosis of the skin.

**scrotocele** (*skrō-tō-sēl*). Hernia in the scrotum.

**scrotum** (*skrō'-tum*). The bag which holds the testicles.

**scruple** (*skroo-pel*). A weight equal to 20 gr apothecaries' weight, or 1·296 grams.

**scurf** (*skerf*). Dandruff. Large aggregates of exfoliating epidermal cells.

**scurvy** (*sker-vi*). Syndrome of extreme vitamin C deficiency, *see* VITAMINS. Principal features are haemorrhage into the tissues and swelling of mucous membranes.

**scybala** (*ski-bu-la*). Faeces passed as hard dry masses.

**sebaceous** (*se-bā-shus*). Fatty, secreting oily matter. *S. glands.* Of skin, secrete fatty material called sebum. *S. cysts.* Dilatation of one of these glands, due to blocking of its opening on to the skin. A cyst is filled with sebum.

**seborrhoea** (*se-bo-rēa*). Excessive secretion of the sebaceous glands.

**sebum** (*sē-bum*). The oil of the skin, secreted by the sebaceous glands.

**secondary areola** (*a-rē-ō-la*). Hyperpigmentation of the skin surrounding the nipple during pregnancy.

**secondary disease.** A disease consequent on another disease already active.

**secondary haemorrhage** (*he-mo-rāg*). *See* HAEMORRHAGE.

**second intention.** The healing of a wound by means of granulation, and the growing of new skin.

**second stage of labour.** Phase of childbirth between the completion of cervical dilation and the delivery of the infant. It normally lasts up to 2 hours and is marked by strong contractions of the uterus and the instinctive desire of the mother to push in a way to expel the baby.

**secretin** (*se-krē-tin*). A hormone formed in the mucous membrane of the duodenum. It is carried by the blood to the pancreas, exciting it to activity. It also stimulates the secretion of bile.

**secretion** (*se-krē-shon*). The active production, filtering or extrusion of material from cells. Certain cells have specialized secretory activity (gland cells).

**section** (*sek-shon*). Usually applied to thin slices of tissue cut for microscopical examination.

**sedative** (*se'-da-tiv*). Allaying excitement or pain.

**sedimentation rate.** *See* ESR.

**segment** (*seg'-ment*). A small piece; section; a subdivision.

**segregation** (*seg-re-gā'-shon*). A setting apart. Isolation.

**sella turcica** (*se-la ter-ki-ka*). Pituitary fossa of the sphenoid bone.

**semen** (*sē-men*). The fluid emission which contains the spermatozoa.

**semicircular canals** (*se-mi-ser-kū-la ca-nals*). Three canals of the internal ear, the sense organs of equilibrium or balance. *See* EAR.

**semilunar cartilages** (*se-mi-lū-na kah-ti-lā-jes*). Two crescentic cartilages, an internal and an external, lying in the knee joint between the femur and tibia. These may be torn and displaced, giving rise to pain and deformity and fluid in the knee joint. Usually removed by operation.

**seminal** (*se-mi-nal*). Relating to the semen. *S. vesicles.* Saclike storage organs for semen.

**seminoma** (*se-mi-nō'-ma*). Malignant neoplasm of the testicular cells.

**senescence** (*se-nes'-ens*). The process of growing old.

**Sengstaken tube** (*seng'-sta-ken tūb*). Oesophageal tube used to compress bleeding varices.

**senility** (*se-ni'-li-ti*). Degenerative changes due to advanced age.

**sensible** (*sen'-si-bl*). Perceptible.

**sensitive** (*sen'-si-tiv*). Able to react to a stimulus.

**sensitization** (*sen-si-ti-zā'-shon*). Act of producing an immunological state in which there is a disproportionately adverse reaction to a substance (antigen or hapten).

**sensory nerves** (*sen-so-ri nervs*). Afferent nerves carrying sensory information to the central nervous system, *cf.* motor nerve.

**sentinel pile** (*sen-ti-nel pīl*). Small external haemorrhoid, sometimes associated with fissure in ano.

**sepsis** (*sep'-sis*). The condition of being infected by pyogenic bacteria.

**septate uterus and vagina** (*sep-tāt ū-te-rus, va-jī-na*). Developmental abnormality of the uterus and/or vagina in which a longitudinal septum divides the organ into two parts.

**septic** (*sep'-tik*). Pertaining to sepsis.

**septicaemia** (*sep-ti-sē-mi-a*). The circulation and multiplication of micro-organisms in the blood. It is a very serious condition if a suitable antibiotic is not available.

**septum** (*sep'-tum*). The division between two cavities; such as s. *ventriculorum*, which separates the right ventricle of the heart from the left.

**sequelae** (*se-kwe-lē*). Morbid conditions remaining after, and consequent on, some former illness.

**sequestrectomy** (*se-kwes-trek'-to-mi*). Operation to remove sequestrum.

**sequestrum** (*se-kwes-trum*). A fragment of dead bone.

**serosa** (*se-rō-sa*). A serous membrane. Serous membranes line the large lymph spaces, *e.g.* pleural, pericardial, peritoneal cavities.

**serositis** (*se-rō-sī'-tis*). An inflamed serous membrane.

**serotonin** (*sē-rō-tō'-nin*). 5-hydroxytryptamine, an amine found in blood platelets, the intestines and brain substance, inactivated by monoamine oxidase.

**serpiginous** (*ser-pi'-ji-nus*). Serpent-like in shape.

**serrated** (*se-rā-ted*). With a saw-like edge.

**serum** (*sār-um*). That part of the blood which remains after the cells, platelets and fibrinogen have been removed, usually by allowing the blood to clot. It consists of a saline solution containing a number of proteins and lipids. Of particular interest are serum albumin and globulin.

**sesamoid bones** (*se-sa-moyd*). Small foci of bone formation in the tendons of muscles. The patella is the largest.

**sessile** (*ses-sīl*). Having no stem, applied to tumours.

**sex chromosomes** (*seks krō-mō-sōms*). These are defined as chromosomes of which there is a homologous pair in the nuclei of one sex and a heterologous pair in the nuclei of the other. In humans the homogametic sex (XX) is female and the heterogametic sex (XY) is male.

**sex-linkage** (*seks lin-kāj*). This refers to genes whose locus is on one of the sex chromosomes.

**sexually transmitted diseases.** The venereal diseases. Infectious diseases transmitted during sexual intercourse, *e.g.* gonorrhoea, syphilis, etc.

**Sheehan's syndrome** (*shē-ans sin'-drōm*). Panhypopituitarism resulting from thrombosis of the pituitary blood supply occurring in association with post-partum haemorrhage.

**Shiga's bacillus** (*shē-gus ba-si-lus*). The *Shigella dysenteriae*.

**shingles.** *See* HERPES ZOSTER.

**shock.** Severe circulatory disturbance characterized by fall in blood pressure, weak rapid pulse, thirst, and pallor. The usual cause is rapid diminution in the blood volume.

**short circuit** (*shawt ser-kit*). Anastomosis between gut or blood vessels which allows the contents to bypass a section of the normal pathway.

**short-sighted** (*shawt-sī-ted*). Myopic.

**shoulder presentation.** A form of transverse lie which must be converted into breech or vertex before delivery is possible.

**show** (*shō*). Popular term for the discharge of slightly blood-stained mucus common at the beginning of labour.

**sialectasis** (*sī-a-lek'-ta-sis*). Dilatation of salivary gland due to obstruction to the flow of saliva.

**sialogogue** (*sī-a-lo-gog*). Substance which stimulates salivation.

**sialolith** (*sī-a-lō-lith*). A salivary calculus.

**sibilus** (*si-bi-lus*). A hissing

sound heard on auscultation of the chest during respiration in bronchitis, etc.

**sibling** (*sib'-ling*). One of two or more children of the same parent.

**sickle-cell anaemia** (*si-kel-sel a-nē-mi-a*). Hereditary anaemia found sometimes in negroes. The red blood cells become sickle-shaped or crescentic.

**siderosis** (*si-de-rō-sis*). (1) Inhalation of iron particles causing pneumoconiosis. (2) Excess of iron in the blood.

**sight** (*sīt*). The power of seeing.

**sigmoid** (*sig-moyd*). Like the Greek letter sigma, applied especially to a bend in the pelvic colon just before it becomes the rectum.

**sigmoidoscope** (*sig-moy-do-'skōp*). An instrument for viewing the interior of the rectum and sigmoid flexure of the colon.

**sigmoidostomy** (*sig-moyd-os'-to-mi*). Opening into sigmoid colon.

**sign** (*sīn*). An indication of the presence of disease.

**signatura** (*sig-na-tū-ra*). A label.

**silicones** (*si'-li-kōnz*). Polymers consisting of alternate silicon and oxygen atoms, with organic groups sometimes attached to the silicon atoms.

**silicosis** (*si-li-kō-sis*). Lung disease due to the inhalation of very fine particles of silica which irritate the lungs causing fibrotic changes. *See* PNEUMOCONIOSIS.

**silkworm gut** (*silk-werm*). A suture material much used by surgeons for sewing up abdominal wounds. It is very strong, not absorbed, and can be sterilized by boiling.

**Simmond's disease** (*si-mons di-sēz*). *See* PANHYPOPITUITARISM.

**simple fracture.** *See* FRACTURE.

**Sim's position.** The patient lies in the semi-prone position across the bed. The buttocks are brought to the edge of the bed. The right knee is flexed more than the left. Used for vaginal examination.

**sinciput** (*sin-ci-put*). The upper fore part of the head.

**sinew** (*si-nū*). A tendon uniting a muscle to a bone.

**sinistral** (*si-ni-stral*). Pertaining to the left side.

**sinuatrial node** (*sī-nu-ā-tri-al nod*). Cells found in the heart at the junction of the superior vena cava and the right atrium. The node is the pacemaker of the heart.

**sinus** (*sī-nus*). (1) A passage leading from an abscess, or some inner part, to an external opening. (2) A dilated channel for venous blood, *e.g. lateral s.*, a large venous channel on the inner side of the skull. It passes near the mastoid antrum and empties itself into the jugular vein. (3) Air sinuses, hollow cavities in the skull bones which communicate with the nose. They are the frontal, maxillary, ethmoidal and sphenoidal sinuses.

**sinus arrythmia** (*sī-nus a-rith-mi-a*). Irregular cardiac rhythm due to the controlling effect of the vagus on the sinuatrial node. The heart rate increases in inspiration and slows during expiration.

**sinusitis** (*sī-nus-ī-tis*). Inflammation of an air sinus.

**sinusoid** (*si-nu-soyd*). Like a sinus. Channels for small blood vessels as found in the liver, suprarenal glands, etc.

**siphonage** (*sī-fo-nāj*). Method of drawing fluid from one vessel to another by means of a bent tube and the use of atmospheric pressure.

**situs inversus viscerum** (*sē-tus in-ver-sus vī-ser-um*). A developmental anomaly in which there is complete transposition of the organs from right to left and vice versa.

**Sjögren's syndrome** (*sher-grens sin'-drōm*). Syndrome characterized by dry mouth, defective lacrimation and rheumatoid arthritis.

**skatole** (*skā-tol*). A nitrogenous compound found in the faeces.

**skeleton** (*ske-le-ton*). The bony framework of the body.

**Skene's glands** (*skēns glans*). These open into the posterior wall of the female urethra, just within the orifice; almost always infected in acute gonorrhoea.

**skin.** Outer covering of the body consisting of epidermis and its appendages (hair, sweat glands) supported by specialized dermal connective tissue.

**skull.** The bony framework of the head.

**sleeping sickness.** (1) Tropical disease due to a trypanosome. The tsetse fly carries the organisms which are transferred to healthy individuals by the bite of the fly. (2) *See* ENCEPHALITIS LETHARGICA.

**slough** (*sluf*). Dead matter thrown off by gangrene or ulcers.

**smallpox** (*smawl-poks*). Variola. A highly infectious disease caused by a virus. Incubation period 12–14 days. Smallpox has been almost eradicated on a world scale by vaccination and enforcement of quarantine regulations.

**smegma** (*smeg-mer*). Thick white secretion forming under the prepuce.

**Smith-Petersen nail** (*smith-pē-ter-sen nāl*). Inserted to fix the two fragments of bone in a fracture of the neck of the femur.

**snare** (*snār*). A looped wire instrument for encircling and strangling some piece of tissue which it is desired to remove, *e.g.* a nasal polypus.

**Snellen's test types** (*sne-lens test tīps*). A chart showing letters of different size and used for testing vision. The patient sits at a distance of 6 metres from it. If only the large top letter can be seen the patient's vision is termed 6/60, *i.e.* he can see at 6 metres what the normal eye can see at a distance of 60 metres.

**snow blindness.** Ophthalmia with photophobia caused by the glare from snow.

**sodium chloride** (*sō-di-um klaw-rīd*). *See* SALINE.

**soft sore.** A venereal sore not due to syphilis. Also known as *chancroid*, and *non-infecting sore*. The causative organism is Ducrey's bacillus.

**solar plexus** (*sō-la plek-sus*). A plexus of nerves and ganglia in the upper region of the abdomen.

**soleus** (*sō-lē-us*). A muscle in the calf of the leg.

**solution** (*so-lū-shon*). A liquid containing a solid which has been dissolved in it.

**solvent** (*sol'-vent*). A liquid able to dissolve another substance.

**somatic** (*sō-ma'-tik*). Pertaining to the body.

**somnambulism** (*som-nam-bū-lism*). Walking and carrying out other activities whilst asleep.

**Sonne dysentery** (*so-nĕ di-sen-te-ri*). Dysentery caused by bacteria of one of the Shigella group.

**soporific** (*sō-po-ri-fik*). Agent causing sleep.

**sordes** (*saw-dēs*). Brown crusts which form on the lips of patients with consistently high temperature or those who are dehydrated.

**souffle** (*soofl*). A soft blowing sound. During late pregnancy the *funic souffle* can sometimes be heard by auscultation of the maternal abdomen, a sound synchronous with the fetal heart and supposed to be produced in the umbilical cord. The *uterine souffle* is a blowing murmur heard over the uterus due to pulsations in the maternal arteries.

**sound** (*sownd*). A probe-like instrument used for exploring cavities, such as the uterus, bladder, etc.

**Southey's tubes** (*su-thēs*). Small perforated metal tubes, used to drain oedematous tissue.

**Spaldings sign** (*spawl-dings sīn*). Sign of fetal death. There is overlapping of the skull bones in x-ray pictures of the skull.

**spasm.** (1) Sudden convulsive involuntary movement. (2) Sudden contraction of a muscle or muscles, especially of the unstriped muscle coats of arteries, intestines, heart, bronchi, etc. The effect of such spasm depends on the part affected: thus asthma is believed to be due to spasm of the muscular coats of the smaller bronchi; and renal colic is due to spasm of the muscle coat of the ureter.

**spasmolytic** (*spas-mō-li-tik*). Substance which relieves spasm.

**spasmus nutans** (*spas-mus nū-tans*). A condition known as nodding spasm in babies, in which the head is continually nodding or turning from side to side.

**spastic** (*spas'-tik*). (1) In a state of spasm. (2) Popular term for cerebral palsy. In patients with this disease the muscles are often spastic, *i.e.* hypertonic, and there is excessive neuromuscular excitability.

**spasticity** (*spas-ti'-si-ti*). The condition of being spastic.

Occurs in upper motor neurone lesions.

**spatula** (*spa'-tū-la*). (1) A flat, flexible, blunt knife, used for spreading ointments and poultices. (2) A tongue depressor.

**species** (*spē-sēs*). A group of organisms having many of the same characteristics. In natural history various species form a genus or class of animals.

**specific** (*spe-si'-fik*). Applied to a medicine or treatment, it means the particular remedy for a certain disease; applied to a disease, it means due to a distinct specific microorganism which causes that disease alone.

**specific gravity** (*spe-si'-fik gra-vi-ti*). By this is meant the ratio between the weight of a substance and the weight of an equal volume of water, the latter being taken, as a matter of convenience, to be $1 \cdot 000$. The specific gravity of a liquid depends on the amount of solid in solution.

**spectroscope** (*spek-tro-skōp*). An instrument for the production and examination of spectra in luminous bodies.

**spectrum** (*spek'-trum*). The band of colours formed when rays of white light are passed through a prism.

**speculum** (*spe-kū-lum*). A polished instrument for examining the interior cavities of the body, especially the vagina, the rectum, the ear, and the nose.

**speech.** The power of speaking; conveying a meaning by vocal sounds.

**speech centre.** The part of the brain controlling speech.

**speech therapist.** One trained to treat defects and disorders of language, voice and speech.

**Spencer-Wells forceps.** The usual forceps for haemostasis during operations.

**sperm.** *See* SPERMATOZOA.

**spermatic cord** (*sper-ma'-tik*). Composed of arteries, veins, lymphatics and nerves, and the vas deferens, the duct of the testicle; it suspends the testicle from the abdomen.

**spermatocele** (*sper-ma-tō-sēl*). A unilocular retention cyst from some portion of the epididymis.

**spermatogenesis** (*sper-ma-tō-je-ne-sis*). The process of formation of sperm. *See* MEIOSIS.

**spermatozoa** (*sper-ma-tō-zō-a*). The male generative cells; minute animated cells found in the semen, which are possessed of the power of self-propulsion by means of a flagellum, and which can fertilize the ovum, or female germ cell.

**spermicide** (*sper-mi-sīd*). Substance destroying spermatozoa.

**sphenoid** (*sfē-noyd*). Wedge-shaped. The name of one of the bones forming the base of the skull.

**sphenoidal** (*sfē-noy-dal*). Pertaining to the sphenoid bone.

**sphincter** (*sfink-ter*). A circular muscle which contracts the orifice of an organ.

**sphincterotomy** (*sfink-te-ro'-to-mi*). Division of sphincter muscles.

**sphygmocardiograph** (*sfig-mō-kar-di-ō-grahf*). Apparatus recording both pulse and heart beats.

**sphygmograph** (*sfig-mō-grahf*). An instrument affixed to the wrist, which moves with the beat of the pulse and registers the rate and character of the beats.

**sphygmomanometer** (*sfig-mō-ma-no'-me-ter*). An instrument for measuring the arterial tension (blood pressure) of the circulation.

**spica** (*spī-ka*). A spiral bandage done with a roller in a series of figure eights. Most used for the shoulder, groin, thumb, and great toe.

**spicule** (*spi'-kūl*). Fragment of bone.

**'spider' naevus** (*spī-der nē-vus*). Dilatation of small blood vessels arising from a central arteriole. These may occur in the skin during pregnancy or under oestrogen stimulation. The distribution of the vessels gives the spots the appearance of a spider.

**spigot** (*spi-got*). Wooden or plastic peg closing a tube.

**spina bifida** (*spī-na bi-fi-da*). Malformation due to failure of the neural arch of one or more of the vertebrae to fuse in the mid-line. As a result the vertebral canal is exposed at this site and may herniate through the opening. *See* MENINGOCELE. The defect most commonly occurs in the lumbo-sacral region. *Spina bifida occulta.* Incomplete closure of the neural arch which may be indicated by a pigmented or hairy patch over the affected part of the spine.

**spinal analgesia** or **anaesthesia** (*spī-nal a-nal-jē-si-a, an-es-thē-si-a*). Infiltration of local anaesthetic agents into the cerebrospinal fluid by means of a lumbar puncture. This procedure results in a block to the nerves below the level of the injection.

**spinal column** (*spī-nal ko-lum*). The backbone. It is composed of seven cervical, twelve thoracic and five lumbar vertebrae and the sacrum with its five fused vertebrae and the coccyx or tailbone.

**spinal cord** (*spī-nal kawd*). The portion of the central nervous system within the spine. It contains many nerve cells and bundles of nerve fibres connecting the various levels of the spinal cord with the brain. Thirty-one pairs of nerves form the connections with the peripheral nervous system of the trunk and limbs. *See also* NERVE ROOT.

**spinal curvature** (*spī-nal kerva-tūr*). The *normal* curvature of the spine is divided

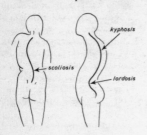

45. *Spinal curvature*

into primary curvature (giving an ape-like stooping posture) and secondary curvatures (cervical and lumbar). For abnormal spinal curvature *see* SCOLIOSIS, KYPHOSIS, LORDOSIS.

**spine** (*spīn*). The backbone or spinal column.

**spirillum** (*spī-ri-lum*). Corkscrew-shaped bacteria.

**spirochaetaemia** (*spī-rō-kē-tē-mi-a*). The presence of spirochaetes in the blood.

**spirochaete** (*spī'-rō-kēt*). Elongated spiral bacteria which move by flexions of the body. Pathogenic spirochaetes cause diseases such as syphilis and Weil's disease.

**spirograph** (*spī-rō-graf*). Instrument for recording respirations.

**spirometer** (*spī-rō'-me-ter*). An instrument for measuring the capacity of the lungs.

**splanchnic** (*splank'-nik*). Pertaining to the viscera. *S. nerves.* Group of sympathetic nerve fibres which supply the viscera.

**splanchnicectomy** (*splank-ni-sek-to-mi*). Surgical removal of the splanchnic ganglia and transection of the splanchnic nerves.

**splanchnology** (*splank-no'-lo-ji*). The study of the viscera.

**splay foot.** Flatfoot. Pes planus.

**spleen.** A mass of lymphoid tissue situated in the mesentery of the abdomen. Unlike the lymph nodes the spleen acts as a filtration organ for blood. The spleen forms an important part of the reticulo-endothelial system and is the generative centre for the formation of many lymphocytes. The spleen is largely responsible for the removal of red blood cells at the end of their life-span.

**splenectomy** (*sple-nek-to-mi*). Removal of the spleen.

**splenic anaemia** (*sple'-nik a-nē'-mi-a*). Banti's syndrome. It is characterized by anaemia and splenomegaly associated with portal hypertension due to hepatic cirrhosis.

**splenic flexure** (*sple-nik fleksūr*). Bend of the colon on the left side, near the spleen.

**spleniculus** (*sple-ni-kū-lus*). Name given to accessory spleen, several of which may be present.

**splenitis** (*sple-nī-tis*). Inflammation of the spleen.

**splenomegaly** (*sple-nŏ-me-ga-li*). An enlarged spleen.

**'splinter' haemorrhages** (*splin'-ter he-mo-rā-jes*). Haemorrhage from longitudinal capillaries in the nail bed giving the appearance of splinters under the nail. Characteristically occur in subacute bacterial endocarditis.

**splints.** Used to immobilize a limb in the case of a fracture, disease or deformity.

**spondyle** (*spon-dīl*). A vertebra.

**spondylitis** (*spon-di-lī-tis*). Inflammation of a vertebra

or vertebrae. *Ankylosing s.* Condition of unknown origin occurring characteristically in young men and comprising the ossification of spinal ligaments with ankylosis of the cervical and sacro-iliac joints.

**spondylolisthesis** (*spon-di-lō-lis-thē'-sis*). The vertebral arch of the fifth lumbar vertebra gives way so that the body of the affected vertebra becomes displaced.

**spondylosis** (*spon-di-lō'-sis*). Term used to describe nonspecific degenerative changes in the intervertebral discs with peripheral ossification. Known as osteoarthritis of the spine.

**spontaneous fracture** (*spon-tā-nē-us frak-tūr*). Fracture due to disease affecting the bone, either abnormality of development or rarefaction of the bone from other causes.

**spontaneous version** (*spon-tā-nē-us ver-shon*). The unaided conversion of a transverse lie into a cephalic or podalic one.

**sporadic** (*spo-ra'-dik*). A disease which is not epidemic, but occurs in one or two isolated cases in a district.

**spore** (*spaw*). Reproductive body which gives rise to new individual organism.

Produced by protozoa, fungi and bacteria, spores constitute a method of wide dispersal of population and a means of survival through unfavourable conditions. Important spore-forming bacteria are *Clostridium welchii* and *Clostridium botulinum*.

**sporotrichosis** (*spo-rō-tri-kō-sis*). Fungus infection giving rise to intradermal granulomas.

**spotted fever** (*spo-ted fē-ver*). (1) Meningococcal bacteraemia giving rise to meningitis and foci of infection in dermal blood vessels. (2) Rocky Mountain spotted fever is a rickettsial disease transmitted by the dog tick.

**sprain** (*sprān*). Severe strain of a joint without fracture or dislocation, but with swelling and often with effusion into joint; may be associated damage to ligaments.

**Sprengel's deformity** (*sprengels de-faw'-mi-ti*). Congenital upward displacement of the scapula.

**sprue** (*sproo*). A disease of tropical climates which causes inflammation of the mucous membrane of the alimentary canal, characterized by soreness of tongue and mouth, chronic diarrhoea, wasting and anaemia.

**spurious pains** (*spū-ri-us pāns*). False labour pains, leading to no result, and sometimes occurring several days before confinement.

**sputum** (*spū-tum*). Expectorated matter. Different types are: *Mucoid*, which occurs in the early stage of irritation. *Muco-purulent*, develops at a later stage, pus is mixed with mucus. *Rusty*, tenacious sputum, occurs in lobar pneumonia. Copious foul-smelling sputum occurs in bronchiectasis. *Foaming*, occurs in oedema of the lung. Separate pellets or nummular sputum occurs in pulmonary tuberculosis. It may be streaked with blood.

**squamous** (*skwā-mus*). Scaly.

**squint** (*skwint*). *See* STRABISMUS.

**staccato** or **scanning speech** (*sta-kah-to, ska-ning*). Hesitation between syllables, and when the sound comes it comes explosively. It is a type of inco-ordination, and occurs in cerebellar lesions.

**Stacke's operation.** Operation used in chronic infection to join the middle ear cavity with that of the mastoid cells.

**stages of labour.** *See* LABOUR.

**stain** (*stān*). Coloured compound used to dye tissues for microscopical examination, *e.g.* eosin, haematoxylin.

**stamina** (*sta'-mi-na*). Vigour. Staying power.

**Stanford-Binet test.** A test of intelligence.

**stapedius** (*sta-pē-di-us*). A muscle of the middle ear.

**stapes** (*stā-pēs*). One of the three ossicles of the middle ear; stirrup-shaped. *See* EAR.

**Staphylococcus** (*sta-fi-lō-ko'-kus*). Genus of Gram positive bacteria which grow in clusters in culture (Greek *staphyle* = bunch of grapes). Many staphs are commensals on the skin. Some are serious pathogens and several strains have evolved which are insensitive to penicillin and other antibiotics.

**staphyloma** (*sta-fi-lō'-ma*). Any protrusion of the sclerotic or corneal coats of the eyeball due to inflammation.

**staphylorrhaphy** (*sta-fi-lo'-ra-fi*). Operation to suture cleft soft palate.

**starch.** Carbohydrate made up of a chain of monosaccharide sugars, *i.e.* a polysaccharide.

**Starr valve.** Artificial heart valve.

**stasis** (*stā-sis*). Standing still. Most commonly used for arrest of the circulation of either blood or lymph, but also for intestinal stasis, a holding up of the contents of the bowel.

**status asthmaticus** (*stā-tus as-ma'-ti-kus*). Severe asthmatic attack lasting for more than 24 hours.

**status epilepticus** (*stā-tus e-pi-lep'-ti-kus*). When a series of major epileptic fits occur without intervening recovery of consciousness the patient is said to be in status epilepticus.

**status lymphaticus** (*stā-tus lim-fa'-ti-kus*). Also termed status thymo-lymphaticus; lymphatism. Sudden death from apparently trivial cause associated with hyperplastic lymphatic tissue. The existence of this syndrome has been disputed.

**steapsin** (*stē-ap'-sin*). Lipase.

**steatoma** (*stē-a-tō-ma*). Tumour composed of fatty tissue.

**steatorrhoea** (*stē-a-to-rē-a*). The passage of pale, bulky, offensive stools with a high fat content and which tend to float on water. Often the first symptom of any malabsorption syndrome.

**steatosis** (*stē-a-tō'-sis*). Fatty degeneration.

**Stegomyia** (*ste-go-mī-a*). Variety of mosquito.

**Stein-Leventhal syndrome** (*stīn-le-ven-thal sin'-drōm*). Syndrome characterized by obesity and sterility in women. The ovaries are enlarged and polycystic, menstruation is anovular, irregular and abnormal, and there is some virilization.

**Steinmann's pin** (*stīn-mans*). A fixation pin inserted through a bone in order to apply extension in the case of fractures. *See* EXTENSION.

**stellate ganglion** (*stel-lāt gan'-gli-on*). Star-shaped sympathetic ganglion situated in the neck. *See* SYMPATHETIC SYSTEM.

**stenosis** (*ste-nō'-sis*). Contraction of a canal or an orifice.

**Stensen's duct** (*sten'-sens dukt*). The duct of the parotid salivary gland, the opening of which is opposite the upper first molar tooth.

**stercobilin** (*ster-kō-bi'-lin*). The colouring matter of the faeces. It is derived from bile pigment.

**stercolith** (*ster-kō-lith*). Faecolith. Compacted mass of faeces.

**stereognosis** (*stār-ē-og-nō-sis*). Recognition of the form of bodies by handling them.

**sterile** (*ste'-rīl*). Barren; unable to have children. In *surgical practice*, sterile means entirely free from germs of all kinds, a result brought about by heat or by antiseptic chemicals or ionizing radiation.

**sterility** (*ste-ri-li-ti*). The condition of being sterile.

**sterilization** (*ste-ri-lī-zā'-shon*).

(1) Made incapable of progeny, *e.g.* by removal of ovaries, tying the Fallopian tubes, hysterectomy or, in the male, vasectomy or tying the vas deferens. (2) Rendering germ-free.

**sternal puncture** (*ster-nal pung-cher*). Technique employed to obtain sample of red bone marrow for investigation. A needle is inserted into the sternum under local anaesthesia, and a small amount of the marrow aspirated.

**sternomastoid muscle** (*ster-nō-mas-toyd mu-sel*). Muscle of neck, running from the inner end of the clavicle and upper border of the sternum to behind the ear. *See* TORTICOLLIS.

**sternum** (*ster-num*). The breastbone.

**steroids** (*stē-royds*). A group of substances with a common basic structure. Slight differences in the chemical configuration produce greatly divergent biological effects, *e.g. see* ADRENAL CORTEX.

**sterols** (*ste-rols*). Steroids with an alcohol (—OH) side group, *e.g.* Cortisol (= hydrocortisone).

**stertor** (*ster-tor*). Snoring type of respiration.

**stethoscope** (*ste-thos-kōp*).

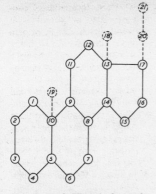

46. *Steroids. Figure shows the basic chemical structure of steroids with the carbon atoms numbered. The distinguishing groups are attached in positions 18 to 21*

Instrument for listening to sounds, *e.g.* heart sounds, respiratory sounds.

**Stevens-Johnson syndrome** (*stē-vens-jon-son sin'-drōm*). Severe form of erythema multiforme in which mucous membranes may be extensively involved.

**sthenic** (*sthe'-nik*). Strong, active.

**stigma** (*stig'-ma*) (pl. **stigmata**). Mark on the skin. Also any permanent condition indicative of some constitutional peculiarity.

**stilette** (*sti-let'*). A sharp probe.

**stillborn** (*stil-bawn*). Any baby born dead after more than 28 weeks gestation.

**Still's disease.** A form of rheumatoid arthritis occurring in children. The syndrome is characterized by polyarthritis, lymphadenopathy and splenomegaly.

**stimulant** (*sti'-mū-lant*). Substance causing an increase in the activity of living material.

**stimulus** (*sti'-mū-lus*). An agent provoking activity.

**stitch** (*stitch*). (1) Suture. (2) Pain in the side due to spasm of the diaphragm.

**Stokes-Adams syndrome** (*stōks-a-dams sin'-drōm*). Syncope due to cerebral hypoxia resulting from heartblock.

**stoma** (*stō-ma*). The mouth.

**stomach** (*stu'-muk*). The dilated portion of the intestinal canal into which the food passes from the oesophagus, and where it undergoes partial digestion.

**stomach pump** (*stu'-muk pump*). Apparatus used to aspirate the contents of the stomach.

**stomatitis** (*stō-ma-tī'-tis*). Inflammation of the mouth.

**stone** (*stōn*). (1) A measure of weight, 14 pounds. (2) A concretion.

**stools.** Discharge of faeces from the bowels.

**strabismus** (*stra-bis'-mus*). Squint; *divergent* when the eye turns out; *convergent* when it turns in.

**strabotomy** (*stra-bo'-to-mi*). Operation to remedy squinting.

**strain** (*strān*). (1) To filter. (2) Condition resulting from unsuitable use of a part.

**strangulated** (*stran'-gū-lā-ted*). Constricted, so that the blood supply is cut off. *See* HERNIA.

**strangury** (*stran'-gu-ri*). Painful micturition.

**strapping** (*stra'-ping*). Material used to bind up injuries.

**stratified** (*stra'-ti-fīd*). In layers.

**stratum** (*stra'-tum*). A layer.

**Streptococcus** (*strep-tō-ko'-kus*). Genus of Gram positive bacteria which grow in chains. Pathogenic cocci produce toxins responsible for scarlet fever, rheumatic fever and acute glomerulonephritis.

**Streptothrix** (*strep-to-thriks*). Filamentous bacteria.

**stress incontinence.** Incontinence of urine or faeces when the intra-abdominal pressure is raised as in coughing or sneezing, etc.

**striae** (*stri-ā*). Lineae albicantes. Scars on the abdomen and thighs due to stretching of the dermis during rapid expansion of the abdomen. Frequently this is seen in association with pregnancy.

**striated muscle** (*stri-ā-ted mu-sel*). Striped voluntary muscle, *cf.* smooth muscle.

**stricture** (*strik'-tūr*). Contraction. Usually applied to the urethra, with consequent inability to pass urine.

**stridor** (*strī'-dor*). A harsh sound during breathing, caused by obstruction to the passage of air.

**stroke** (*strōk*). Cerebrovascular accident. *See also* HEAT-STROKE.

**stroma** (*strō'-ma*). The connective tissue.

**stupor** (*stū-por*). State of unconsciousness.

**Sturge-Weber syndrome** (*sterj-we-ber sin'-drōm*). Syndrome characterized by capillary naevus on the face in the distribution of the fifth cranial nerve associated with angiomas of the cerebral cortex which may cause focal epilepsy, hemiparesis and mental deficiency.

**stye** (*stī*). Suppuration around an eyelash follicle.

**styptic** (*stip'-tik*). Agent which arrests bleeding.

**sub.** A prefix denoting beneath or under.

**subacute** (*su-ba-kūt*). Less than acute, *i.e.* fairly gradual onset, *cf.* chronic, long in duration.

**subacute bacterial endocarditis** (*sub-a-kūt bak-tār-i-al en-dō-kar-dī'-tis*). Bacterial colonization of defective heart valves with consequent bacteraemia and distribution of septic emboli throughout the body.

**subacute combined degeneration of the cord.** Degeneration of the posterior and lateral columns of the spinal cord due to vitamin B$_{12}$ deficiency.

**subarachnoid haemorrhage** (*sub-a-rak-noyd he-mo-rāj*). Haemorrhage into the subarachnoid space.

**subarachnoid space** (*sub-a-rak-noyd spās*). The space between the arachnoid membrane and the pia mater. It contains cerebrospinal fluid.

**subclavian** (*sub-klā-vi-an*). Under the clavicle: thus the subclavian artery and vein are vessels passing under the clavicle.

**subclinical** (*sub-kli'-ni-kal*). Without any obvious signs of the disease.

**subconscious** (*sub-kon'-shus*). Thought processes which occur without the awareness of the individual, *i.e.* he is unconscious of these processes (equals unconscious 'mind'). It must be assumed that most of the neuronal activity in the central nervous system is subconscious. Only some of the products of nerve activity reach awareness. This consciousness of thought is probably a quantitative measure of the number of neurons conducting complementary impulses. The mechanism of 'awareness' is, however, a philosophical problem.

**subcutaneous** (*sub-kū-tā'-nē-us*). Under the skin.

**subinvolution** (*sub-in-vo-lū'-shon*). Failure of involution.

**subjacent** (*sub-jā'-sent*). Lying below.

**subjective** (*sub-jek'-tiv*). Internal: pertaining to one's self.

**subliminal** (*sub-li'-mi-nal*). Below the threshold.

**sublingual** (*sub-lin'-gwal*). Under the tongue.

**subluxation** (*sub-luk-sā'-shon*). Less than dislocated, *i.e.* partial dislocation.

**submaxillary** (*sub-mak-si'-la-ri*). Beneath the maxilla.

**submucous** (*sub-mū-kus*). Beneath a mucous membrane.

**subnormal** (*sub-naw-mal*). Below normal.

**subphrenic** (*sub-fre'-nik*). Under the diaphragm. *S. abscess*. A collection of pus beneath the diaphragm.

**substrate** (*sub-strāt*). Compound on which an enzyme acts.

**subtotal hysterectomy** (*sub-tō-tal his-te-rek-to-mi*). The removal of the uterus, excluding the cervix. Now rarely performed.

**succenturiate placenta** (*suk-sen-tū-ri-āt pla-sen-ta*). An accessory placenta.

**succus entericus** (*su-kus en-te'-ri-kus*). The digestive juice secreted by the glands in the small intestine.

**succussion** (*su-ku-shon*). Sound made on shaking a patient if fluid is present in a hollow cavity.

**sudamina** (*sū-da-mi-na*). Sweat rash.

**sudorific** (*sū-do-ri-fik*). An agent causing perspiration.

**suffused** (*su-fūsd*). Congested. Blood-shot.

**suggestibility** (*su-jes-ti-bi-li-ti*). A state when the patient readily accepts other people's ideas and influences.

**suicide** (*su'-i-sīd*). To kill oneself.

**sulcus** (*sul-kus*). A furrow.

**sulphonamides** (*sul-fo'-na-mīds*). A group of drugs which have bacteriostatic properties used in the treatment of certain infections.

**sunstroke** (*sun'-strōk*). *See* HEATSTROKE.

**superciliary** (*sū-per-si-li-a-ri*). Having to do with the eyebrows.

**supercilium** (*sū-per-si-li-um*). The eyebrow.

**superego** (*sū-per-e'-gō*). A Freudian term. Control from within of instinctive acts such as aggression. Possibly an adoption of parental attitudes taught in childhood.

**superfecundation** (*sū-per-fe-kun-dā'-shon*). The fertilization of two ova discharged at the same ovulation by two distinct acts of insemination effected at a short interval.

**superfetation** (*sū-per-fē-tā-shon*). Condition of doubtful authenticity in which twins are derived from separate ovulations and separate acts of coitus during different intermenstrual periods.

**superior** (*sū-pār-i-or*). Above. The upper of two organs.

**supination** (*sū-pi-nā-shon*). Turning the palm of the hand upwards.

**supine** (*sū-pīn*). Lying face upwards; in the case of the forearm, having the palm uppermost.

**supplemental air** (*su-ple-men'-tal*). That part of the residual air of the lung which after the tidal air has been expelled may be driven out by forced respiration.

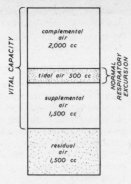

47. *Lung volumes*

the position of structures beneath it.

**surgery** (*ser'-je-ri*). (1) The part of medicine concerned with diseases needing treatment by operation. (2) A physician or surgeon's consulting room.

**surgical** (*ser'-ji-kal*). Pertaining to surgery.

**susceptible** (*su-sep-ti-bel*). Liable to, *e.g.* infection.

**suspension** (*sus-pen'-shon*). (1) Hanging. (2) Undissolved particles dispersed in a liquid.

**suspensory bandage** (*sus-pen-so-ri ban-dāj*). A bandage to support the testicles.

**sutures** (*soo-tūrs*). (1) Silk, thread, catgut, nylon, etc., used to sew a wound. (2) The union of flat bones by their margins, *e.g.* bones of the skull.

**swabs.** Small pieces of wool, gauze over wool, or gauze only, used for cleansing wounds and for removing blood at operations.

**sweat** (*swet*). Perspiration. The fluid secreted on to the skin by the sweat glands.

**sycosis** (*sī-kō'-sis*). Inflammation of the hair follicles, especially of the beard and whiskers.

**symbiosis** (*sim-bī-ō'-sis*). The living together of two organisms, whose mutual

**suppository** (*su-po-si-ta-ri*). Rectally administered cones containing a medicament in a base which is soluble at body temperature.

**suppression** (*sup-pre-shon*). To prevent some activity, *e.g.* glandular secretion, cough, etc.

**suppuration** (*su-pū-rā'-shon*). The formation of pus.

**supra-orbital** (*sū-pra-aw-bi-tāl*). Above the orbit.

**suprapubic** (*sū-pra-pū'-bik*). Above the pubes.

**suprarenal** (*sū-pra-rē-nal*). Above the kidney. *S. glands. See* ADRENAL GLANDS.

**sural** (*sū-ral*). Relating to the calf of the leg.

**surface** (*ser'-fās*). The outer part. *S. markings.* Lines drawn on the skin to show association is necessary to each, although neither is parasitic on the other.

**symblepharon** (*sim-ble'-fa-ron*). Adhesion of the eyelids to the eyeball.

**Syme's amputation** (*sīms*). Amputation through the ankle joint.

**sympathectomy** (*sim-pa-thek'-to-mi*). Surgical transection of sympathetic nerves usually with excision of part of the sympathetic chain.

**sympathetic system.** Part of the *autonomic nervous system*. The pre-ganglionic fibres leave the spinal cord between segments T1–L2 and synapse in the various ganglia. The postganglionic fibres are unmyelinated. Some sympathetic fibres leave the CNS in the cranial nerves.

**symphysiotomy** (*sim-fi-si-o-to-mi*). The operation of dividing the symphysis pubis (of the mother) so as to facilitate delivery in certain cases of contracted pelvis.

**symphysis** (*sim-fi-sis*). Growing of bones together. The *symphysis pubis* is the bony mass bounding the front of the pelvis, at the lower end of the abdomen. *See* PELVIS.

**symptom** (*simp'-tom*). A noticeable change in the body and its functions, evidence of disease. Usually meaning the change complained of by the patient.

**symptomatology** (*simp-to-ma-to'-lo-ji*). A study of the symptoms of disease.

**synapse** (*sī-naps*). Region where nerve cells communicate. There is no continuity between the neurons and impulses are transmitted from one nerve cell to another by the passage of chemical messengers which stimulate the post-synaptic nerve cell.

**synarthrosis** (*si-nar-thrō'-sis*). Immovable union of bones, *e.g.* the cranial bones.

**synchondrosis** (*sin-kon-drō'-sis*). A joint whose surfaces are united by cartilage.

**synchysis** (*sin-ki-sis*). Softening of the vitreous humour of the eye. *S. scintillans*. Bright particles found in the vitreous humour.

**synclitism** (*sin-kli-tism*). Descent of the fetal head through the pelvis with its planes parallel to those of the pelvis.

**syncope** (*sin'-ko-pē*). Transient loss of consciousness.

**syndactyly** (*sin-dak-ti-li*). Webbed fingers.

**syndesmitis** (*sin-des-mī'-tis*). Inflammation of ligaments.

**syndrome** (*sin'-drōm*). Collection of symptoms and/or signs which comprise a recognizable pattern of disease.

**synechia** (*sī'-ne-ki-a*). Adhesion of the iris to the cornea, or to the crystalline lens.

**synergy** (*si'-ner-ji*). The working together of two or more agents.

**synonyms** (*si-nō-nims*). Different words having the same meaning.

**synostosis** (*si-nos-tō'-sis*). Abnormal osseous union of bones.

**synovectomy** (*sī-nō-vek'-to-mi*). Operation to remove synovial membrane.

**synovial fluid** (*sī-nō-vi-al floo-id*). The liquid which lubricates the joints.

**synovial membrane** (*sī-nō-vi-al mem-brān*). That lining a joint cavity but not covering the articular surfaces.

**synovitis** (*sī-nō-vī-tis*). Inflammation of the synovial membrane of a joint.

**synthesis** (*sin'-the-sis*). The building up of complex substances by the union and interaction of simpler materials.

**synthetic** (*sin-the'-tik*). Pertaining to synthesis. Artificial.

**syphilide** (*si'-fi-līd*). Lesion of the skin due to syphilis. May be papular, macular, squamous, etc.

**syphilis** (*si'-fi-lis*). One of the sexually transmitted diseases. Now rarely seen. Most common in male homo-sexuals. Caused by a specific spirochaete, the treponema pallidum. *S.* may be congenital or acquired. *Congenital* may be inherited from the mother. The chief symptoms in young babies: wasting, snuffles, rashes, enlargement of liver and spleen. If child survives, he may later show pallor, malnutrition, depressed bridge of nose, rhagades, square skull, thickening of tibiae, corneal opacities, Hutchinson's teeth. *See* RHAGADES, HUTCHINSON'S TEETH. *Acquired* is divided into three stages. (1) First stage or primary *S.* with local symptoms, 2 to 3 weeks after infection. Hard chancre on penis, vulva, or cervix. Inflamed glands in groin. Lesions infective, *see* CHANCRE. (2) Second stage or secondary *S.*, 1 to 2 months after infection, with rashes, sore throat, mucous patches, condylomata, general enlargement of glands, anaemia and fever. Infective, *see* CONDYLOMA. (3) Third stage or tertiary *S.*, 2 to 10 years, or even longer after infection. Non-infective. Manifestations, include gummata, tabes, GPI. *See* GENERAL PARALYSIS.

**syringe** (*si'-rinj*). An instrument for injecting fluids, or for exploring and aspirating cavities.

**syringomyelia** (*si-rin-gō-mī-ē'-li-a*). Progressive degenerative disease affecting the brainstem and spinal cord in which the tracts of fibres subserving pain and temperature are mainly affected.

**syringomyelocele** (*si-rin-gō-mī-el'-ō-sēl*). Form of myelocele in which there is a communication between the mass and the central canal of the spinal cord.

**syringotomy** (*si-rin-go'-to-mi*). Cutting open a fistula.

**system** (*sis-tem*). An organized scheme. A series of parts concerned in a basic function such as nutrition by the alimentary system.

**systemic** (*sis-te'-mik*). Affecting the whole body.

**systemic lupus erythematosus** (*sis-te-mik lū-pus e-ri-the-ma-tō-sus*). One of the so-called 'collagen diseases'. *See* LUPUS ERYTHEMATOSUS.

**systole** (*sis-to-lē*). The period when the heart contracts. *See* DIASTOLE.

**systolic blood pressure** (*sis-tō'-lik*). Upper limit of arterial blood pressure, *cf.* diastolic pressure.

**systolic murmur** (*sis-tō-lik mer-mer*). Adventitious sound heard during systole.

**T**

**TAB.** Triple vaccine to prevent typhoid, paratyphoid A and paratyphoid B.

**T bandage.** A special bandage used for keeping dressing on the perineum.

**tabes** (*tā-bēz*). Wasting. *T. dorsalis* (locomotor ataxia). Syphylis affecting the posterior columns of the spinal cord which carry the sensory fibres from the trunk and limb. Sometimes it is associated with general paralysis of the insane when the syndrome is known as *taboparesis. T. mesenterica.* Tuberculosis of peritoneal glands.

**tachycardia** (*ta-kē-kar'-di-a*). Increased heart rate.

**tactile** (*tak'-tīl*). Relating to touch.

**Taenia** (*tē'-ni-a*). Tapeworm. *T. solium, T. saginata* and *T. echinococcus* are parasitic to man.

**talc.** French chalk. Used as dusting powder.

**talipes** (*ta'-li-pēz*). Clubfoot. Term used to cover a group of foot deformities in which the sole of the foot is no longer plantigrade. The term talipes is qualified by four adjectives which describe the elements of the deformity. These are equinus, valgus, varus and calcaneus. The commonest deformities are *T. equino-varus* and *T. calcaneo-valgus*.

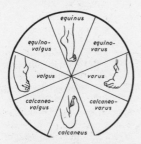

*48. Deformities in talipes*

**talus** (*tā-lŭs*). The ankle.

**tampon** (*tam'-pon*). A plug of wool or gauze introduced into the vagina. Commonly used by women during menstruation.

**tamponade** (*tam-pō-nāde*). Compression. Usually *cardiac t.* in which the action of the heart is impeded by the presence of fluid in the pericardium.

**tantalum** (*tan'-ta-lum*). A resistant metal sometimes used in bone surgery for plates or wire.

**tapeworm** (*tāp'-werm*). *See* TAENIA.

**tapping.** *See* ASPIRATION.

**tar** (*tah*). Dark liquid obtained from pine-wood. It has antipyretic and antiseptic properties. *Coal-tar.* Black liquid distilled from coal. It contains benzene, phenol, cresols, naphthalene, etc.

**target cell** (*tah'-get sel*). Erythrocyte with dark central area and dark peripheral ring, seen in forms of anaemia.

**tarsal** (*tar'-sal*). Bones of the ankle, *cf.* carpal bones. There are seven in man forming a group which articulate with the tibia and fibula and the metatarsal bones.

**tarsalgia** (*tah-sal'-ji-a*). Pain in the foot.

**tarsectomy** (*tah-sek-to-mi*). Excision of part of the tarsal group of bones.

**tarsoplasty** (*tah-sō-plas'-ti*). Plastic surgery of the eyelid.

**tarsorrhaphy** (*tah-so'-ra-fi*). Stitching the eyelids together.

**tarsus** (*tar'-sus*). (1) The seven small bones of the foot. (2) The cartilaginous framework of the eyelid.

**tartar** (*tar'-ta*). Deposit on the teeth of calcium salts derived from saliva.

**taste bud.** Specialized sensory end organ, situated on the tongue and oral mucosa, which is sensitive to taste.

**taurocholic acid** (*taw-rō-kō-lik a'-sid*). One of the bile acids.

**taxis** (*tak'-sis*). Locomotion of an organism or a cell in response to a directional stimulus, *cf.* kinesis.

**Tay-Sachs' disease** (*tā-saks*). Amaurotic familial idiocy. Degenerative disease of infancy affecting the brain and optic nerves. Most commonly found in Jewish families and may be inherited by a recessive gene.

**t.d.s.** *Ter die sumendum*, to be taken three times a day.

**tears** (*tārs*). Secretion of the lacrimal gland.

**tease** (*tēz*). To divide a tissue into shreds.

**teat** (*tēt*). Nipple.

**technique** (*tek-nē'k*). Method.

**teeth.** Teeth are derived from ectodermal buds. There are two dentitions in man. *Primary dentition* (milk teeth, temporary teeth, deciduous teeth) which erupt in the first two years of life, and *secondary dentition* (permanent teeth) which

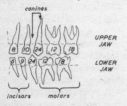

49. *Primary dentition. The teeth are marked with the time of eruption in months*

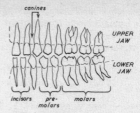

50. *Secondary dentition*

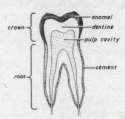

51. *A section of a tooth*

erupt from about the sixth year onwards with corresponding shedding of the primary teeth. Each tooth is composed of dentine which is surrounded by a material known as 'cement' except the erupted portion which is covered by a hard material called 'enamel'. The blood supply and nerve supply of the tooth is contained in the central pulp cavity.

**tegument** (*te'-gŭ-ment*). The skin.

**tela** (*tā-la*). Tissue formed like a web.

**telangiectasis, telangioma** (*te-*

*lan-ji-ek'-ta-sis*, *te-lan-ji-ō'-ma*). Lesion consisting of a number of tortuous dilated capillaries which have a web-like appearance.

**telepathy** (*te-le'-pa-thi*). The transference of thought from one person to another. There is considerable doubt as to whether this is possible and the question is under investigation.

**temper tantrums** (*tem'-per tan'trums*). Behaviour disorder in children. Particularly common around the age of 2 years.

**temperament** (*tem'-pe-ra-ment*). A person's mental outlook.

**temperature** (*tem'-pe-ra-tūr*). A measurement of the degree of heat. The average normal temperature of the human body is 37°C (98·6°F). The average temperature of a sick-room should be about 16°C (65°F).

**temples** (*tem'-plz*). The part of the forehead between the outer corner of the eye and the hair.

**temporal** (*tem'-por-ral*). Relating to the temple. Thus *t.* artery, *t.* bone, *t.* lobe of the brain.

**temporal arteritis.** Giant cell arteritis. A disease of unknown aetiology characterized by general malaise, aches and muscle pains and acute inflammation of the arteries, particularly those of the scalp.

**tendinitis** (*ten-di-nī'-tis*). Inflammation of a tendon.

**tendo Achilles** (*ten-do a'-ki-lēs*). The stout tendon of the calf muscles at the back of the heel.

**tendon** (*ten'-don*). A sinew, a cord of fibrous white tissue by which a muscle is attached to a bone or other structure.

**tendovaginitis, stenosing** (*ten-dō-va-gi-nī-tis ste'-nō-zing*). Stenosing tenosynovitis, de Quervain's disease. Fibrous thickening of tendon sheath most commonly affecting the tendons of the abductor muscles of the thumb.

**tenesmus** (*te-nes'-mus*). Painful straining to empty the bowel. May be a symptom of a neoplasm in the rectum.

**tennis elbow** (*ten'-nis el'bō*). Painful disorder affecting the fibres by which the extensor muscles of the forearm are attached to the external epicondyle. The precise nature of the disorder is not known.

**tenoplasty** (*te-nō-plas'-ti*). Plastic surgery to a tendon.

**tenorrhaphy** (*te-no'-ra-fi*). Operation to suture a tendon.

**tenosynovitis** (*te'-nō-sī-nō-vī'-tis*). Inflammation in the sheath of a tendon.

**tenotomy** (*te-no'-to-mē*). Cutting a tendon.

**tension** (*ten'-shon*). The act of stretching.

**tensor** (*ten'-sor*). A muscle which stretches.

**tent, oxygen.** Enclosure in which the patient is surrounded by an atmosphere of high oxygen content.

**tent, steam.** Tent erected around a bed to provide a moist atmosphere. Screens and an old sheet of blanket are used. Steam is directed inside from a kettle. Temperature of tent, 70°F (21°C).

**tentorium cerebelli** (*ten-to'-ri-um se-ri-bel-li*). The part of the dura mater which separates the cerebral spheres from the cerebellum.

**tepid** (*te'-pid*). Just warm.

**teratogen** (*te-ra'-tō-jen*). Agent inducing fetal malformation.

**teratoma** (*te-ra-tō'-ma*). A neoplasm arising from totipotent cells, *i.e.* cells which like the cells of an early embryo possess the ability to differentiate into all the components of the body. The origin of these cells is disputed. An example of a teratoma is a 'dermoid' tumour which may contain hair, muscle, teeth, glandular structures, etc.

**teres** (*te'-rās*). Round and smooth. *Ligamentum t.* Ligament of the head of the femur.

**terminology** (*ter-mi-no'-lo-ji*). Nomenclature.

**tertian** (*ter'-shan*). *See* MALARIA.

**tertiary syphilis** (*ter'-she-rē*). *See* SYPHILIS.

**test.** (1) Trial. (2) A reaction distinguishing one substance from another.

**test meal.** *See* FRACTIONAL TEST MEAL.

**testicles** (*tes'-ti-kls*). The testes.

**testis** (*tes'-tis*). (pl. **testes**). Organ which produces spermatozoa.

**testosterone** (*tes-tos'-te-rōn*). A steroid hormone with androgenic properties, *see* ANDROGEN. Probably the principal sex hormone secreted by the testes.

**tetanus** (*te'-ta-nus*). Lock-jaw. Disease caused by *Clostridium tetani* characterized by rigidity and spasm of the muscles. The causative organism is anaerobic and thrives in wounds contaminated by soil or road dust containing the spores. A powerful toxin is produced by the Clostridium which reaches the spinal cord by retrograde spread up the motor nerves, and is responsible for the clinical features. Infants usually have a course of immunization against tetanus and a booster dose can be given after an accident.

**tetany** (*te'-ta-ni*). A condition marked by spasms of the extremities, particularly of hands and feet (carpopedal spasm) due to faulty calcium metabolism. It may be due to dysfunction of the parathyroid glands, alkalosis, rickets.

**tetracyclines.** Group of chemically related antibiotics which include Aureomycin (chlortetracycline), Terramycin (oxytetracycline) and Achromycin (tetracycline hydrochloride), etc.

**tetralogy of Fallot** (*te'-tra'-lo-ji*). *See* FALLOT'S TETRALOGY.

**tetraplegia** (*te-tra-plē'-ji-a*). Paralysis of all four limbs.

**thalamus** (*tha-la-mus*). Collection of neurons in the forebrain which serves as a major co-ordinating region for sensory information.

**thalassaemia** (*tha-las-sē-mi-a*). Genetically determined abnormality in which there is continued production of fetal haemoglobin. The clinical features are those of a haemolytic anaemia. Two forms are recognized; one in which the condition is homozygous (thalassaemia major), and the other heterozygous (thalassaemia minor). The latter is generally symptomless.

**thalidomide** (*tha-li'dō-mīd*). Non-barbiturate sedative found to induce fetal malformations if taken by pregnant women.

**thaumatrope** (*thaw'-ma-trōp*). Instrument demonstrating persistence of visual impressions: images printed on opposite sides of a card appear to fuse when it is rotated rapidly so that each side is presented alternately.

**theca** (*thē'-ka*). A sheath. Examples are the meninges of the spinal cord, and the synovial sheaths of the flexor tendons of the fingers.

**thecoma** (*thē-kō'-ma*). Benign tumour of ovarian theca mainly fibromatous, but includes fatty and sometimes epithelial elements.

**thenar** (*thē'-nar*). Relating to the palm of the hand at the base of the thumb.

**theory** (*thē-o-ri*). Logical principles relating to a subject.

**therapeutics** (*the-ra-pū'-tiks*). Branch of medicine which deals with treatment.

**therm** (*therm*). A unit of heat. The amount of heat required to raise one gram of water through one degree centigrade.

**thermography** (*ther-mo'-gra-fi*).

Study of temperature variations in parts of the body by scanning infra-radiations emitted by skin. Used to detect vascular disorders and tumours of soft tissues such as the breast.

**thermolabile** (*ther'mō-lā'-bīl*). Describing a substance which undergoes change with temperature.

**thermometer** (*ther-mo'-me-ter*). An instrument used to record variations of temperature. *Clinical t.* A small thermometer used for taking the temperature of the body. It is graduated from 35°C (95°F) to 43·5°C (110°F). It is made so that the mercury does not fall when the thermometer is taken from the patient. After the temperature has been recorded the mercury is shaken down. *Low reading t.* Necessary for detecting hypothermia. *See* TEMPERATURE, and p. 13.

**thermophilic** (*ther-mō-fi'-lik*). Describing an organism which flourishes at high temperatures.

**thermostat** (*ther'-mō-stat*). Apparatus which is made to regulate heat automatically.

**thiamine** (*thī'-a-min*). Aneurine, vitamin $B_1$, thiamine diphosphate (cocarboxylase) is an important co-enzyme concerned in carbohydrate metabolism. Thiamine deficiency causes beri-beri.

**Thiersch** (*tersh*). Type of skin graft in which the epidermis and upper part of the dermis is employed, *cf.* full thickness graft.

**thigh** (*thī*). Part of lower limb above the knee.

**Thomas's splint.** (1) Knee splint for immobilizing a fractured femur or tibia and fibula. It consists of two sidepieces of metal with a crosspiece at foot, and an oblique ring for fixation in groin. Leg is kept in position by pieces of material slung between sidepieces and adjusted to the fracture. (2) Hip splint used for immobilization of the hip.

**Thomsen's disease** (*tom-senz di-sēz*). Myotonia congenita.

**thoracic** (*tho-ra'-sik*). Pertaining to the thorax.

**thoracic duct.** The largest lymphatic vessel. It receives the fat absorbed from the intestine and the lymph from the greater part of the body. It ascends from the abdomen through the thorax to the left side of the neck, where it empties itself into the angle of union between the left internal jugular vein and the subclavian vein.

**thoracocentesis** (*tho'-ra-ko-*

*sen-tē'-sis*). Puncture of the thorax, *e.g.* aspiration of pleural effusion.

**thoracolysis** (*thor-a-kō-lī'-sis*). The severing of adhesions between the two layers of the pleura.

**thoracoplasty** (*tho'-ra-kō-plas-ti*). Operation in which part of the chest wall is resected in order to collapse the underlying lung. Formerly used in the treatment of tuberculosis.

**thoracotomy** (*tho-ra-ko'-to-mi*). Operation of opening the thorax.

**thorax** (*tho'-raks*). The chest; the cavity which holds the heart and lungs.

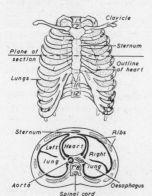

*52. The thorax*

**Thorium X** (*thaw'-ri-um eks*).

Radioactive isotope of radium ($^{224}$R) which is primarily an emitter of $\alpha$ particles which penetrate about 1 mm in tissues.

**threadworm** (*thred'-werm*). *Oxyuris vermicularis*. Small worm parasitic in the rectum; common in children.

**threonine** (*thrē'-ō-nēn*). An amino-acid.

**threshold** (*thresh'-hōld*). The intensity of a stimulus below which there is no response by a given irritable system.

**thrill** (*thril*). A vibratory impulse perceived by palpation.

**thrombectomy** (*throm-bek'-to-mi*). Removal of a blood clot.

**thrombin** (*throm'-bin*). Essential factor required in the blood clotting mechanism. *See* BLOOD COAGULATION.

**thrombo-angiitis** (*throm-bō-an-ji-ī'-tis*). Inflamed blood vessel with formation of a blood clot. *T. obliterans.* Inflammatory, obliterative disease of the blood vessels, especially in the limbs.

**thrombo-arteritis** (*throm-bō-ar-te-rī'-tis*). Arteritis with thrombosis.

**thrombocytes** (*throm'-bō-sīts*). Blood platelets.

**thrombocytopenia** (*throm-bō-sī-tō-pē-ni-a*). Deficiency of platelets in the blood.

**thromboendarterectomy** (*throm'-bō-end-ar-ter-ek'-to-mi*). Operation to remove a clot from a blood vessel.

**thrombokinase** (*throm-bō-kī'-nāz*). The active principle of a substance liberated when the blood platelets are disintegrated. It is necessary for the clotting of blood.

**thrombolytic** (*throm-bō-li'-tik*). An agency which breaks down clots.

**thrombophlebitis** (*throm-bō-fle-bī'-tis*). Inflammation of a vein with thrombosis.

**thrombophlebitis migrans.** Recurrent thrombophlebitis affecting superficial veins in different sites. There is sometimes an association with carcinoma of the pancreas or stomach.

**thromboplastin** (*throm-bō-plas'-tin*). Thrombokinase.

**thrombosis** (*throm-bō'-sis*). Coagulation of blood in the vessels. The clot thus formed is termed a *thrombus*.

**thrombus** (*throm'-bus*). (plu. **thrombi**). A clot of blood found in the heart or in a blood vessel.

**thrush** (*thru'-sh*). Infection of mucous membrane, *e.g.* mouth or vagina, by *Candida albicans*. This fungus infection gives rise to white patches on the membrane.

**thymectomy** (*thī-mek'-to-mi*). Operation to remove the thymus gland. Sometimes performed for myasthenia gravis.

**thymoma** (*thī'-mō-ma*). Malignant neoplasm of the thymus.

**thymus** (*thī'-mus*). A gland at the root of the neck. It is largest in children and then gradually atrophies. The function of the thymus is not clear. It appears to be concerned with the immunological mechanisms of the body. It has been suggested that it acts as a 'priming station' for lymphocytes where they are selected for release into the general circulation. However, at the present time it is not possible to be certain of its function. The gland, which is situated in the anterior mediastinum reaches its maximum size at puberty and thereafter slowly atrophies.

**thyroglossal cyst** (*thī'-rō-glo-sal*). Cyst in the thyroglossal duct which is the embryonic canal formed by the migration of the presumptive thyroid cells from the surface of the tongue.

**thyroid cartilage** (*thī'-royd*). The large cartilage of the larynx forming the 'Adam's apple'.

**thyroid crisis.** Acute severe thyrotoxicosis which may follow subtotal thyroidectomy in the absence of pre-operative antithyroid treatment.

**thyroidectomy** (*thī-roy-dek'-to-mi*). Operative removal of the thyroid gland.

**thyroid gland** (*thī'-royd gland*). A bi-lobed ductless gland lying in front of the trachea. Its secretion, thyroxine, controls metabolism, growth and development. Congenital lack causes cretinism. Under-secretion in later life causes myxoedema. Excessive secretion causes thyrotoxicosis.

**thyrotoxicosis** (*thī-rō-tok-si-kō'-sis*). Hyperthyroidism, a syndrome due to an excessive production of thyroid hormone which has the effect of uncoupling oxidative phosphorylation, *i.e.* reducing the production of ATP by oxidative metabolism, in the cells. As a result the metabolic rate is speeded up in an attempt to maintain the yield of ATP. Clinically, hyperthyroidism is characterized by tachycardia, sweating, tremor, weight loss and increased appetite. Hyperthyroidism may be *primary* when the thyroid is at fault, or *secondary* when there is excessive stimulation of the thyroid by TSH from the pituitary. Recently a gamma globulin with thyroid stimulatory properties has been identified and is known as long-acting thyroid stimulant (LATS) which is considered to be the cause of the exophthalmos often associated with hyperthyroidism.

**thyrotrophic** (*thī-rō-trō'-fik*). Stimulating the thyroid. *T. hormone* is produced by the pituitary.

**thyroxine** (*thī-rok'-sin*). The active principle of the secretion of the thyroid gland. A substance rich in iodine.

**tibia** (*ti'-bi-a*). The shin bone; the larger bone of the leg below the knee. *See* SKELETON.

**tic.** Spasmodic twitching of muscles; usually of face and neck.

**tic douloureux** (*tik doo-loo-rer*). Trigeminal neuralgia.

**tick** (*tik*). A blood-sucking parasite. *T. fever*. (1) Relapsing fever. (2) Rocky Mountain fever, a rickettsial fever.

**tidal air** (*tī-dal ā-r*). That which is inspired and expired during normal breathing.

**tincture** (*tink-tūr*). An alcoholic solution of a drug.

**tinea** (*ti'-ni-a*). Ringworm.

**tinnitus aurium** (*tin-ni'-tus aw'-ri-um*). A ringing in the ears.

**tissue** (*ti'-shū*). An aggregate of similar cells performing a similar function.

**tissue culture.** Method by which cells and tissues are grown under artificial conditions after their removal from the parent organism.

**titration** (*tī-trā'-shon*). Quantitative analysis by volume by means of standard solutions.

**titre** (*tē-ter*). A standard of purity or strength.

**tocography** (*to-ko'-gra-fi*). Method of recording alterations in the intra-uterine pressure.

**tocopherol** (*to-ko'-fe-rol*). Vitamin E. Its precise function is unknown but it is widely used as an antioxidant in medical preparations.

**tolerance** (*to'-le-rans*). Ability to tolerate a substance. Usually applied to (a) *immunological tolerance*, in which there is no immunological reaction to a potential antigen or (b) *tolerance to drugs*, *e.g.* barbiturates, morphine, etc. when the dose requires to be increased to achieve the same effect. The mechanism of this is not clear but it has been suggested that there is an increased synthesis of the enzymes responsible for the breakdown of the drug.

**tomography** (*to-mo'-gra-fi*). Technique in radiography which brings into focus only

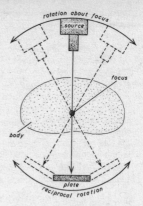

53. *Tomography*

those objects lying in the plane of interest, while blurring structures on either side of the object's plane; also known as body section radiography.

**tone** (*tōn*). (1) State of tension as found in muscles. (2) Quality of sound.

**tongue** (*tung*). The muscular organ which lies in the floor of the mouth, and whose chief functions are to assist in the mastication and tasting of food and in vocalization.

**tongue tie** (*tung' tī*). Extremely rare condition in which the tongue is rendered immobile by adhesions to the floor of the mouth. Minor degrees of tongue tie are common and

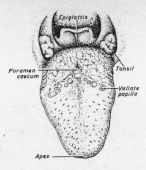

54. *The tongue*

are not a cause for delayed speech.

**tonic** (*to'-nik*). (1) A traditional medicine which was thought to increase general physical well-being after an illness. (2) Term applied to continuous spasms, *cf.* clonic.

**tonometer** (*to-no'-me-ter*). Instrument for measuring tension such as that used to measure intra-ocular tension.

**tonsillectomy** (*ton-si-lek'-to-mi*). Operative removal of the tonsils.

**tonsillitis** (*ton-si-lī'-tis*). Inflammation of tonsils.

**tonsillotome** (*ton-sil'-ō-tōm*). Instrument for cutting off a tonsil.

**tonsils** (*ton'sils*). Two oval bodies of lymphoid tissue on either side of the throat at the opening of the pharynx.

**toothed** (*tootht*). Dentate. Possessing teeth.

**tophus** (*tō-fus*). Concretion of uric acid salts found on the ear lobes characteristic of gout.

**topical** (*to'-pi-kal*). Pertaining to a particular locality. Local.

**topography** (*to-po'-gra-fi*). A study of the various areas of the body.

**torpor** (*tor'-per*). Lethargy.

**torsion** (*tor'-shon*). Twisting.

**torso** (*tor'-sō*). The trunk.

**torticollis** (*tor-tē-kol'-lis*). Wry-neck. The head is flexed and drawn to one side as the result of contraction of the sternomastoid muscles either due to spasm or fibrosis in the body of the muscle.

**tourniquet** (*tor'-nē-kā*). An instrument used to exert pressure on an artery and so arrest bleeding.

**toxaemia** (*tok-sē'-mi-a*). Toxins in the circulation. *See also* PRE-ECLAMPSIA, PRE-ECLAMPTIC TOXAEMIA.

**toxic** (*tok'-sik*). Poisonous.

**toxicology** (*tok-si-ko'-lo-ji*). The study of poisons.

**toxicosis** (*tok-si-kō'-sis*). Any disease due to poisoning.

**toxin** (*tok'-sin*). A poison, usually of bacterial origin.

**toxoid** (*tok'-soyd*). A non-poisonous modification of a toxin. Sometimes used to immunize against disease.

**toxoid-antitoxin** (*tok'-soyd-an-ti-tok'-sin*). A mixture of toxoid and its antitoxin.

**toxoplasmosis** (*tok'-sō-plas-mō'-sis*). Infection by *Toxoplasma gondii*. The clinical manifestations vary in severity. In infants severe encephalitis may occur. Other results of infection include nephritis, pneumonia, rashes and lymphadenopathy.

**trabecula** (*tra-be'-kū-la*). A septum extending into an organ from its capsule or wall.

**trace elements** (*trās e'-le-menz*). Mineral substances whose presence in minute amounts in the diet is necessary for the maintenance of health, *e.g.* cobalt, copper, manganese, etc.

**tracer** (*trā-ser*). Radioactive isotope or substance containing a radioactive isotope which enables the substance to be traced in metabolic systems.

**trachea** (*tra'-kē-a*). The windpipe; the air passage from the larynx to the bronchi. *See* BRONCHI.

**tracheitis** (*tra-kē-ī'-tis*). Inflammation of the trachea.

**trachelorrhaphy** (*tra-ke-lo'-ra-fi*). The operation of suturing a torn cervix uteri.

**tracheobronchitis** (*tra-ki-o-bron-kī'-tis*). Inflammation of trachea and bronchi.

**tracheostomy** (*tra-kē-os'-to'-mi*). Incision into the trachea to provide an accessory airway.

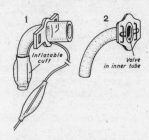

*55. Tracheostomy tubes*
*(1) Cuffed plastic tube*
*(2) Silver valved tube (Negus)*

**tracheotomy** (*trak-ē-o'-to-mi*). Incision of the trachea.

**trachoma** (*tra-kō'-ma*). Virus mediated conjunctivitis which untreated results in blindness.

**traction** (*trak'-shon*). Pulling, as for example in traction of a limb to facilitate correct apposition.

**tragus** (*trā'-gus*). The small eminence just inside the ear.

**trait** (*trā*). A special characteristic of the individual.

**trance** (*trahn'-s*). State of unnatural sleep; catalepsy.

**tranquillizer** (*tran'-qwil-lī-zer*).

Drug with sedative and tranquillizing action, such as chlorpromazine. Used to relieve anxiety, tension and agitation in mental illness. May be useful in the control of pain during a terminal illness. While the patient is taking this drug, the action of a hypnotic or analgesic is made more powerful.

**transaminase** (*tran-sa'-mi-nāz*). Enzyme which transfers amino (—NH₂) groups from one substance to another. Enzymes of this type are liberated into the bloodstream from damaged cells, particularly muscle cells, and the estimation of the *serum transaminases* (glutamic-oxaloacetic transaminase or GOT and glutamic-pyruvic transaminase or GPT) is sometimes helpful in the diagnosis of conditions in which there is muscle damage, *e.g.* myocardial infarction, dermatomyositis, etc.

**transference** (*trans'-fe-renz*). A psycho-analytical term. The patient transfers his own emotions on to the analyst, *e.g.* he may develop an intense love or hatred of him. Also used if the patient transfers his own emotions on to someone else as when he blames someone else for what he has done himself.

**transfusion** (*trans-fū'-shon*). *See* BLOOD TRANSFUSION.

**transillumination** (*tranz-i-lū-mi-nā'-shon*). The method whereby suppuration in the maxillary or frontal sinus is detected. The patient is placed in a completely darkened room, and a bright light placed in the mouth. The affected side is not so highly illuminated as the sound side.

**transmigration** (*tranz'-mī-grā'-shon*). The passage of cells through a membrane.

**transperitoneal** (*tranz-pe-ri-to-nē'-al*). Through the peritoneum.

**transplantation** (*tranz-plan-tā'-shon*). Operation to remove a portion of tissue from one part of the body to another.

**transposition of vessels** (*tranz-po-zi'-shon*). Defect of development in which the pulmonary artery arises from the left ventricle and the aorta from the right ventricle.

**transudation** (*tran-sū-dā'-shon*). Oozing of fluid through a membrane or from a tissue.

**transurethal** (*tranz-ū-rē'-thral*). Via the uretha.

**transverse** (*trans'-vers*). Across. A tranverse incision is from side to side. *T. process.* Lateral projection of the neural arch of a vertebra with which the head of a rib articulates.

**transvestism** (*trans'-ves-tizm*). Psychiatric condition in which there exists an anomaly of instinct. The patient wears the clothes characteristic of the opposite sex. Transvestites may identify themselves completely with the opposite sex and develop delusional convictions of this kind.

**trapezium** (*tra-pē'-zi-um*). First bone in second row of the carpal bones.

**trapezius** (*tra-pē'-zi-us*). A large muscle, running from the nape of the neck and the upper part of the spine, to the clavicle and scapula.

**trapezoid** (*tra-pē'-zoyd*). Second bone in second row of the carpal bones.

**trauma** (*traw'-ma*). Injury.

**treatment** (*trēt'-ment*). A way of curing a disease. *Conservative t.* Treatment by rest and drugs rather than by surgery. In dentistry, treatment of a tooth without extracting it. *Palliative t.* An attempt to alleviate pain, etc. but not a cure for the disease. *Prophylactic t.* A means of preventing the disease such as by immunization against it, etc.

**Trematoda** (*tre-ma-to'-da*).

Parasites which infect man, causing bilharzia.

**tremor** (*tre'-mor*). Involuntary trembling.

**Trendelenburg's operation** (*tren-de'-len-bergs o-pe-rā'-shon*). Used to treat varicose veins. The long saphenous vein is ligated in the groin, *T.'s position.* Operation position with patient supine tilted with the head down. *T.'s sign.* Test of the ability of the abductor muscles of the hip to steady the pelvis when one leg is raised from the ground.

**trephining** (*tre-fī'-ning*). Removing a circular piece of tissue to gain access to the enclosed structure, *e.g.* trephining the bone of the skull.

**Treponema pallidum** (*tre-pō-nē'-ma pa'-li-dum*). The infecting agent of syphilis.

**trial of labour.** Attempt to achieve spontaneous delivery in any case where there is doubt about a normal delivery; always done in hospital where there may be speedy intervention if necessary.

**triangular bandage** (*trī-an'-gū-la*). Made by cutting a 36-inch square of linen diagonally across. It is very useful in emergencies and for minor casualties.

**triceps** (*trī'-seps*). Certain muscles with three heads, especially the one at the back of the arm which extends the elbow.

**trichiasis** (*tri-kī'-a-sis*). Inversion of the eyelashes towards the eye.

**trichiniasis** (*tri-ki-nī-a-sis*), **trichinosis** (*tri-ki-nō-sis*). Infection with a parasitic worm, *Trichina spiralis*, which is parasitic in pigs and sometimes in man.

**Trichocephalus dispar** (*tri-kō-ke'-fa-lus*). The whipworm. A parasite of the human large intestine.

**Trichomonas vaginalis** (*tri-kō-mō-nas' va-ji-nā'-lis*). A protozoon, motile by means of flagellae. It is a common cause of vaginitis.

**trichonosis** (*tri-kō-nō'-sis*). Abnormality of hair.

**trichophytosis** (*tri-kō-fī-tō'-sis*). Fungus infection of the hair.

**trichuris** (*tri-kū-ris*). Type of threadworm.

**tricuspid valve** (*trī-kus'-pid*). Valve with three cusps, particularly the heart valve between the right atrium and right ventricle.

**trigeminal** (*trī-je'-mi-nal*). Triple.

**trigeminal nerves.** Fifth pair of cranial nerves. They are motor and sensory and each has three branches supplying the skin and structures of the face, tongue and teeth.

**trigeminal neuralgia** (*nū-ral'-ji-a*). Pain in the face of unknown cause. The distribution is confined to branches of the trigeminal nerve. The pain is paroxysmal and precipitated by mild stimuli such as washing the face or eating.

**trigger finger** (*trig'-ger fin'-ger*). A thickening of the tendon sheath at the metacarpophalangeal joint often of the first finger of the right hand. The finger can be bent but not straightened without help.

**trigone** (*trī'-gōn*). A triangle. *T. vesicae.* Triangular space in the bladder, immediately behind the opening to the urethra.

**trimester** (*tri-mes'-ter*). A three-month period.

**triplegia** (*trī-plē-ji-a*). Paralysis of three limbs.

**triplets** (*trip'-lets*). Three children resulting from one pregnancy.

**triploid** (*tri'-ployd*). Having three times the haploid number of chromosomes in a nucleus.

**trismus** (*tris'-mus*). Lock-jaw. Occurs as a reflex in dental caries. Is also a symptom of tetanus.

**trisomy** (*tri'-so-mi*). Presence of additional somatic chromosomes.

**trocar** (*trō'-kar*). The perforating instrument used with a cannula to draw off fluids from the body.

**trochanter** (*tro-kan'-ter*). Two processes at the junction of the neck and shaft of femur.

**trochlear** (*tro'-klē-ar*). (1) Relating to a pulley. (2) Relating to the trochlear nerve.

**trochlear nerves** (*tro'-klē-ar*). The fourth pair of cranial nerves. Motor nerves to the eyes.

**trophic** (*trō'-fik*). Relating to nutrition. Trophic ulcers occur where nutrition is poor, particularly if there is paralysis.

**trophoblast** (*trō'-fō-blarst*). The outer ectodermal layer of the embedding ovum.

**Trousseau's sign** (*troo'-sōs sīn*). Sign of increased nervous excitability due to hypocalcaemia. A sphygmomanometer cuff is inflated above the patient's systolic blood pressure for 3 minutes. Spasm in the flexor muscles produces the classical *main d'accoucheur.*

**trunk.** The torso.

**truss** (*trus*). An apparatus for retaining a hernia in place.

**Trypanosoma** (*tri'-pa-nō-sō-ma*). A genus of microscopic parasites which cause sleeping sickness and other diseases.

**trypanosomiasis** (*tri'-pa-nō-sō-mī'-a-sis*). Infection with trypanosomes.

**trypsin** (*trip'-sin*). A peptidase, which breaks down proteins and peptides at certain peptide links.

**trypsinogen** (*trip-si'-nō-jen*). A precursor of trypsin.

**tryptophane** (*trip'-to-fān*). An essential amino-acid.

**tsetse fly** (*tet'-sē-flī*). Genus of dipteran insects which are carriers of trypanosome diseases such as sleeping sickness.

**tubal** (*tū'-bal*). Relating to a tube, and especially to an oviduct. *T. gestation* or *pregnancy.* Pregnancy in a Fallopian tube. *See* EXTRA-UTERINE GESTATION.

**tubercle** (*tū'-ber-kl*). (1) A small eminence. (2) The small greyish nodule which is the specific lesion of the tubercle bacillus.

**tuberculide** (*tū-ber'-kū-līd*). Any skin rash due to tuberculous infection.

**tuberculin** (*tū-ber'-kū-lin*). A preparation from cultures of the tubercle bacillus used in diagnosis of tuberculosis.

**tuberculoma** (*tū-ber-kū-lō-ma*).

Walled-off region of caseating tuberculosis.

**tuberculosis** (*tū-ber-kū-lō'-sis*). Infection by *Mycobacterium tuberculosis*.

**tuberculous** (*tū-ber'-kū-lus*). Connected with tuberculosis.

**tuberosity** (*tū'-be-ro'-si-ti*). Bony eminence.

**tuberous sclerosis** (*tū'-be-rus skle-rō'-sis*). See EPILOIA.

**tubo-ovarian** (*tū'-bo-ō-vā'-ri-an*). Connected with both the Fallopian tube and the ovary (*e.g.* abscess, cyst).

**tubule** (*tū-būl*). Small tube.

**tularaemia** (*tu-la-rē'-mē-a*). Deer fly fever caused by *Pasteurella tularensis*.

**tumefaction** (*tū-me-fak-shon*). Becoming swollen.

**tumour** (*tū'-mer*). A lump. Frequently used synonymously with neoplasm.

**tunica** (*tū'-ni-ka*). A term applied to several membranes, *e.g. T. vaginalis*, the serous coat of the testicle.

**turbinate bones** (*ter'-bi-nāt bōnz*). Three thin convoluted bones situated on the lateral wall of each nasal fossa.

**turbinectomy** (*ter-bin-ek'-to-mi*). Operation to excise a turbinate bone.

**turgid** (*ter'-jid*). Swollen, distended.

**Turner's syndrome** (*ter-nerz*). Gonadal dysgenesis is caused by an abnormality of the sex chromosomes. There are multiple abnormalities comprising the syndrome webbing of the neck, cubitus valgus, failure of gonad development and often coarctation of the aorta.

**tussis** (*tus'-sis*). A cough.

**twins** (*twii-nz*). Two children from a single pregnancy.

**tylosis** (*tī-lō'-sis*). Thickening of the skin of the soles and palms.

**tympanites** (*tim-pa-nī'-tēz*). A distended state of the abdomen caused by gas in the intestines.

**tympanitis** (*tim-pan-ī'-tis*). Otitis media.

**tympanoplasty** (*tim'-pan-ō-plas'-ti*). Operation to reconstruct sound-conducting mechanism in middle ear.

**tympanum** (*tim'-pa-num*). Also called tympanic cavity. A part of the middle ear, and comprises a cavity in the temporal bone deep to the tympanic membrane. *T. membrane.* The membrane separating the middle from the external ear, commonly called the eardrum.

**typhoid fever** (*tī'-foyd fē-ver*). An acute infectious disease which flourishes where the standard of hygiene is poor. Caused by ingestion of the *Salmonella typhi* from contaminated food or water supplies. The germs reach the intestines and through the lymph channels produce a bacteraemia. After the first week the germs settle in the spleen, liver and intestines, especially the ileum. Here the lymph follicles known as Peyer's patches are attacked. They become inflamed, raised, and eventually the tissue of the follicle sloughs off. It is at this stage that intestinal haemorrhage or perforation may occur. Incubation period for the disease is 12–14 days and the patient remains infectious until bacteriological tests are negative. The onset is gradual. For 4 or 5 days the temperature is of the step-ladder type. If untreated, the patient becomes very ill during the second week with high temperature and slow pulse and the stools are often pea-soup in character. Rose-coloured spots, in crops, appear on the abdomen, chest and between the shoulder blades. By the third week, if untreated, the patient is delirious. Treatment is with co-trimoxazole, chloramphenicol, usually with dramatic improvement. *See also* ENTERIC FEVER.

**typhus fever** (*tī'-fus fē-ver*). A highly infectious fever characterized by a petechial rash, high temperature and great prostration. It is caused by Rickettsia bodies from infected lice or rat fleas.

**tyrosine** (*tī-rō-sin*). An essential amino-acid.

# U

**ulcer** (*ul'-ser*). Region in which there is a breach in the continuity of an epithelium.

**ulcerative** (*ul'-se-ra-tiv*). Pertaining to ulceration. *U. colitis*. A disease with inflammation and ulceration of the colon. There is diarrhoea, and mucus and blood are passed in the stools. The patient is anaemic. The disease may be mild or severe and pathogenic organisms appear not to cause it, though emotional stress seems to precipitate it.

**ulna** (*ul'-na*). The inner bone of the forearm.

**ulnar.** The name of an artery, a vein and a nerve running beside the ulna.

**ultramicroscopic** (*ul-tra-mī-krō-sko'-pik*). Too small to be seen with a microscope.

**ultra-violet rays.** Photons with higher frequency distribution than the violet end of the visible spectrum. *See* RADIATION.

**umbilical cord** (*um-bi'-lī'-kal*

*kord*). The funis; the cord connecting the fetus with the placenta.

**umbilicated** (*um-bi'-li-kā-ted*). With an appearance like the umbilicus.

**umbilicus** (*um-bi-lī'-kus*). Region of attachment of the umbilical cord. A small depressed scar on the anterior abdominal wall.

**unciform** (*un'-si-form*). The hook-shaped bone of the wrist.

**uncinariasis** (*un'-si-na-rī'-a-sis*). Infection with hook-worm.

**unconsciousness** (*un-kon'-shus-nes*). A state of being insensible as when anaesthetized.

**undulant** (*un'-dū-lant*). Wave-like. *U. fever. See* BRUCEL-LOSIS.

**unguentum** (*un-goo-en'-tum*). An ointment; abbreviation, *ung.*

**unguis** (*ung'-gwis*). A finger-nail.

**unicellular** (*ū-ni-sel'-lū-la*). Composed of one cell.

**unilateral** (*ū-ni-la'-te-ral*). Found only on one side.

**uniocular** (*ū-ni-o'-kū-la*). Relating to one eye.

**union** (*ū'-nē-on*). Joining together to form one. Esp., union of fracture.

**uniovular** (*ū-ni-o'-vū-la*). With one ovum. Identical twins come from the same ovum.

**uniparous** (*ū-ni'-pa-rus*). Having borne only one child.

**unit** (*ū'-nit*). An individual thing or group forming a complete whole. A standard of measurement.

**urachus** (*ū'-rā-kus*). A fibrous cord in the fetus from the bladder to the umbilicus. It becomes the median umbilical ligament.

**uraemia** (*ū-rē'-mi-a*). Strictly this means an elevation of the urea concentration in the blood above its normal value of about 5 mmol/litre. Generally, however, it is used to describe a syndrome resulting from impaired renal function which may be due to *renal* or *extrarenal* causes, *e.g.* dehydration. There are disturbances of salt and water balance and acid–base equilibrium in addition to the elevation of the blood urea.

**uraniscorrhaphy** (*ū-ra-nis-ko'-ra-fi*). Suture of a cleft palate.

**urate** (*ū-rāt*). Salt of uric acid.

**urea** (*ū-rē-a*). Principal excretory product of protein catabolism. It is water soluble and has the chemical structure:

$$O=C<^{NH_2}_{NH_2}$$

**urea concentration test** (*ū'-rē-a kon-sen-trā'-shon test*). The normal amount of urea in urine is 2 per cent. If a definite quantity of urea, 15 grams in 100 ml water, is given to a fasting subject, the amount of urea eliminated by the kidneys can be estimated by specimens taken 1, 2 and 3 hours after. The proper excretion of urea shows an adequately functioning kidney. The percentage should rise to 3 or 4. This test is used to estimate renal efficiency.

**uresis** (*ū-rē-sis*). Urination.

**ureter** (*ū'-re-ter*). The canal between the kidney and the bladder, down which the urine passes.

**ureteral** (*ū-rē'-te-ral*). Pertaining to the ureter.

**ureterectomy** (*ū-rē-te-rek'-to-mi*). Excision of a ureter.

**ureteric** (*ū-rē-te'-rik*). Pertaining to a ureter. *U. reflux*. The flow of urine up the ureters at the same time as voiding to the exterior; can be a contributory cause to recurrent urinary infection in childhood.

**ureteritis** (*ū-rē-te-rī-tis*). Inflammation of a ureter.

**ureterocele** (*ū-rē-te-rō-sēl*). The result of congenital atresia of a ureteric orifice which causes a cystic enlargement of the portion of the ureter situated in the bladder wall.

**ureterolith** (*ū-rē'-te-rō-lith'*). Stone in a ureter.

**ureterolithotomy** (*ū-rē'-te-ro-li'-tho-to-mi*). Operation for the removal of a stone impacted in the ureter.

**ureterosigmoidostomy** (*ū-rē'-te-rō-sig-moy-dos'-to-mi*). Implantation of a ureter into the sigmoid colon.

**ureterovaginal** (*ū-rē-te-rō-va-jī'-nal*). Pertaining to a ureter and the vagina.

**ureterovesical** (*ū-rē-te-rō-ve-sī'-kal*). Pertaining to a ureter and the bladder.

**urethra** (*ū-rē'-thra*). The canal between the bladder and the exterior through which the urine is discharged.

**urethral** (*ū-rē'-thral*). Pertaining to the urethra.

**urethritis** (*ū-rē-thrī'-tis*). Inflammation of the urethra.

**urethrocele** (*ū-rē'-thrō-sēl*). Urethral diverticulum. A small pouch in the wall of the urethra more common in women than in men. The origin is probably the result of a developmental defect.

**urethrography** (*ū-rē-thro'-gra-fi*). X-ray examination of the urethra by means of retrograde injection of a radio-opaque dye.

**urethroplasty** (*ū-rē-thrō-plas'-ti*). Plastic repair to the urethra.

**urethroscope** (*ū-rē-thro-skōp*). An instrument for viewing the interior of the urethra.

**urethrotomy** (*ū-rē-thro'-to-mi*).

Incision of the urethra to remedy stricture; the instrument used being a urethrotome.

**uric acid** (*ū'-rik a'-sid*). Complex nitrogen-containing organic compound only slightly water-soluble. Formed in the breakdown of nucleic acids. It is excreted by primates and Dalmatian dogs but not by other mammals. Patients with gout accumulate uric acid salts in the blood and tissues.

**uridine** (*ū'-ri-dēn*). A nitrogenous base present in RNA.

**urinalysis** (*ū-ri-na'-li-sis*). Analysis of urine.

**urinary** (*ū'-ri-na-ri*). Pertaining to the urine. *U. organs.* These include the kidneys, ureters, bladder and urethra.

**urination** (*ū-ri-nā'-shon*). Micturition. The act of discharging urine.

**urine** (*ū'-rin*). Excretory product of the kidneys.

**uriniferous tubules** (*ū-ri-ni'-fe'-rus*). *See* NEPHRON.

**urinometer** (*ū-ri-no'-me-ter*). A small glass instrument with a graduated stem, used for measuring the specific gravity of urine.

**urobilin** (*ū-rō-bi'-lin*). Pigmented derivative of urobilinogen.

**urobilinogen** (*ū-rō-bi'-li'-no-jen*). Derivative of bilirubin

which is made in the intestine by the gut bacteria. Some of it is absorbed and, in circumstances in which there is impaired liver function, may be excreted in the urine.

**urochrome** (*ū-rō-krōm*). Pigment colouring urine.

**urogenital sinus** (*ū-rō-je'-ni-tal sī-nus*). Part of the developing genitalia which forms the bladder and urethra. It develops as a ventral diverticulum from the hind gut.

**urography** (*ū-ro'-gra-fi*). X-ray examination of the urinary tract.

**urolith** (*ū-rō-lith'*). A stone found in the urine.

**urologist** (*ū-ro'-lo-jist*). A specialist in urology.

**urology** (*ū-ro'-lo-ji*). The study of diseases of the urinary tract.

**uroscopy** (*ū-ros'-ko-pi*). Examination of the urine.

**urticaria** (*er-ti-kā'-ri-a*). Nettle rash: hives. Allergic reaction affecting the permeability of small blood vessels. Characterized clinically by erythema and the formation of wheals.

**uterine** (*ū-te-rīn*). Relating to the uterus.

**uterogestation** (*ū-te-rō-jes-tā'-shon*). The period of pregnancy.

**uterovesical** (*ū'-ter-ō-ve-sī-kal*). Relating to the uterus and the bladder.

**uterus** (*ū-te-rus*). Womb. Muscular hollow pelvic organ. In the resting state it measures about 3 in by 2 in and is triangular in shape with a cervix about 1 in which projects into the vagina. It is connected bilaterally

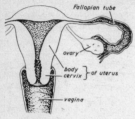

*56. The uterus*

to the oviducts (Fallopian tubes). The uterus has a glandular epithelium lining it and the whole structure is under the control of sex hormones, in particular oestrogens and progesterone. *See* MENSTRUATION. The uterus is the normal site of implantation of the trophoblast. During pregnancy the uterus grows out of the pelvis to occupy much of the abdominal cavity. After delivery, when contraction of the smooth muscle in the wall expels the fetus and placenta, the uterus diminishes in size, returning to its resting state. *See* INVOLUTION.

**utricle** (*ū'-trikl*). (1) The larger sac of membrane in the vestibule of the internal ear. (2) The prostatic vesicle.

**uvea** (*ū-vē-a*), **uveal tract.** The middle coat of the eyeball. The choroid, ciliary body and iris as a whole.

**uveitis** (*ū-vi-ī'-tis*). Inflammation of the uvea.

**uvula** (*ū'-vū-la*). A small fleshy body hanging down at the back of the soft palate.

**uvulectomy** (*ū-vū-lek'-to-mi*). Excision of uvula.

**uvulitis** (*ū-vū-lī'-tis*). Inflammation of the uvula.

# V

**vaccination** (*vak-si-nā-shon*). (1) Inoculation of cowpox lymph into the arm as a protection from smallpox. No longer done routinely on babies. (2) Protective inoculation with any vaccine.

**vaccine** (*vak-sēn*). An extract or suspension of attenuated or killed organisms. The antigenic properties of the organism are retained and the vaccine is used to immunize the recipient.

**vaccinia** (*vak-si'-ni-a*). Cowpox. In man, it gives immunity to smallpox and is therefore used in vaccination against that disease.

**vacuole** (*vak-ū-ōl*). Specialized

region within a cell surrounded by plasma membrane. *See also* PHAGOCYTOSIS.

**vagal** (*vā-gal*). Pertaining to the vagus nerve.

**vagina** (*va-jī'-na*). The passage leading from the cervix uteri to the vulva. The lower limit of this canal is formed by the hymen.

**vaginal** (*va-jī'-nal*). Pertaining to the vagina.

**vaginismus** (*va-ji-nis'-mus*). Spasmodic contraction of the vagina whenever the vulva or vagina is touched. May be a cause of painful sexual intercourse.

**vaginitis** (*va-ji-nī'-tis*). Inflammation of the vagina.

**vagotomy** (*vā-go'-to-mi*). Surgical division of the vagus nerve sometimes performed on patients with peptic or duodenal ulcers.

**vagus** (*vā'-gus*). *See* CRANIAL NERVES (10).

**valgus** (*val'-gus*). *See* TALIPES.

**valine** (*vā-lēn*). One of the essential amino-acids.

**valve.** A fold across a channel allowing flow in one direction only.

**valvotomy** (*val-vo'-to-mi*). Incision into a valve, especially HEART VALVE. The purpose of the operation is to widen the orifice of a stenosed valve.

**valvulae conniventes** (*val-vū-lē ko-ni-ven-tēs*). Transverse folds of mucous membrane in the upper part of the small intestine.

**valvulitis** (*val-vū-lī'-tis*). Inflammation of a valve.

**valvulotomy** (*val-vū-lo-to-mi*). *See* VALVOTOMY.

**van den Bergh's test** (*van-den bergs*). Method by which the amounts of conjugated and unconjugated bilirubin are estimated in the serum. This is sometimes helpful in the differential diagnosis of jaundice.

**varicella** (*va-ri-se-la*). Chicken-pox.

**varices** (*va-ri-sēs*) (sing. **varix**). Dilated, twisted veins.

**varicocele** (*va-ri-kō-sēl*). A varicose condition of the veins of the spermatic cord.

**varicose ulcer** (*va-ri-kōs ul'-ser*). Ulceration of the lower legs due to reduction in the blood supply resulting from the increased venous pressure.

**varicose veins** (*va-ri-kōs vāns*). Dilated veins in which the valves have become incompetent. As a result the blood flow may become reversed or static. Most common in the legs where the blood pools by gravitation. Other examples are piles and oesophageal varices.

**varicotomy** (*va-ri-ko'-to-mi*). Excision of varicose vein.

**variola** (*va-ri-ō'-la*). *See* SMALL-POX.

**varioloid** (*va'-ri-ō-loyd*). A mild form of smallpox, sometimes seen in persons who have been previously vaccinated.

**varix** (*vār-iks*). An enlarged and tortuous vein.

**varus** (*vār-us*). *See* TALIPES.

**vas.** A vessel, or duct of the body; as *vas deferens*, the duct of the testis.

**vascular** (*vas-kū-la*). (1) Possessing a blood supply. (2) Concerning the blood vessels and the supply of blood.

**vascular system.** System of the blood vessels.

**vasectomy** (*vā-sek'-to-mi*). Removal of a part of the vas deferens. Used as a method of sterilization of the male.

**vasoconstriction** (*vā-sō-kon-strik'-shon*). Contraction of blood vessels.

**vasodilatation** (*vā-sō-dī-la-tā'-shon*). Dilatation of blood vessels.

**vasomotor** (*vā-sō-mō-tor*). Concerned with constriction of blood vessels. *V. nerves.* Sympathetic nerves which control the tone of the smooth muscle in the walls of blood vessels.

**vasopressin** (*vā-so-pre-sin*). Posterior pituitary extract. *See* PITUITARY GLAND.

**vasospasm** (*va'-so-spasm*). Spasm of the blood vessels.

**vasovagal syndrome** (*vā-sō-vā-gal sin-drōm*). Slowing of the heart rate with a feeling of nausea and grave distress. The attack may last a few minutes or an hour. The cause is unknown.

**Vater's ampulla** (*vah-ters am-poo-la*). Small dilatation in the terminal portion of the common bile duct where it empties into the duodenum.

**VDRL test.** Antigen–antibody test for syphilis. Antibody to syphilis in serum under test is revealed by flocculation of antigen.

**vector** (*vek'-ter*). A carrier. One who conveys the infection to another person.

**vegetations** (*ve-je-tā'-shons*). Concretion of small clots on the diseased valves of the heart which occur in endocarditis.

**vegetative** (*ve'-je-ta-tiv*). Having the power of growth.

**vein** (*vān*). A vessel carrying the blood to the heart.

**vena cava** (*vē-na kā'-va*). The superior vena cava and the inferior vena cava are two large veins which return blood from the head and body and empty it into the right atrium of the heart.

**venepuncture** (*vē-nē-pungk'-cher*). Inserting a needle into a vein.

**venereal** (*ve-nār-ē-al*). Relating to sexual intercourse. *V. diseases*. Infectious diseases transmitted during sexual intercourse, *e.g.* gonorrhoea, syphilis.

**venereology** (*ve-nār-ē-o'-lo-ji*). The study of venereal disease.

**venesection** (*vē-nē-sek'-shon*). Blood-letting. A vein is opened and blood drained off from it. Frequently performed in the past for almost any ailment. There are very few present-day indications for venesection.

**venography** (*vē-no-gra-fi*). X-ray examination of veins following injection of contrast medium opaque to x-rays.

**venous** (*vē-nus*). Relating to the veins.

**ventilation** (*ven-ti-lā'-shon*). (1) The supply of fresh air. (2) The process of breathing.

**ventral** (*ven'-tral*). Relating to the belly.

**ventral root.** Anterior root, motor root. The nerve root containing the motor fibres.

**ventricles** (*ven'-trikls*). The two lower chambers of the heart are known as the right and left ventricles. The cavities in the brain also are known as ventricles.

**ventricular septal defect** (*ven-tri-kū-la dē-fekt*). Defect of development in which a passage remains patent between the two ventricles. Usually causes no disability and may close spontaneously during the early years of life. *See also* FALLOT'S TETRALOGY.

**ventriculography** (*ven-trik'-ū-lo-gra-fi*). X-ray examination of the ventricles of the brain. Air or a radio-opaque dye is introduced into the ventricles enabling their size and position to be observed.

**ventriculostomy** (*ven-trik'-ū-los-to-mi*). Operation to open a ventricle of the brain usually in order to construct a bypass when the flow of cerebrospinal fluid is obstructed.

**ventrofixation** (*ven-trō-fik-sā'-shon*). Operation to suture an abdominal viscus to the anterior abdominal wall.

**ventrosuspension** (*ven-trō-sus-pen-shon*). *See* VENTROFIXATION.

**venule** (*ve'-nūl*). Small vein.

**vermicide** (*ver-mi-sīd*). Substance able to kill worms in the intestine.

**vermiform appendix** (*ver-mi-fawm*). *See* APPENDIX VERMIFORMIS.

**vermifuge** (*ver'-mi-fūj*). Substance used to dispel worms.

**verminous** (*ver-mi-nus*). Infested with parasites, *e.g.* fleas, lice.

**vernix caseosa** (*ver-niks kā-sē-ō-sa*). The sebaceous material which covers the skin of the fetus.

**verruca** (*ve-roo'-ka*). A wart.

**Versene** (*ver'-sēn*). See EDTA.

**version** (*ver'shon*). The manoeuvre of altering the presentation of the fetus in the uterus so as to facilitate its delivery. It may be done with or without an anaesthetic or sedative. *Cephalic version* is turning the fetus, so that the head presents, while *podalic version* brings about a breech presentation. *Bipolar version*, version by acting upon both poles of the fetus.

**vertebrae** (*ver-te-brē*). The thirty-three small bones which form the backbone, or spinal column. *See* SKELETON.

**vertebrobasilar disease** (*ver-te-brō-ba-si-la di-sēz*). Occlusive disease affecting the vertebral and basilar arteries which results in a syndrome characterized by recurrent attacks of blindness, diplopia, vertigo, dysarthria, ataxia, and hemiparesis due to transient cerebral ischaemia.

**vertex** (*ver'-teks*). The crown of the head.

**vertigo** (*ver-tī'-gō*). Giddiness.

**vesica** (*vē'-si-ka*). The bladder.

**vesical** (*ve-sī'-kal*). Relating to the bladder.

**vesicant** (*vē'-si-kant*). A blistering agent.

**vesicle** (*vē'-si-kel*). A small blister. Blisters of greater diameter than 5 mm are termed bullae.

**vesicovaginal** (*ve-sī'-kō-va-jī'-nal*). Relating to the bladder and the vagina.

**vesicular breathing** (*ve-si'-kū-la brē'-thing*). The normal sound of inspiration heard on auscultation.

**vesiculitis** (*ve-si-kū-lī'-tis*). Inflammation of seminal vesicles.

**vestibular neuronitis** (*ves-ti'-bū-la nū-ro-nī'-tis*). Disorder affecting the vestibular nerve which is characterized by extreme vertigo while the hearing is unaffected. May result from streptomycin toxicity.

**vestibule** (*ves'-ti-būl*). (1) A small cavity of the ear into which the cochlea opens. (2) The space between the labia minora.

**vestigial** (*ves-ti'-ji-al*). Rudimentary. Bearing a trace of something now vanished or degenerate.

**viable** (*vī-a-bel*). Able to live.

**Vibrio** (*vib'-ri-ō*). Genus of bacteria with a characteristic

361 VIS

curved shape resembling a comma. One of these causes cholera.

**vicarious** (*vi-kār-i-us*). Substituted.

**villi** (*vi-lī*) (sing. **villus**). Fine soft processes of living cells. *Intestinal v.* in the small intestine, each contains a central vessel or lacteal, surrounded by a plexus of capillaries. *Chorionic v.* Processes arising from the chorion, the outer membrane of the developing ovum. Specialization of a mass of villi ultimately forms the placenta.

**villous** (*vi'-lus*). Resembling villi.

**Vincent's angina** (*vin-sens an-jī'-na*). Infection of the oral mucous epithelium by a symbiotic association of a spirochaete (*Borrelia vincenti*) and a fusiform Gram-negative bacterium (*Fusobacterium planti-vincenti*). Many consider these to be a secondary infection following an unrecognized primary lesion of the mucosa, *e.g.* virus infection, vitamin deficiency, etc.

**viraemia** (*vi-rē'-mi-a*). Presence of viruses in the blood.

**virilism** (*vi'-ri-lism*). The appearance of masculine characteristics in the female.

**virology** (*vī-ro'-lo-ji*). The study of viruses.

**virulence** (*vi-rū-lens*). Ability of an organism to overcome the resistance of the host.

**virus** (*vī-rus*). One of a group of disease-produced parasites which require to be inside the host cell in order to replicate. Some of the larger viruses, *e.g.* vaccinia (about 0·2 micron diameter), have a complex structure. Many of the smaller viruses consist largely of nucleic acid molecules.

**viscera** (*vi'-se-ra*). Plural of viscus.

**visceroptosis** (*vi-se-rop-tō'-sis*). Prolapse of the abdominal viscera.

**viscid** (*vis'-kid*), **viscous** (*vis-kus*). Sticky, thick, adhesive.

**viscus** (*vis'-kus*). An internal organ; *e.g.* the heart, lung, or stomach, etc.

**vision** (*vi'-syon*). The act or faculty of seeing. *Binocular vision*, use of both eyes without seeing double. *Central vision, direct vision*, that performed through the centre of the retina. *Double vision*, diplopia, a failure to fuse the images thrown upon the two retinae at the same time: two images are therefore seen and objects appear double. May be due to defect in muscles of the eye or an error of refraction. It is also a symptom of some nervous diseases, *e.g.* encephalitis lethargica. *Peripheral vision*, *indirect vision*, that performed by the peripheral or circumferential portion of the retina. *Stereoscopic vision*, that which gives perception of distance and solidity.

**visual** (*vi'-zū-al*). Pertaining to vision. *V. field*. The total area which can be seen at the same time without turning the head.

**vital** (*vī'-tal*). Pertaining to life. *V. capacity*. The amount of air that can be breathed out after a complete inspiration. *V. statistics*. Statistics of birth, marriages, deaths and diseases in a population.

**vitallium** (*vi-ta'-li-um*). An alloy used in bone surgery for nails, screws, plates, etc.

**vitamins** (*vi-ta-mins*). Organic substances which an organism requires to ingest from its environment. The reason that vitamins are essential is because the body cannot synthesize these metabolic requirements. At the present time most of the metabolic processes affected by vitamin molecules are unknown. Vitamin deficiencies are recognized by clinical syndromes such as scurvy (vitamin C deficiency). The vitamins presently recognized are as follows:

### Fat-soluble vitamins

**Vitamin A.** A carotene derivative. Plays important role in the regeneration of visual purple in the retina. Effect on cell metabolism unknown. Deficiency: xerophthalmia, follicular hyperkeratosis, night blindness.

**Vitamin D.** Group of sterols. Increase absorption of calcium from the gut. Mode of action not known. Deficiency: rickets, tetany.

**Vitamin E.** Group of tocopherols. Probably important in metabolism as it is found ubiquitously in the body. Function unknown.

**Vitamin K.** Group of substituted naphthaquinones. Plays an important part in the synthesis of prothrombin by the liver. Mode of action unknown. Deficiency: hypo-prothrombinaemia, haemorrhage.

### Water-soluble vitamins

**Vitamin C. Ascorbic acid.** Important factor in production of mucopolysaccharides. Mode of action unknown. Deficiency: scurvy.

**Vitamin $B_1$. Thiamine.** Thiamine diphosphate is an important co-enzyme in carbohydrate metabolism. Deficiency: polyneuritis, beriberi.

**Vitamin B₂. Riboflavin.** Essential part of an important respiratory co-enzyme. Deficiency: non-specific malaise, cerebellar syndromes, glossitis, etc.

**Vitamin B₆.** Pyridoxine derivatives. Deficiency: no distinctive features.

**Nicotinic acid.** Constituent of co-enzymes which act as electron transport substances in conjunction with dehydrogenase enzymes. Deficiency: pellagra (in association with other deficiencies).

**Folic acid group.** Pteroylglutamic acid and derivatives. Important co-factor in transmethylation. Deficiency: megaloblastic anaemia.

**Vitamin B₁₂.** Cyanocobalamin. Function unknown. Deficiency: megaloblastic anaemia, degeneration of the spinal cord.

The vitamins which have been mentioned are present in adequate quantities in the articles of food in a normal omnivorous diet. Dietary restriction, unless the diet is 'balanced', may lead to vitamin deficiency.

**vitelline** (*vi'-te-lēn*). Pertaining to the vitellus, or yolk.

**vitello-intestinal duct** (*vi-te-lō-in-tes-tī-nal dukt*). Embryonic duct between the yolk-sac and the developing gut.

**vitiate** (*vi-shē-āt*). To corrupt, contaminate.

**vitiligo** (*vi-ti-lī'-gō*). Disorder of pigment cells in which patches of depigmented skin arise, often in a symmetrical distribution.

**vitreous chamber of the eye** (*vi'-trē-us chām'-ber*). The region of the eye containing the vitreous humour. *See* EYE.

**vivisection** (*vi-vi-sek'-shon*). Scientific examination of a living animal.

**vocal cords** (*vō'-kal kor'-dz*). Two folds of mucous membrane in the larynx attached behind to the arytenoid cartilages, and in front to the back of the thyroid cartilage. Voice is produced by variation in position of these cords when acted on by small muscles of the larynx, and at the same time forcing through them an expiratory blast of air.

**volatile** (*vo'-la-tīl*). That which evaporates quickly.

**volition** (*vo-li'-shon*). The act or power of willing.

**Volkmann's paralysis** (*volkmans*). *V. contracture*. Fibrosis in a muscle due to prolonged ischaemia. Most often associated with spasm of the brachial artery following fracture of the humerus which leads to contracture of the forearm flexor muscles.

**volt** (*vōlt*). Unit of electrical potential.

**voluntary** (*vo'-lun-ta-ri*). Free. Regulated by choice and desire.

**volvulus** (*vol-vū'-lus*). Twisting of gut about its mesenteric attachment.

**vomer** (*vō'-mer*). A bone of the septum of the nose.

**vomit** (*vo'-mit*). To eject the contents of the stomach through the mouth.

**vomiting of pregnancy.** Early morning vomiting occurring in early pregnancy. Sometimes severe (*hyperemesis gravidarum*). Probably of hormonal origin.

**von Gierke's disease** (*von gerkes di-sēz*). Glycogen storage disease. Recessively inherited defect in the metabolism of glycogen which prevents utilization of glycogen. As a result the tissues become stuffed with glycogen while hyperglycaemia occurs.

**von Recklinghausen's disease** (*von re'-kling-how-zenz*). *See* NEUROFIBROMATOSIS.

**vulnerable** (*vul'-ne-rubl*). Susceptible.

**vulva** (*vul'-va*). Female external genitalia.

**vulvectomy** (*vul-vek'-to-mi*). Excision of vulva.

**vulvitis** (*vul-vī'-tis*). Inflammation of the vulva.

**vulvovaginal** (*vul-vō-va-jī-nal*). Pertaining to the vulva and the vagina.

**vulvovaginitis** (*vul-vō-va-ji-nī'-tis*). Inflammation of both the vulva and the vagina.

## W

**Waldeyer's ring** (*val-dā-yers ring*). Circle of lymphoid tissue in the pharynx formed by the faucial, lingual and pharyngeal tonsils.

**Wallerian degeneration** (*va-lār-i-an dē-je-ne-rā-shon*). Degeneration of a nerve after it has been cut or severed.

**wart** (*wawt*). Hyperplasia of epidermal cells due to a virus infection.

**Wassermann reaction** (*va-serman*). Test for the presence of antibodies to *Treponema pallidum*. Together with the *Kahn test* is useful in the diagnosis of syphilis.

**water-borne.** Spread by water, such as certain diseases, *e.g.* typhoid fever.

**water-brash.** Regurgitation of stomach acid into the oesophagus.

**water-hammer pulse.** *See* CORRIGAN'S PULSE.

**Waterhouse-Friderichsen syn-**

**drome** (*waw-ter-hows frē-de-rik-sen*). Syndrome resulting from bilateral adrenal haemorrhage accompanying the purpura of acute septicaemia, usually meningococcal.

**weal** (*wē-el*). Raised patch on skin due to intradermal effusion. Sometimes spelt wheal.

**wean** (*wēn*). To cease feeding a baby at the breast.

**Weber syndrome** (*we-ber sin'-drōm*). Hemianopia caused by posterior cerebral aneurysm.

**Weil's disease** (*vīls*). Epidemic spirochaetal jaundice. Disease caused by a Leptospira characterized by fever, headache and pains in the limbs. Many patients develop jaundice and purpuric rash.

**Weil-Felix reaction** (*vīl-fē-liks rē-ak'-shon*). An agglutination reaction for typhus.

**wen.** *See* SEBACEOUS CYST.

**Werner's syndrome** (*ver'-nerz sin'-drōm*). Hereditary syndrome comprising cataract, osteoporosis, subnormal growth and sexual development, early onset of arteriosclerosis and premature greying of hair.

**Wernicke's encephalopathy** (*ver-ni-kes en-ke-fa-lo-pa-thi*). Syndrome occurring in association with alcoholic polyneuritis characterized by vertigo, nystagmus, ataxia and stupor. It is considered to be due to thiamine deficiency.

**Wertheim's operation** (*vert-hīms*). A radical operation for uterine cancer, whereby the uterus, tubes, ovaries, broad ligaments, pelvic lymph glands and cellular tissue around ureters are removed *en masse*.

**Wharton's duct** (*waw-tons*). The duct of the submaxillary gland.

**wheal** (*wēl*). Acute local oedema, *e.g.* as occurs in urticaria. *See* WEAL.

**Wheelhouse's operation.** External (perineal) urethrotomy for stricture of the urethra.

**Whipple's disease** (*wi-pels*). Intestinal lipodystrophy. Disease of unknown cause in which there is progressive deposition of mucoprotein in the wall of the small intestine.

**whipworm.** *See* TRICHOCEPHALUS.

**white cell.** *See* BLOOD CELLS.

**white leg.** Thrombosis of deep leg veins.

**whitlow.** *See* PARONYCHIA.

**whooping cough** (*hoo'-ping kof*). Pertussis.

**Widal reaction** (*vē-dal*). Test to identify by an agglutination reaction either typhoid organisms (if serum is known) or typhoid antibodies (in test serum).

**Willebrand's disease** (*wi-le-brans*). Inherited defect of blood vessels and clotting mechanism.

**willpower.** A voluntary effort which directs our actions and can overcome some primary impulse such as fear.

**Wilms's tumour.** *See* NEPHROBLASTOMA.

**Wilson's disease.** A rare metabolic disorder, hepatolenticular degeneration, in which copper accumulates in the liver and certain nuclei of the brain.

**windpipe.** Trachea.

**Winslow's foramen** (*win-slōs fo-rā'-men*). An aperture between the stomach and liver formed by folds of peritoneum. It forms a communication between the greater and lesser peritoneal cavities.

**wisdom teeth.** The posterior molars. They erupt at about 21 years of age.

**withdrawal.** In psychology meaning to 'shrink into oneself'. A normal method of adjustment in a frightening situation. *W. symptoms.* Symptoms which appear when a drug, to which a person has become addicted, is withheld from him.

**Wolffian duct** (*wool-fi-an*). Vertebrate kidney duct which becomes the epididymis and vas deterens.

**womb** (*woom*). The uterus.

**Wood's glass.** Ultra-violet filter used to detect fluorescence of ringworm fungus.

**woolsorters' disease.** *See* ANTHRAX.

**word salad.** Jumble of incomprehensible phrases. A speech defect occurring in some forms of schizophrenia.

**wound** (*woond*). Injury.

**wrist.** The joint between the hand and the forearm.

**writer's cramp** (*rī'-ters kramp*). Spasm of the hand and forearm brought on by efforts to write. Largely due to defective posture when writing.

**wry-neck** (*rī-nek*). *See* TORTICOLLIS.

# X

**xanthelasma** (*zan-the-las'-ma*). Small yellowish nodules located on and near the eyelids.

**xanthine** (*zan'-thēn*). A purine base.

**xanthochromia** (*zan-thō-krō-mi-a*). Term applied to the distinctive yellow colour of cerebrospinal fluid following a subarachnoid haemorrhage. It is due to haemolysis

of the blood in the subarachnoid space.

**xanthoderma** (*zan-thō-der'-ma*). Yellowness of the skin.

**xanthoma** (*zan-thō'-ma*). A cholesterol-containing tumour.

**X chromosome** (*krō-mō-sōm*). The sex chromosome which is paired in the homogametic sex. Unlike the Y chromosome it carries many major genes.

**xenopsylla cheopis** (*ze-nop-sila chē-op'-is*). A rat flea which can transmit plague and typhus.

**xeroderma** (*ze-rō-der-ma*). Excessive dryness of the skin.

**xerophthalmia** (*ze-rof-thal'-mi-a*). Ulceration of the cornea occurring in vitamin A deficiency.

**xeroradiography.** Technique for soft tissue radiography using special equipment giving a positive print.

**xerosis** (*ze-rō'-sis*). Abnormal dryness, *e.g.* of the conjunctiva or the skin.

**xerostomia** (*ze-ros-tō-mi-a*). Dryness of the mouth.

**xiphoid process** (*zī-foyd prō-ses*). Small cartilage at the lower end of the sternum.

**x-rays.** Photons with a frequency distribution higher than the ultra-violet range of the electromagnetic spectrum. *See* RADIATION.

**Y**

**yaws.** Framboesia. Tropical disease which resembles syphilis, caused by *Treponema pertenue.*

**Y chromosome.** Sex chromosome found only in the heterogametic sex (male). It is shorter than the X chromosome and usually carries few major genes.

**yeast** (*yēst*). Unicellular fungi (Ascomycetes) which possess enzymes capable of converting sugars into ethanol with the release of carbon dioxide. Yeasts are also used as sources of protein and vitamins.

**yellow fever.** Virus-mediated disease, transmitted by mosquitoes, characterized by fever, prostration, jaundice and gastrointestinal haemorrhage.

**Z**

**zero** (*zār-ō*). Nought, nothing.

**Ziehl-Neelsen's stain** (*zēl-nēl-son*). Staining technique used to identify tubercle bacilli by their ability to retain the stain when treated with acid; hence acid-fast bacilli.

**Zollinger–Ellison syndrome** (*zo-ling-er el-li-son*). Increased production of acid gastric juice in response to gastrin secreted by pancreatic neoplasm, resulting in peptic ulceration and in-activation of enzymes of the small intestine which operate only in the alkaline range.

**zona** (*zō-na*). Literally a girdle and applied to mean shingles. *See* HERPES. *Z. pellucida.* Membrane surrounding the ovum.

**zonula ciliaris** (*zo'-nū-la si-li-a-ris*). Suspensory ligament of lens of the eye.

**zoogloea layer** (*zoo-glē-a lār*). Colonies of bacteria in a jelly-like layer. Found on the top of a sand filter bed. This layer contains algae and protozoa and helps in water purification.

**zoology** (*zoo-o-lo-ji*). That part of biology which deals with the study of animal life.

**zoosperm** (*zō-ō-sperm*). Spermatozoa.

**zoster** (*zos'-ter*). Shingles. *See* HERPES.

**zygoma** (*zi-gō-ma*). The cheekbone.

**zygote** (*zī-gōt*). The cell formed by combination of ovum with spermatozoon.

# APPENDIX 1

## Blood

The figures given below represent the approximate ranges of normal values for the constituents of the peripheral blood.

### RED CELLS

| | |
|---|---|
| Haemoglobin | 12 to 18 g/dl |
| Red cells | 3·9 to 6·5 × $10^{12}$/litre |
| Reticulocytes (newly formed red cells) | less than 1 per cent of total red cells |
| Mean cell volume (MCV) | 75 to 95 fl |
| Packed cell volume (PCV or Haematocrit) | 0·41 |
| Mean cell diameter (MCD) | 6·7 to 7·7 μm |
| Mean cell haemoglobin concentration (MCHC) | 30 to 35 g/dl |

### WHITE CELLS

| | |
|---|---|
| Total white cells | 4·0 to 10·0 × $10^9$/litre |
| Neutrophils | 60 to 70 per cent |
| Lymphocytes | 25 to 35 per cent |
| Basophils | 1 per cent |
| Eosinophils | 1 to 4 per cent |
| Monocytes | 4 to 8 per cent |
| Platelets (thrombocytes) | 150 to 400 × $10^9$/litre |

## BLOOD CHEMISTRY

| | |
|---|---|
| Urea | 2·5 to 6·6 mmol/litre |
| Uric acid (men) | 0·15 to 0·4 mmol/litre |
| Uric acid (women) | 0·1 to 0·35 mmol/litre |
| Cholesterol | 3·6 to 7·8 mmol/litre |
| Bilirubin | less than 17 $\mu$mol/litre |
| Calcium | 2·25 to 2·6 mmol/litre |
| Phosphate | 0·8 to 1·45 mmol/litre |
| Bicarbonate ($CO_2$) | |
|     (Adults) | 23 to 31 mmol/litre |
|     (Children) | 18 to 23 mmol/litre |
| Fasting blood sugar | |
|   (glucose) | |
|     (Adults) | 3·6 to 5·6 mmol/litre (65 to 100 mg/100 ml) |
|     (Children) | 2·2 to 5·6 mmol/litre (40 to 100 mg/100 ml) |
| Potassium | 3·5 to 5·5 mmol/litre |
| Sodium | 133 to 144 mmol/litre |
| Chloride | 96 to 106 mmol/litre |
| Total plasma proteins | 62 to 82 g/litre |
|   Albumin | 36 to 52 g/litre |
|   Globulin | 24 to 37 g/litre |
|   Fibrinogen | 1·5 to 4·0 g/litre |

# APPENDIX 2

## A Guide to the use of Drugs

### Control over the use of drugs

Modern drugs are often powerful synthetic products which can be highly effective in the treatment or control of human diseases, but may also be dangerous if used inexpertly. New drugs are first studied in animals, and are used medicinally only after such studies have shown that the compounds have an acceptably low toxicity, as no drug is completely without side-effects. Some side-effects may become apparent only after some years of use, and the risks to the fetus must always be kept in mind if a drug is taken during pregnancy. Infrequent side-effects can only be linked with the causative drug if a careful record is kept of all unexpected signs and symptoms occurring during treatment of an illness with any drug.

The use of a number of drugs at the same time may complicate the identification of side-effects, but may also conceal the interaction of one drug with another. The possibility of addiction to, or dependence on, a drug must also be considered. It has long been known that dependence on powerful narcotics such as morphine and diamorphine can develop, but dependence can occur with many other drugs, such as the barbiturates and the widely prescribed tranquillizers. Prescribed drugs may be misused in various ways by patients. Doses may be taken in the wrong amounts and at the wrong times, and treatment may be stopped too soon; adequate information should be given to patients to ensure full compliance with therapy. It should be remembered that tranquillizers, antidepressants, sedatives and analgesics may be taken in overdose as part of a suicidal intent.

**Descriptions of drugs**

The availability of drugs changes as new drugs come into use, and the proprietary names of many drugs differ from one country to another. In most countries full information on drugs and their doses are available in official publications. No attempt will be made here to give a comprehensive list of drugs, but some indication is given of the types of drugs in general use.

**Dosage of drugs**

The recommended dose of any proprietary drug will normally be provided by the manufacturer, and may be given as a total dose to be taken over 24 hours, or expressed as a stated number of mg or ml to be taken at intervals during the day.

There are idiosyncrasies in the absorption of drugs, and the same dose may produce different blood levels in patients of the same weight. It must also be remembered that diseases of the liver and kidneys may slow down the metabolism and excretion of drugs from the body, and so cause dangerously high drug blood levels. In such cases, the dose of drug should be reduced accordingly.

## DRUGS ACTING AGAINST INFECTION

There are now drugs which are active against most bacteria, although drug-resistant bacteria are an increasing problem, and the potent antibacterial drugs now in use may have side-effects as well as showing interaction with other drugs.

The main groups of antibiotics include the penicillins, the cephalosporins, the aminoglycosides and the tetracyclines.

The *penicillins* act by interfering with the formation of the bacterial cell wall, and are used chiefly in infections with penicillin-sensitive Gram-positive organisms. The dose depends on the type and site of infection and the particular penicillin being used. Some penicillins are effective orally, others may be given by intramuscular injection, or in some cases intravenously. The penicillins in use include benzylpenicillin, cloxacillin, amoxycillin and ampicillin, but others are available. Penicillins active in pseudomonal infections are represented by ticarcillin and carbenicillin. The most serious side-effect of penicillin is hypersensitivity, which can cause rash, an anaphylactic reaction or death. Once a person has developed a hypersensitivity to a penicillin, the hypersensitivity will extend to all other penicillins, and the susceptible patient should be informed, and his case records should be clearly marked.

The *cephalosporins* act in a similar way to the penicillins, but are active against both Gram-negative as well as Gram-positive organisms. Those in use include cephalosporin, cephradine and cephamandole, to name a few. They are often the first alternative drugs used if the infection is penicillin-resistant.

Hypersensitivity is the main side-effect, and some patients who are sensitive to the penicillins may also be sensitive to the cephalosporins.

The *aminoglycosides* are active against Gram-negative and Gram-positive infections, but are more toxic than the penicillins and cephalosporins. They are represented by gentamicin, kanamycin, amikacin and tobramycin. (Streptomycin, although an aminoglycoside, is now used almost exclusively for the treatment of tuberculosis.)

Toxic effects include deafness and kidney damage, and they should be avoided in cases of renal impairment, in the elderly, and during pregnancy.

The *tetracyclines* are wide-range antibiotics, and include tetracycline, oxytetracycline, and chlortetracycline. Their use has declined as a result of increasing bacterial resistance, and they are contra-indicated in renal disease as they exacerbate renal failure.

Tetracyclines are laid down in bones and teeth, and can cause discolouration of the teeth. They should not be given to children or pregnant women. Changes in the bacterial content of the bowel caused by the tetracyclines may lead to a troublesome diarrhoea.

## Other groups of antibiotics

The *macrolides*, of which erythromycin is the only important member. It is active mainly against Gram-positive organisms, and is useful in respiratory and middle ear infections. Also useful in penicillin-sensitive patients.

The *lincomycins* include lincomysin and clindamycin. They are active against Gram-positive organisms and resistant staphylococci, and are used in bone and joint infections. Their value is limited, as a serious side-effect is pseudomembranous colitis, and the drugs should be withdrawn if any diarrhoea develops.

*Chloramphenicol* is a potentially dangerous antibiotic as it may cause a fatal aplastic anaemia. It should be used only in the treatment of typhoid fever, or in severe infections with *H. influenzae*.

*Acrosoxacin and spectinomycin* are antibiotics used in the treatment of penicillin-resistant gonorrhoea.

The *sulphonamides* are not antibiotics, but synthetic antibacterial agents. Their action is bacteriostatic rather than bactericidal. Their use has now declined, but sulphadimidine and sulphafurazole are representative products used in urinary infections. Co-trimoxazole contains a sulphonamide with trimethoprim, also used for urinary and respiratory infections, although trimethoprim is being increasingly used alone, as it has fewer side-effects. The side-effects of the sulphonamides generally include rash, renal failure, bone marrow depression and agranulocytosis.

## ANTIFUNGAL AGENTS

*Griseofulvin* is given orally for the extended treatment of fungal infections of the hair and nails.

*Nystatin* is used in the local treatment of candida infections of the skin and mucous membranes.

*Flucytosine* is given orally or by injection for systemic yeast infections, but it may cause bone marrow depression, and resistance may develop during treatment.

*Ketoconazole* represents a new class of orally active antifungal agents for superficial as well as systemic fungal infections, and of value in prophylaxis in immunocompromised patients. It may cause some hepatic impairment, and care is necessary in pregnancy.

## ANTIVIRAL AGENTS

Viral infections are not susceptible to treatment with antibiotics, and most superficial infections heal spontaneously with general nursing care. The few antiviral agents in use include idoxuridine, which is used locally for herpes simplex lesions and shingles, and as eye drops for dendritic corneal ulcers. Vidarabine is also used locally for eye infections, and by injection for herpes simplex infections in immunocompromised patients, but side-effects include anorexia, vomiting and confusion, as well as disturbances of bone marrow and kidney function.

*Acyclovir* is a highly active antiviral agent used orally and topically in herpes simplex infections, and intravenously in immunocompromised patients. Side-effects include rash, neurological disturbances, and the dose should be reduced in renal impairment.

*Inosine pranobex* is effective orally in herpes simplex infections, and has the additional advantage of stimulating the natural immune defence system.

## ANTITUBERCULAR AGENTS

Rifampicin, isoniazid, ethambutol and streptomycin are the main drugs used in the treatment of tuberculosis. Initially, a combination of three drugs is given, usually rifampicin, isoniazid and/or ethambutol/streptomycin, and continued for eight weeks. After reports on the drug sensitivity of the causative organisms, treatment is continued with two drugs, one of which is normally isoniazid. Extended treatment over nine months or more is necessary to eliminate the infection. Secondary antitubercular drugs include capreomycin and cycloserine; pyrazinamide is of particular value in tuberculous meningitis.

## ANTI-AMOEBIC AGENTS

Metronidazole is most commonly used for acute amoebic dysentery, and diloxanide for chronic infections. Metronidazole is also effective in amoebic liver abscess, but emetine is now rarely used on account of the low margin between therapeutic and toxic doses. Chloroquine is also used in liver abscess, but the action is slower and less reliable than that of metronidazole.

## ANTIMALARIALS

*Treatment:* Chloroquine is frequently used for the initial treatment of most forms of malaria. Some strains of the causative organism are becoming resistant to chloroquine, and seriously ill patients from S.E. Asia, where resistance is increasingly common, should be treated with intravenous injections of quinine. After initial treatment, primaquine is used mainly for the eradication of benign tertian malaria.

Chloroquine, primaquine, proguanil and pyrimethamine are

used for *prophylaxis*, but the drug of choice depends largely on the area to be visited, and whether resistant organisms are present or not. Treatment should be selected in accordance with current reports from the World Health Organization, and commenced before reaching a malarial zone, and continued for at least 30 days after leaving it.

## ANTHELMINTICS

*Tapeworms:* Niclosamide kills the worms, which are then partially digested and excreted.

*Roundworms:* Piperazine is the most widely used drug for the treatment of roundworm infestation in both adults and children. Alternative drugs include bephenium, mebendazole, thiabendazole and pyrantel.

*Hookworms:* Tetrachlorethylene and bephenium are widely used, with mebendazole and pyrantel as effective alternatives. The anaemia often associated with hookworm infestation must also be treated.

*Threadworms:* These are common in children, and cause itching round the anus at night. Anthelmintics are generally less effective in threadworm infestation, but piperazine and thiabendazole are widely used. In all cases, the entire family should be treated, and a high degree of personal hygiene is essential to prevent reinfestation.

*Filariasis:* Diethylcarbamazine is the drug of choice in filariasis, but death of the parasites may be associated with allergic reactions. Antihistamines may be necessary, or topical corticosteroids for severe skin irritation.

## DRUGS ACTING ON THE ALIMENTARY SYSTEM

### Antacids

These are the most effective drugs for the immediate relief of the pain due to gastric inflammation or ulceration. The most commonly used are aluminium hydroxide, magnesium trisilicate, magnesium hydroxide or carbonate, and sodium bicarbonate. Mixtures of these antacids are also frequently used, but they are essentially palliative and not curative.

## Ulcer healing drugs

Carbenoxolone is a synthetic drug related to a constituent of liquorice, and is of value in gastric and duodenal ulceration. It has many side-effects, including salt and water retention, and monitoring of the blood pressure, electrolyte balance and weight are necessary during treatment.

Cimetidine and ranitidine reduce the secretion of gastric acid by a blocking action on $H_2$-receptors, and so have an indirect healing action. They have powerful ulcer-healing properties, but it should be remembered that they may disguise the symptoms of gastric cancer, and careful diagnosis is necessary before treatment is commenced.

*Antispasmodics* cause a reduction in gastric secretions and gastro-intestinal motility. Dicyclomine and propantheline are widely used, but many similar drugs are available. Side-effects include blurred vision, and dryness of the mouth, and in the elderly there is the risk that they may precipitate glaucoma.

## Pancreatin

Strong pancreatin preparations are used to make up for reduced or absent secretions from the pancreas which can occur following surgical removal of the pancreas or in cystic fibrosis in infants.

## Drugs used to relieve diarrhoea

Antibiotics are of no great value in the treatment of diarrhoea, as in the UK most simple diarrhoeas are viral in origin. The most important part of treatment, especially in infants and the elderly, is the replacement of lost fluid and electrolytes. Drugs used to reduce intestinal hurry and so control the symptoms of diarrhoea include codeine phosphate, diphenoxylate and loperamide, but these drugs are preferably avoided in children and the elderly. Kaolin is a useful adsorbent for controlling the symptoms of diarrhoea, and methylcellulose may be of value in decreasing faecal fluidity.

## Laxatives

Laxatives are frequently misused, and many patients with constipation would be treated more suitably by changing the diet to increase the bulk and amount of dietary fibre. Stimulant laxatives are represented by bisacodyl and danthron; faecal softeners include docusate and liquid paraffin. Irritant laxatives are represented by cascara. Lactulose is a semi-synthetic sugar that is not absorbed, and produces a laxative effect by osmosis. It also inhibits to some extent the growth of ammonia-producing organisms, and is of value in hepatic encephalopathy.

**Drugs acting on the rectum and anus**

Prednisolone and sulphasalazine enemas are useful in the supplementary treatment of ulcerative colitis. Itching of the anus should be diagnosed before treatment is commenced, but the symptoms can often be controlled by the use of a locally applied corticosteroid-containing ointment, or a suppository of similar composition. Local anaesthetic preparations are suitable for short-term use, but continued use may cause skin sensitisation.

# DRUGS ACTING ON THE CARDIOVASCULAR SYSTEM

**Heart failure**

Digoxin is the most widely used cardiac glycoside in cases of heart failure. It increases the force of the contraction of the heart muscle, reduces the heart rate and promotes a secondary diuresis. In excessive doses it may cause nausea, loss of appetite and slowing of the heart rate.

**Diuretics**

Retention of fluid in the tissues is often caused by heart failure, but it may also be caused by other diseases including liver or kidney failure.

The thiazides, represented by hydrochlorothiazide and bendrofluazide, act mainly on the distal tubule, are highly effective diuretics, but they may bring about an excessive loss of potassium, and supplementary potassium therapy may be required. The more powerful and rapidly acting loop diuretics include frusemide and bumetanide. These drugs inhibit resorption from the ascending loop of Henle, and care must be taken that the diuresis is not so great as to cause hypotension.

## Drugs which decrease myocardial excitability

When there is an irregularity of the heart beat, drugs should be used only after a precise diagnosis of the nature of the irregularity has been made. Drugs used in ventricular arrhythmias include lignocaine, mexiletine, procainamide, disopyramide, practolol and quinidine. In supraventricular tachycardia, amiodarone, verapamil, atropine and beta-adrenoceptor blocking agents such as propranolol are used.

## Drugs reducing blood pressure or antihypertensives

There are many views about how frequently and to what extent a raised blood pressure should be reduced by drugs. In the elderly, the disadvantages may outweigh the advantages, and a reduction in weight and giving up cigarette smoking may be more beneficial than the use of drugs.

Drugs in common use include beta-adrenoceptor blocking agents such as propranolol, acebutolol, oxprenolol and labetolol, which may be used in association with a diuretic; centrally acting drugs exemplified by clonidine and methyldopa; adrenergic neurone blocking agents such as bethanidine and guanethidine, and alpha-adrenoceptor blocking agents represented by indoramin and prazosin. The doses of all these drugs should be assessed at frequent intervals by regular blood pressure readings.

## Drugs used for angina pectoris

Glyceryl trinitrate is still one of the most effective drugs for the rapid relief of the pain of angina pectoris. It may be used as sublingual tablets, but more recently an ointment and a plaster containing the drug have been introduced. It is valuable as a prophylactic if taken before any activity likely to provoke an anginal attack. Perhexiline and nifedipine are also used prophylactically.

## Anticoagulants

These drugs are used mainly for controlling venous rather than arterial thrombosis. They may be used prophylactically to prevent clotting, or for treatment. For a rapid action, heparin may be given intravenously, followed by an oral anticoagulant such as warfarin. Dose is based on the prothrombin time. Ancrod is sometimes used as an alternative to heparin, but its use requires care, and resistance may develop.

## DRUGS ACTING ON
## THE RESPIRATORY SYSTEM

### Expectorants and cough suppressants

Expectorants are said to promote the expulsion of bronchial secretions, and ipecacuanha and ammonium chloride have long been used for that purpose. Cough suppressants are occasionally useful in the control of dry and useless cough, and representative drugs include codeine phosphate, pholcodine and isoaminile. Constipation is a side-effect of most cough suppressants.

### Bronchodilators

The drugs now in most frequent use are the selective beta-adrenoceptor stimulants such as salbutamol and terbutaline. The non-selective isoprenaline is now used less frequently. These drugs are best given by metered-dose aerosol products for oral inhalation, but patients may require full instructions to obtain the optimum response. They may also be given orally for a slower and more prolonged action, or by injection for very severe conditions. Xanthine bronchodilators such as aminophylline may also be given orally, or by suppository when a prolonged action is required. For the prophylactic treatment of asthma, sodium cromoglycate is the drug of choice, but has the disadvantage that it must be given as a powder by oral inhalation. It appears to prevent the release of spasmogens by stabilising mast cells. Ketotifen is a newer drug, active by mouth, but must be given for about four weeks to evoke a full prophylactic response.

### Corticosteroid drugs

These drugs may sometimes be life-saving when given as hydrocortisone intravenously in the treatment of severe asthma or status asthmaticus, usually together with an injection of salbutamol. Patients with less severe asthma may be given short courses of oral prednisolone, and then transferred to oral aerosol therapy with drugs such as betamethasone or budesonide.

## DRUGS ACTING ON
## THE NERVOUS SYSTEM

### Analgesics

These may be of the following kinds:

1. Non-narcotic analgesics used for mild or moderate pain.
2. Narcotic analgesics used for moderate to severe pain.
3. Analgesics acting at a specific site, such as ergotamine tartrate for migraine.
4. Anti-inflammatory analgesics.

#### NON-NARCOTIC ANALGESICS

Aspirin is the best known drug of this group, and it also has anti-inflammatory and antipyretic properties. Side-effects include indigestion, gastric irritation and damage, and anaemia caused by the consequent acute or chronic blood loss. Hypersensitivity to aspirin may precipitate severe asthma.

Paracetamol is a similar mild analgesic, and is generally well tolerated, but it has no anti-inflammatory action. Overdose may cause serious liver damage. Benorylate is a compound from which aspirin and paracetamol are released when the drug is metabolized, and may be better tolerated.

#### NARCOTIC ANALGESICS

This group includes analgesics of varying potency. Dihydrocodeine is an analgesic of moderate potency, and may be given orally or by injection. Pentazocine is more potent by injection, and the response to oral therapy may be less satisfactory. Dextropropoxyphene alone is much less potent, but is more active when given with paracetamol as in Distalgesic, but in overdose the combined reactions may be more difficult to treat. In severe pain, morphine is very effective by injection, but it may cause respiratory depression, and is potentially a drug of addiction. Diamorphine is a more powerful but shorter-acting analgesic, and is best used for the pain of terminal illness where the problems of addiction do not occur. Alternative powerful analgesics include pethidine, levorphanol and buprenorphine. Papaveretum is a preparation of all the alkaloids of opium.

SITE-SPECIFIC PAIN RELIEF

Ergotamine tartrate is used solely for the relief of pain in migraine. Clonidine, methysergide and pizotifen are used in prophylaxis, not treatment.

ANTI-INFLAMMATORY ANALGESICS

The non-steroidal anti-inflammatory drugs (NSAIDs) are widely used in the treatment of rheumatoid conditions. Aspirin is a drug of this type, but the newer agents may be more active and sometimes better tolerated. However, NSAIDS should be used with care in all cases of gastric ulceration, asthma and allergic disorders, where renal or hepatic impairment is present, and during pregnancy. Side-effects include nausea, headache, tinnitus and hypersensitivity reactions. Naproxen, ibuprofen, indomethacin and fenoprofen are representatives of the many drugs now available. Phenylbutazone, once widely used, is now reserved for the *hospital* treatment of ankylosing spondylitis.

### Hypnotics, sedatives and minor tranquillizers

Sleep difficulties are best resolved by finding and treating the cause than by giving drugs. Barbiturates are effective hypnotics, but their use is now discouraged, as more effective and safer drugs are available. Dependence and tolerance to barbiturates may occur, and rapid withdrawal may precipitate severe withdrawal symptoms. The benzodiazepines are now the preferred drugs, as they have an anxiolytic as well as an hypnotic action, and they are much less dangerous in overdose. A wide range of benzodiazepines is now in use. Those used as hypnotics include nitrazepam, flurazepam, temazepam and diazepam. Other sedatives include chloral preparations, and some antihistamines have useful sedative properties.

### Major tranquillizers

These drugs are used in psychotic mental illness, and some are of particular value in schizophrenia. The most important group is the phenothiazines, which includes chlorpromazine, prochlorperazine and trifluoroperazine. Some have more marked sedative and extrapyramidal side-effects than others, and selection of a particular drug depends on the degree of sedation as well as the antipsychotic effect required. Chlorpromazine is of value as supplementary treatment with analgesics in controlling the severe pain of terminal illness. Lithium salts are used in some types of manic depression.

## Antidepressants

*Tricyclic antidepressants* are used in the control of severe depression not requiring electroconvulsive therapy. Representative drugs include imipramine, amitriptyline and mianserin. Response to treatment may be slow and relief of symptoms may not occur for two to three weeks or more. Side-effects include dryness of the mouth and other anticholinergic responses, and care is necessary in urinary retention, and in hypertension.

*Monoamine oxidase inhibitors* (MAOI) such as phenelzine and isocarboxazid are now used less frequently, as they have many side-effects, and may cause dangerous hypertensive episodes with some amine-containing foods such as cheese. Tricyclic depressants should not be given until at least 14 days have elapsed after the withdrawal of MAOI therapy.

## Anticonvulsants

If possible an accurate diagnosis of the type of epilepsy should be made before treatment is started. Patients must be supervised regularly to make sure that the fits are controlled without causing unpleasant side-effects. Phenobarbitone is still used, as it has a long action, but for grand mal seizures much reliance is placed on phenytoin or carbamazepine, with sodium valproate and ethotoin as alternatives. Sodium valproate and ethosuximide are used in the control of petit mal, especially in children. Other drugs used in all forms of epilepsy include clonazepam and sulthiame. Status epilepticus may be treated with intravenous diazepam or clonazepam, bearing in mind the risks of respiratory depression and venous thrombosis.

Paraldehyde remains useful, as if required it may be given rectally as well as by intramuscular injection.

## Drugs used in parkinsonism

Drugs are used to restore an improved balance between the dopamine and cholinergic effects in the brain. Levodopa, a precursor of dopamine, is widely used often in conjunction with a dopacarboxylase inhibitor such as carbidopa or benserazide. Selegiline also has an inhibitory action, but bromocriptine appears to act by stimulating remaining dopamine receptor functions. Amantadine is a second-line drug. Drugs that have a mainly anticholinergic effect include benzhexol, orphenadrine and procyclidine.

## ORAL CONTRACEPTIVES

These are tablets containing an oestrogen or a progestogen which, when taken orally for the required number of days each month, prevent conception. A combination of these drugs is more effective than either alone. The amount of oestrogen in each tablet should not exceed 50 micrograms and many preparations contain 30 micrograms.

Oral contraceptives increase the risk of vascular thrombosis particularly in women over the age of 35 years, those who are overweight and those who are cigarette smokers.

## DRUGS AFFECTING ALLERGIC REACTIONS

In acute allergic reactions such as anaphylactic shock and severe asthma adrenaline should be given by intramuscular injection, repeated every 15 minutes as required. Slow intravenous injection of chlorpheniramine or other antihistamine is useful supplementary therapy. Corticosteroids may also be given intravenously, but the onset of action may take some hours to develop.

In allergic conditions such as hay fever and allergic rhinitis and drug allergies, oral antihistamines may be given, but may cause drowsiness. Car-driving patients should be warned of that risk, although some of the newer antihistamines, such as terfenadine, cause less sedation. Locally applied corticosteroid preparations are useful in allergic conditions of the eye and nose and skin. Some corticosteroids are also of value orally in suppressing allergic reactions.

## ENDOCRINOLOGICAL PREPARATIONS

### Thyroid

*Thyroid hormones* are used in the congenital or acquired, including surgical, loss of the secretion from the thyroid gland.

Thyroxine sodium or liothyronine sodium are most commonly used.

*Antithyroid substances* are used to counteract the effects of an overactive thyroid gland. The drugs used include carbimazole, propylthiouracil, propranolol and potassium perchlorate.

## Adrenal cortex

When secretion from this area fails due to Addison's disease or surgical removal, the deficiency may be controlled by hydrocortisone tablets, or fludrocortisone. In acute failure of the adrenal cortex cortisone injections may be used for a limited time.

If the secretion from the adrenal cortex is excessive, it may be controlled by dexamethasone or metyrapone.

Good control of either a deficiency or excess needs very careful control.

## Insulin

A deficiency of insulin secretion from the pancreas causes diabetes mellitus with impaired digestion of food stuffs, particularly of carbohydrates. The deficiency can sometimes be counteracted by reducing the amount of carbohydrate in the diet but diabetes which occurs in children, young adults and sometimes older adults will need insulin replacement for control of the disease.

Insulin is produced mainly from the pancreas of an animal and is usually of mixed cow and pig origin, but human insulin is now available.

Insulin must be injected subcutaneously, and besides short-acting soluble insulin, modified insulins with an intermediate and long-action are also available. For emergency use, as in diabetic coma, soluble insulin is the only form that can be injected intravenously.

### ORAL HYPOGLYCAEMIC PREPARATIONS

These may be used if diet alone does not control diabetes mellitus in older and usually overweight patients. They are active only when some residual pancreatic insulin-producing tissue is present.

Chlorpropamide represents a number of available sulphonylurea drugs, with the advantage that a single daily dose is usually sufficient, whereas tolbutamide is usually given twice a day. The biguanides such as metformin, act mainly by increasing the use of peripheral glucose. A side-effect of the biguanides is an unpredictable lactic acidosis, and for that reason phenformin is no longer in use.

**Female sex hormones**

Oestrogen, represented by ethinyloestradiol, is used in a variety of menstrual disorders. It is no longer used routinely in menopausal conditions, although it is useful when given for short periods for the control of hot flushes and other menopausal vasomotor symptoms. Topically, it is used in the treatment of senile vaginitis and associated symptoms. Large doses may be of value in some neoplastic conditions, and stilboestrol, a synthetic oestrogen, is used in prostatic carcinoma. Stilboestrol, once used for the suppression of lactation, has been replaced for that purpose by bromocriptine.

**Male sex hormones**

Androgens may be given after castration, or in other cases of hypogonadism. Methyltestosterone may be given as sublingual tablets, but for a long action, injections of a depot form of testosterone are preferred.

**Posterior pituitary preparations**

If the antidiuretic hormone or vasopressin is not produced by the posterior pituitary the result will be diabetes insipidus. Vasopressin can be given in various ways including nasally as desmopressin. Paradoxically, chlorpropamide may reduce the polyuria of diabetes insipidus.

## APPETITE SUPPRESSANTS

These drugs should not be used for the control of overweight; it is better to instruct the patient about different eating habits. Fenfluramine may be given for a limited time but is best avoided. Amphetamines must never be used because they can cause addiction.

## DRUGS FOR THE MANAGEMENT OF MALIGNANT DISEASE

Groups of drugs which can be used are cytotoxic drugs, cytotoxic antibiotics, sex hormones and corticosteroids.

## Cytotoxic drugs

These drugs interfere with the reproduction of both cancer cells and normal body cells. A careful watch must be kept on the cells in the blood while such drugs are being used. The drugs in this group include cyclophosphamide, mercaptopurine, methotrexate, vincristine, chlorambucil and cytarabine. It is usual to give short controlled courses of different combinations of these drugs.

## Cytotoxic antibiotics

Some antibiotics have cytotoxic properties, and doxorubicin is now widely used in the control of active leukaemia, and various lymphomas. In common with most cytotoxic drugs, it produces some depression of the bone marrow, and another side-effect is alopecia. Mitomycin and amsacrine have similar properties. Bleomycin is used mainly in lymphoma, and is exceptional in not causing bone marrow depression.

## Sex hormones

Cancer of the prostate can usually be controlled by stilboestrol.

Some cancers of the breast may be helped by nandrolone which is a type of androgen.

## Corticosteroids

Prednisone may be used in the acute leukaemias or in breast cancer which has metastasised.

# DRUGS USED IN THE TREATMENT OF ANAEMIA

The type of anaemia and, if possible, its cause must be diagnosed before treatment is started with drugs. Ferrous sulphate or ferrous gluconate may be given in iron deficiency anaemias.

For megaloblastic anaemia, vitamin $B_{12}$ is necessary and can be given as hydroxocobalamin or cyanocobalamin by injection. Folic acid may be necessary to correct some types of anaemia.

# APPENDIX 3

## Desirable Weights of Adults according to Height and Frame

### MEN

| height without shoes (cm) | ft in | small frame kg | lb | medium frame kg | lb | large frame kg | lb |
|---|---|---|---|---|---|---|---|
| 155·0 | 5 1 | 50·8–54·4 | 112–120 | 53·5–58·5 | 118–129 | 57·2–64·0 | 126–141 |
| 157·5 | 5 2 | 52·2–55·8 | 115–123 | 54·9–60·3 | 121–133 | 58·5–65·3 | 129–144 |
| 160·0 | 5 3 | 53·5–57·2 | 118–126 | 56·2–61·7 | 124–136 | 59·9–67·1 | 132–148 |
| 162·5 | 5 4 | 54·9–58·5 | 121–129 | 57·6–63·0 | 127–139 | 61·2–68·9 | 135–152 |
| 165·0 | 5 5 | 56·2–60·3 | 124–133 | 59·0–64·9 | 130–143 | 62·6–70·8 | 138–156 |
| 167·5 | 5 6 | 58·1–62·1 | 128–137 | 60·8–66·7 | 134–147 | 64·4–73·0 | 142–161 |
| 170·0 | 5 7 | 59·9–64·0 | 132–141 | 62·6–68·9 | 138–152 | 66·7–75·3 | 147–166 |
| 172·5 | 5 8 | 61·7–65·8 | 136–145 | 64·4–70·8 | 142–156 | 68·5–77·1 | 151–170 |
| 175·0 | 5 9 | 63·5–68·0 | 140–150 | 66·2–72·6 | 146–160 | 70·3–78·9 | 155–174 |
| 177·5 | 5 10 | 65·3–69·9 | 144–154 | 68·0–74·8 | 150–165 | 72·1–81·2 | 159–179 |
| 180·0 | 5 11 | 67·1–71·7 | 148–158 | 69·9–77·1 | 154–170 | 74·4–83·5 | 164–184 |
| 182·5 | 6 0 | 68·9–73·5 | 152–162 | 71·7–79·4 | 158–175 | 76·2–85·7 | 169–189 |
| 185·0 | 6 1 | 70·8–75·7 | 156–167 | 73·5–81·6 | 162–180 | 78·5–88·0 | 173–194 |
| 187·5 | 6 2 | 72·6–77·6 | 160–171 | 75·7–83·9 | 167–185 | 80·7–90·3 | 178–199 |
| 190·0 | 6 3 | 74·4–79·4 | 164–175 | 78·0–86·2 | 172–190 | 82·6–92·5 | 182–204 |

## WOMEN

| height without shoes | | small frame | | medium frame | | large frame | |
|---|---|---|---|---|---|---|---|
| (cm) | ft in | kg | lb | kg | lb | kg | lb |
| 142·5 | 4 8 | 41·8–44·5 | 92–98 | 43·5–48·5 | 96–107 | 47·2–54·0 | 104–119 |
| 145·0 | 4 9 | 42·7–45·9 | 94–101 | 44·5–49·9 | 98–110 | 48·1–55·3 | 106–122 |
| 147·5 | 4 10 | 43·6–47·2 | 96–104 | 45·8–51·3 | 101–113 | 49·4–56·7 | 109–125 |
| 150·0 | 4 11 | 44·9–48·5 | 99–107 | 47·2–52·6 | 104–116 | 50·8–58·1 | 112–128 |
| 152·5 | 5 0 | 46·3–49·9 | 102–110 | 48·5–54·0 | 107–119 | 52·2–59·4 | 115–131 |
| 155·0 | 5 1 | 47·6–51·3 | 105–113 | 49·9–55·3 | 110–122 | 53·5–60·8 | 118–134 |
| 157·5 | 5 2 | 49·0–52·6 | 108–116 | 51·3–57·2 | 113–126 | 54·9–62·6 | 121–138 |
| 160·0 | 5 3 | 50·3–54·0 | 111–119 | 52·6–59·0 | 116–130 | 56·7–64·4 | 125–142 |
| 162·5 | 5 4 | 51·7–55·8 | 114–123 | 54·4–61·2 | 120–135 | 58·5–66·2 | 129–146 |
| 165·0 | 5 5 | 53·5–57·6 | 118–127 | 56·2–63·0 | 124–139 | 60·3–68·0 | 133–150 |
| 167·5 | 5 6 | 55·3–59·4 | 122–131 | 58·1–64·9 | 128–143 | 62·1–69·9 | 137–154 |
| 170·0 | 5 7 | 57·2–61·2 | 126–135 | 59·9–66·7 | 132–147 | 64·0–71·7 | 141–158 |
| 172·5 | 5 8 | 59·0–63·5 | 130–140 | 61·6–68·5 | 136–151 | 65·8–73·9 | 145–163 |
| 175·0 | 5 9 | 60·8–65·3 | 134–144 | 63·5–70·3 | 140–155 | 67·6–76·2 | 149–168 |
| 177·5 | 5 10 | 62·6–67·1 | 138–148 | 65·3–72·1 | 144–159 | 69·4–78·5 | 153–173 |

# APPENDIX 4

## Diet

The human does not eat nutrients but food and the type of food eaten varies a great deal from culture to culture. However, certain basic nutrients are necessary for the production of energy, for adequate growth, the replacement of tissues and the maintenance of health.

The basic nutrients include:

1. Carbohydrates
2. Proteins
3. Fats
4. Vitamins
5. Minerals

### 1. Carbohydrates

These contain carbon, hydrogen, and oxygen. Carbohydrates may be eaten as starch or as sugars. Sugars may be disaccharides or monosaccharides. The disaccharides are sucrose, containing one molecule of glucose and one of fructose; maltose, which contains two molecules of glucose, and lactose, which contains glucose and galactose. During digestion carbohydrates are broken down to the monosaccharides, glucose, fructose and galactose. These are used in the body for the production of energy or stored as glycogen.

Carbohydrate is the only nutrient in sugar but is also present in such foods as bread, potatoes, rice and pasta. In these foods there are other nutrients including protein and vitamins.

The carbohydrates in the food supply from 50 per cent to 80 per cent of the total daily intake of calories. In wealthier countries fat and protein account for a relatively greater number of calories but in poorer countries a larger proportion of calories is obtained from carbohydrates.

## 2. Proteins

These contain oxygen, hydrogen, nitrogen and sometimes sulphur. They are necessary to the body for growth and repair. Opinions about the amount of protein necessary daily for a human differ widely and the amount suggested has varied from 40 grams to 100 grams. At present in the United Kingdom it is recommended that a fully grown adult should eat between 60 and 70 grams of protein a day which will supply about 10 per cent of his total daily intake of calories. It is possible that humans would be healthier with a smaller amount of protein in the diet. Pregnant and lactating mothers need more protein than other adults.

Protein is made up of twenty-three amino acids and of these eight are called 'essential' amino acids and a further two are 'essential' in children. The term 'essential' is used because the body is unable to synthesize these amino acids and must have them in the food. Proteins were formerly known as first class, or animal, proteins which contained all the essential amino acids, and second class or vegetable proteins which contained some of the essential amino acids. This categorization has now stopped because it is realized that a varied intake of vegetable proteins including cereals and pulses can contain all the essential amino acids. The quantity of vegetable protein that needs to be eaten is very much greater than animal protein and this can be a disadvantage.

Protein is used in the body for growth and repair and any excess is used up for energy or stored as fat.


## 3. Fats

All fats are made up of a mixture of glycerol and fatty acids but the characteristics of the fatty acids differ. A fatty acid is formed from a chain of carbon atoms with hydrogen and oxygen. A saturated fatty acid is one in which all the bonds between the carbon atoms are single. A mono-saturated fatty acid is one in which one bond is double; a poly-unsaturated fatty acid is one in which there are two or more double bonds.

Fat is found in dairy products such as milk, cream, cheese and butter; but it is also present in and around meat, in nuts, pulses and in some fish including herring and salmon.

There are three poly-unsaturated fatty acids essential for health and these are linoleic acid, linolenic acid and arachidonic acid.

The amount of fat that is necessary in the diet for health is not known. Cultural factors and the family income cause a wide variation in intake.

Fats are emulsified by the bile salts in the digestive tract and then broken down by lipase into glycerides, glycerol and fatty acids.

Fats form the main supply of stored energy in the body. When it is metabolized one gram of fat produces twice as many calories as a gram of protein or a gram of carbohydrate. Fat is also a source of vitamins A, D, E and K.

## 4. Vitamins

These are a small but necessary part of the diet. The results of vitamin deficiencies were recognized in most cases before the chemical structure of the vitamin had been established. They were called A, B, C etc., but this, in the light of later knowledge, has led to some confusion in the nomenclature.

### FAT SOLUBLE VITAMINS

*Vitamin A* is supplied to the body in food as retinol and carotene. It is present in animal fats such as halibut and cod liver oil, milk, butter and cheese. It is also present in carrots and green vegetables with dark green leaves such as spinach.

2 500 International Units (IU) are necessary each day. Deficiency causes night blindness, hardening of the skin and the covering of eye which can cause blindness. A deficiency is rare in the developed countries.

An excess of vitamin A, which can occur if children are given too large an amount, can cause irritability, loss of appetite, an itching skin and swellings over the bones.

*Vitamin D* is supplied to the body in animal fats including milk, butter and cheese. It can also be made by the body when the skin is exposed to ultraviolet light.

The recommended daily intake of vitamin D for infants is 400 International Units and for adults 100 International Units.

A deficiency of vitamin D in children causes rickets; and in malnourished women who have a number of pregnancies it can cause osteomalacia.

An excess of vitamin D occurs through overdosage of small children and can cause irritability, loss of appetite, loss of weight and occasionally death.

*Vitamin E* is associated with fertility in rats but in humans its use is still uncertain.

*Vitamin K*. A deficiency of vitamin K in the human is associated with impaired clotting of the blood. The deficiency is unlikely to be caused by a low intake and is probably due to a defect in its use by the body.

## THE WATER SOLUBLE VITAMINS

*Vitamin B* is now known to be a collection of different vitamins.

*Vitamin $B_1$* or thiamine is necessary for the metabolism of glucose in the body and is probably of particular importance in the nourishment of nerve cells. A regular supply of this vitamin is needed because very little is stored in the body. It is present in a wide variety of foods including unrefined cereals, potatoes, green vegetables and milk.

A deficiency of this vitamin is very rare in the United Kingdom unless a patient is not taking food. A deficiency is common in poorer countries particularly if rice or other cereals are refined. Beriberi is the result of deficiency.

There used to be a vitamin known as $B_2$ but it is now known to be a group of vitamins of which the most important is riboflavine. Its source and use are similar to those of thiamine. Deficiency, which is rare in the United Kingdom, causes cracks at the corners of the mouth, a sore, red tongue and a dry, scaly skin.

*Nicotinic acid* is present in unrefined cereals and dairy products. Deficiency is most common in rice-eating countries and causes pellagra. Exposed areas of the skin become pigmented and scaly, there is diarrhoea and there may be severe mental symptoms including depression.

*Vitamin $B_6$* is rather like vitamin E. Its use is established in animals but in humans it is not yet understood. It is widely available in vegetables.

*Vitamin $B_{12}$* is present in meat and is necessary for the formation of blood cells.

A deficiency occurs because it is not absorbed through the stomach wall and its lack causes pernicious anaemia. Replacement must be by repeated injections.

*Folic acid* is also necessary for the formation of blood cells and it is widely available in vegetables.

A deficiency may occur in pregnant women and iron and

folic acid may be given routinely during pregnancy to prevent anaemia.

*Vitamin C* or ascorbic acid is necessary for the healthy development of collagen in the body; this includes bones, teeth and the lining of blood vessels.

It is present in all fruits and vegetables particularly citrus fruits.

The human adult needs about 30mg a day and in the United Kingdom a quarter of this amount is normally supplied by potatoes.

A deficiency of vitamin C causes scurvy and the disease is most commonly seen in elderly people who have an insufficient dietary intake.

## 5. Minerals

These, like vitamins, are essential in the human diet for normal development and health; less, however, is known about many of them than about some vitamins.

*Sodium or salt* is to be found in all body fluids and the greater amount of it is in the extra-cellular fluid. The amount remains constant in the healthy adult. Sodium acts with potassium to stabilize the acid base balance.

The daily intake necessary is about 1g but some people who like salty food may eat up to 10g.

*Potassium* acts with sodium to keep a constant acid base balance in the body. Potassium is found mostly in intra-cellular fluid. Potassium is present in most foods that humans eat including fruit, vegetables and cereals.

A deficiency is unlikely to be due to a low intake but to an excessive loss from the body as may occur in severe diarrhoea or while taking diuretics.

*Calcium* is present in the greatest quantity of all minerals in the body. Most of it is in the teeth and bones.

The daily intake necessary is probably about 500mg but it has been suggested that 1 000mg could be necessary. It is present in large amounts in dairy foods, particularly cheese, and in hard water and in many vegetables.

A deficiency of calcium is seldom due to a lack in the dietary intake but to a failure of absorption, as may occur in steatorrhoea, or to defective use in the body as may occur in diseases of the parathyroid.

*Phosphorus* forms compounds with calcium in the bones and

teeth. It also takes part in cell metabolism and reproduction. It is widely available in the diet and the body can deal with an excess by excretion in the stools or urine.

*Iron* is necessary in the body for the formation of haemoglobin. The daily intake needs to be about 10mg and probably up to 20mg in pregnant women. It is present in meat, liver, bread and vegetables.

A deficiency intake causes one type of anaemia but in the United Kingdom this type of anaemia is more often due to an acute or chronic loss of blood than to a low intake of iron.

*Iodine* is vital to the body for the production of thyroxin by the thyroid gland. In most parts of the world it is present in the earth and water and vegetables in the diet have absorbed it. In areas where there is a shortage of iodine in the soil, humans may develop enlargement of the thyroid gland.

*Fluorine* occurs naturally in some soils and therefore in some water supplies. If it is present in a quantity of about one part per million of water it lessens the incidence of dental caries. If present in amounts of 4 or 5 p.p.m. it can cause mottling of the teeth.


## DIET FOR OBESITY

The problem of being overweight is largely one of more affluent countries. It is usually caused by eating more than is necessary coupled with a sedentary way of life. Crash diets are of little use and a change in eating habits is necessary for the maintenance of permanent weight reduction.

During weight reduction the total intake of calories should be limited to 1 000 calories a day and a steady weight loss of 1 to 2lb a week is sufficient.

A normal pattern of eating should be observed and the total calories divided between three or four meals. The following foods should be omitted entirely:

    Sugar, cakes, biscuits, sweet puddings
    Alcohol
    Fried foods
    Chocolate, sweets, etc
    Jam, honey, marmalade, syrup, etc
    Dried fruits

Potato crisps
Sweet canned or bottled drinks

When the target weight has been reached the daily diet may be increased but the above foods are better omitted. A weekly check should be kept and a stricter diet started if the weight is increasing.

It is wise to seek medical advice before starting a reducing diet, and essential if the person is not in good health.

## DIABETIC DIETS

The principles of any diabetic diet are the restriction of starches and sugars. The quantity allowed in the diet each day must be eaten and at regular intervals; this is important if insulin is being used. In children it is more difficult to keep an exact control of these foods but it is best to encourage the diabetic child to take an early, responsible share in the management of his diet.

In all diabetic diets it is usual to aim at a daily fixed total calorie intake which may be about 1800 kcal. This amount will vary with the sex, size and occupation of the patient. The diet is usually made up of about 210g of carbohydrate, 80g of protein and 70g of fat.

Carbohydrate is the nutrient which must be most carefully controlled and it is common to work out a system of dietary 'exchanges' based on the quantity of a food which contains 10g of carbohydrate.

The daily intake of milk will be controlled at about $\frac{3}{4}$ pint and of butter at $\frac{1}{2}$oz.

It is usual to give the patient guidance about the following groups of foods which may also be controlled by the 'exchange' system:

1. Foods which may be eaten in an unlimited quantity, including tea and coffee without sugar and with milk from the daily allowance, clear soups, cheese, fish, meat, eggs and most vegetables.
2. Foods which may be eaten in moderation including all carbohydrate foods, fresh and dried fruit, pasta, thick soups, 'diabetic' foods and dry wines and sherry.
3. Foods to be avoided include sugar, sweets, jam, syrup, sweet puddings, ice-cream, sweet wines and sherry, spirits and liqueurs.

## HIGH FIBRE DIET

This diet is increasingly used in constipation and in diverticulitis. It should include a large proportion of foods which are rich in fibres and relatively low in calories. These foods include:

Porridge and muesli
Bran which can be used in baking
Wholemeal flour and bread
Fresh and dried fruit
Vegetables and pulses
Unrefined rice

## GLUTEN FREE DIET

This diet is used in the management of coeliac disease and in other conditions in which the bowel is unable to deal with gluten. Gluten, a plant protein, is found in wheat, rye and barley. It is made of two parts, glutenin and gliadin, and it is the latter which is harmful. Flour can be produced which is free of gluten and this flour must be used in all baking for a patient who is unable to tolerate gluten. Very small amounts of gluten can be harmful. All cereals which are not gluten free, e.g. cakes, biscuits, tinned foods, sauces, etc. which contain normal flour must be excluded from the diet.

## LOW SATURATED FAT DIET

This diet may be used in the management of diseases of the blood vessels and in multiple sclerosis. Fats to be avoided are those of animal origin and those which are solid at room temperature. Structurally the fats to be avoided are those that are saturated and the fats to be included in the diet are the mono-unsaturated or preferably the poly-unsaturated fats. The fats to be avoided are fat on meat, butter, lard, cream, cheese and bacon. Milk should be skimmed and not more than two eggs should be eaten a week.

Sunflower seed oil is the best oil to use in the preparation of food and one of the varieties of poly-unsaturated margarine must be used instead of butter on bread and in baking.

Fatty fishes to be avoided include mackerel, herring and salmon; also all fish canned in oil such as sardines and tuna fish.

# LOW RESIDUE AND HIGH PROTEIN DIET

This diet may be used in the management of ulcerative colitis. All foods that are high in fibre content should be avoided. These include unrefined cereals, wholemeal bread, vegetables, fruit and dried fruit and nuts. Fried food should also be avoided.

There should be an increased intake of lean meat, milk, fish, cheese (apart from cream cheese), eggs and refined cereals.

# INTRAVENOUS FLUIDS

Fluids may be given intravenously to replace losses of body fluid, to replace lost blood and to keep a balance of fluid and electrolytes in those patients who are unable to take solid or liquid food by mouth.

Great care must be taken in children and in those patients with heart or kidney disease when giving intravenous fluids.

For infants and children the exact requirements of fluid must be calculated from the child's weight and the composition of the fluid must be adjusted in association with the acid base balance of the blood which should be monitored every 4 hours, together with the electrolyte measurements.

The following intravenous solutions may be used in adults according to need:

1. Sodium chloride solution when there is fluid and salt loss. Sodium lactate may be added.
2. Dextrose 5% solution can be used to replace water loss and provide some nourishment. Sodium chloride and dextrose may be used together.
3. Potassium chloride may be added to sodium chloride or dextrose solution to replace potassium lost in the urine or in diarrhoea.
4. Sodium bicarbonate solution and sodium lactate are used to correct acidosis after estimation of the acid base balance in the blood.
5. Dextran solution can be used for the emergency increase of the blood volume after haemorrhage and when blood is not immediately available.

If intravenous feeding needs to be continued for a period of time the calorie needs of the patient can be supplied by the addition of a solution of synthetic amino acids and emulsified fats to the intravenous fluids.

Some drugs can be added to intravenous fluids; others have undesirable side-effects or lose their potency when added to intravenous fluids. These actions should be checked before any drug is added in this way.

# APPENDIX 5

## First Aid

The AIMS of first aid are:

1. To save life.
2. To prevent the injury and the effects of the injury getting worse.
3. To get a live patient to hospital or into other medical care.
4. To reduce the anxiety of the patient.

First aid may be done by a doctor but can be done effectively by anybody trained in the art of giving first aid and practised in applying it.

ALCOHOL should never be given.

NO DRINKS should be given to any patient apart from the conscious severely burned adult.

### Priorities

The first aider must identify and treat urgently all life-threatening conditions. To this end the following questions should be asked about each casualty and answered as rapidly and accurately as possible in order that the appropriate steps may be instigated.

1. Should the patient be removed from a position of danger such as a live source of electricity?
2. Is the patient breathing or not breathing? The brain can live for only about 4 minutes without a supply of oxygen reaching it in the blood. Do not waste time splinting or bandaging a patient who is not breathing. A hospital can treat a live casualty but not a dead one.
3. Is the patient bleeding severely? Both internal and external bleeding need to be recognized and immediate attention paid to stopping any visible bleeding; a casualty with internal bleeding needs urgent transfer to hospital.

4. Is the patient conscious or unconscious? Diagnosing the cause of unconsciousness is not of immediate concern to the first aider but the correct positioning of the patient will save life and must be practised by all those who study first aid

### REMOVING THE PATIENT FROM A POSITION OF DANGER

This may involve turning off an electric supply with a well-insulated device or dragging the patient out of water. A casualty trapped in a car should be left until a doctor and, if possible, the fire brigade arrive. The first aider should only attempt to carry out this manoeuvre if the car is on fire. If you are dragging a casualty out of water, artificial respiration can and should be started before you have the patient in an ideal place and position.

### IS THE PATIENT BREATHING?

If the casualty is not breathing artificial respiration should be started with the minimum delay. The following measures should be carried out as rapidly as possible because there is no time to waste.

a. Put the casualty flat on his back, arch his neck and lift his lower jaw upwards and forwards. This will lift his tongue away from the back of his throat and provide an airway (Figs. 57 and 58).
b. Clear the mouth of any debris including pieces of food and false teeth.
c. Keeping the jaw in the correct position with one hand under the patient's chin, take a deep breath in. Place your open mouth firmly over the patient's nose while keeping his mouth shut with upward pressure under his chin. Breathe out steadily and firmly

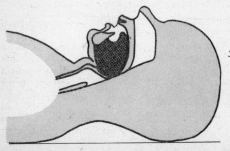

57. *The tongue blocking the throat of an unconscious patient*

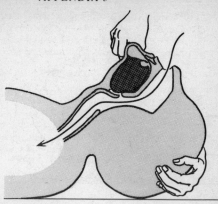

58. *The lower jaw lifted upwards and forwards thus lifting the tongue from the back of the throat*

until you see the patient's chest rise. Lift your head, turn it to one side, take a deep breath in and repeat the manoeuvre (Figs. 59 and 60). If mouth-to-nose respiration is impossible mouth-to-mouth respiration should be carried out.

d. Artificial respiration should be continued until either the patient breathes spontaneously, or a doctor says that he is dead, or if a doctor is not available it should be continued for at least an hour.

The most common cause of difficulty in getting air into the lungs is an obstruction in the air passages; the most common obstruction

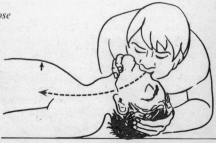

59. *Mouth-to-nose respiration. The chest of the casualty rises as it fills with air*

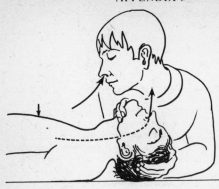

60. *Operator takes away his mouth and breathes in himself. The chest of the casualty falls on expiration*

is the tongue which due to the malpositioning of the head falls backwards and effectively blocks the passage at the back of the nose and mouth. Have a quick look in the mouth to make sure that no further debris has appeared and then lift the lower jaw and pull it forward. Correct the extension of the neck by putting one hand under the nape of the neck and pulling the head backwards with the other hand. Continue mouth-to-nose or mouth-to-mouth respiration.

If you are using this method of artificial respiration on a child, care must be taken in the amount of air blown into the lungs. The chest must be watched constantly because damage can be done to the lungs by over-vigorous inflation. If the patient is a small child it is usually easier for the first aider to put his mouth over the child's nose and mouth.

Vomiting may occur while artificial respiration is being carried out. The patient's head should be turned immediately to one side and the mouth rapidly cleaned out before artificial respiration is continued.

Mouth-to-nose or mouth-to-mouth respiration is the most effective method of artificial respiration available to the first aider. It is impossible to practise on a live person but should be practised on one of the models available for this purpose.

IS THE PATIENT BLEEDING SEVERELY?

Bleeding may be external or internal.

External bleeding can be seen on the outside of the body.

Internal bleeding may be hidden within the body or show its presence when passed in urine, coughed up, etc. Internal bleeding may be severe around a fracture, particularly that of the femur or thigh bone.

The diagnosis of severe bleeding must be made quickly because the loss of a litre of blood is serious.

*External bleeding* will be seen if looked for. Press on the area from which the blood is coming. A sterile pad is best but a bare hand is better than nothing. Put a pad over the area and bandage firmly. Raise the limb which is injured in order to decrease the blood supply to it. If blood appears through the bandage, do not remove the dressing but put another on top and bandage again more firmly.

If there are pieces of glass or other foreign bodies in a wound remove the loose ones but do not touch those that are firmly embedded. If you think that there may be a fracture under the wound build up a pad around the wound before bandaging firmly.

*Internal bleeding.* The patient will be pale, cold and sweating. There may be swelling from an injury such as a fractured femur. No time should be lost trying to make an accurate diagnosis. The casualty should be sent to hospital because he will need replacement of the blood lost as well as treatment of his injuries.

IS THE PATIENT CONSCIOUS OR UNCONSCIOUS?

A conscious patient makes some effort to answer a question or obey a command.

If a casualty is breathing but unconscious he should be put in the recovery position (Fig. 61). Clear the debris from the patient's mouth. Turn the patient on to his front and his face towards you. Bend his leg, nearest to you, at the knee and bring it towards you over the other leg. Bend the arm nearest to you, at the elbow and bring the forearm towards you and let it rest on the ground parallel to the casualty's face. Finally lift his chin upwards. If possible arrange the casualty so that he has a slight head down tip.

An unconscious patient must not be left alone. A constant watch

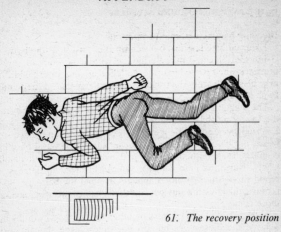

*61. The recovery position*

must be kept to make sure that he continues to breathe, does not choke and is gently controlled if he becomes restless.

If the patient is unconscious and not breathing artificial respiration must be commenced immediately. If he starts breathing but remains unconscious he must then be put in the unconscious position.

ALL CASUALTIES who have needed treatment for FAILURE TO BREATHE or for UNCONSCIOUSNESS must be seen by a doctor at a hospital.

### Organization

At some point while dealing with a number of casualties who have life-threatening conditions you must also get an estimate of the total number of casualties and send somebody to arrange for ambulances and a doctor if possible. You will need to decide which patients need hospital treatment most urgently. Use all the available help in carrying out this organization. Calm organization is an important function of a trained first aider.

**Burns**

After life-saving measures have been applied, burns must be given first aid treatment. The seriousness of a burn depends to a large extent on the amount of the surface area of the body affected.

TREATMENT

1. *Extinguish the fire.* If necessary lay the casualty down and roll him in a blanket or rug to put out flames.
2. *Cool* the burnt area with cold water, if available, for at least ten minutes. This procedure lessens the damage done to the body tissues by the burn area and also relieves the pain.
3. *Cover the burnt area.* Use a sterile dressing if possible; if such dressing are not available use any clean pieces of cloth.

DO NOT USE ANY OINTMENT OR LOTION.
DO NOT BURST ANY BLISTERS.

Keep the casualty lying down until he reaches hospital. A large amount of fluid is lost from burnt areas and to remedy this loss conscious adult casualties should be given frequent small drinks of liquid.

DO NOT GIVE ALCOHOL.

*Burns of the eye* should be washed gently under running water for at least ten minutes and then covered with a clean dry dressing until medical help can be obtained.

A SEVERELY BURNT PATIENT NEEDS QUIET, CALM HANDLING AND A GREAT DEAL OF REASSURANCE.

**Fractures and dislocations**

A fracture is any break or crack in a bone. A fracture may be either closed or open.

1. *A closed fracture.* The skin is intact over the area of the fracture.
2. *An open fracture.* The skin is broken over the area of the fracture. This is important because germs can enter and cause infection.

A dislocation is the disruption of a joint and occurs most commonly at the shoulder joint and the jaw. Again this may be closed or open.

*Diagnosis* of a fracture or dislocation can only be made conclusively by an x-ray. This is beyond the scope of the first aider but the following signs are suggestive:

1. History of a fall or other violent injury
2. Pain
3. Tenderness on examination
4. Swelling
5. Loss of power
6. Deformity

TREATMENT

Always remember that the fracture of a large bone such as the femur can be a major cause of blood loss and a blood transfusion may be the most urgent treatment. Never waste time on elaborate splinting; concentrate on getting a live patient to hospital but remember the following principles:

1. A closed fracture must never become an open fracture through careless handling.
2. An open fracture must be covered to prevent infection.
3. The fracture must be prevented from getting worse during the journey to hospital.
4. *Never* cause the casualty greater pain during the diagnosis or treatment. The fractured area will be very tender and must be handled with great care.
5. No attempt must be made to restore a dislocated joint to its normal position.

*The two basic principles* to be observed in the treatment of all fractures and dislocations are:

1. Immobilization to increase the comfort of the patient and prevent the injury getting worse.
2. Speedy removal to hospital for expert diagnosis and treatment.

If you are in doubt about the diagnosis of a fracture treat the injury as a fracture.

If one arm or one leg is fractured the uninjured limb can be used as a standard of normality and the injured limb compared with it for size and shape. Elaborate splinting is unnecessary and may do more harm than good by causing undue movement of the casualty and delaying his removal to hospital.

BASIC PRINCIPLES OF SPLINTING

1. The site of the fracture must be immobilised together with the joints above and below it.
2. The natural contours of the body should be levelled out by soft padding or a rolled up woollen scarf, rags, etc.
3. No bandages should be put on so tightly that the blood circulation is hindered.

*Fractures of the shoulder blade and upper arm*: Loose padding should be put between the arm and the body. The chest can be used as a splint and the arm placed in the most comfortable position against it—usually with the elbow bent and the forearm in a sling. This position immobilizes both the shoulder and elbow joints.

*Fractures of the elbow and lower arm*: Padding should be placed between the arm and the body but the elbow should not be bent. The casualty will usually be more comfortable lying on a stretcher with the injured arm gently tied to the side of his body.

*Fractures of the wrist and hand*: The elbow can be bent and a sling used to keep the forearm and hand immobilized against the front of the chest.

*Fractures of the thigh bone or femur*: These are serious injuries because of the large amount of blood that can be lost around the site of the fracture. It is important that the casualty should be sent to hospital as soon as possible. Lay the casualty flat on a stretcher. Put padding between the knees, ankles and contours of the legs. Gentleness is important. Tie the feet together with a figure-of-eight bandage (Fig. 62). Tie the knees together and place bandages around both legs above and below the fracture. Always remember

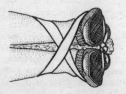

62. *A figure of eight bandage around the feet and ankles*

that the casualty will be severely ill with this fracture and be gentle, calm and reassuring.

*Fractures below the knee*: Remember that in all fractures of the shin bone or tibia the injury is likely to be or to become an open fracture. If one leg is fractured the sound leg may be used as a splint for the injured one. Lay the casualty flat. Place padding between the thighs, knees and ankles. Tie the feet together with a figure-of-eight bandage. Tie the knees together and both legs together with bandages above and below the fracture.

If both legs are fractured the injury is a very severe one. If possible two long splints should be used, one on each side of the body, long enough to reach from the armpits to beyond the feet. If such splints are not available one splint should be used from the level of the groin to beyond the feet and put between the two legs. Padding should be placed between the long splints or the shorter splint and the contours of the body and around the knees and ankles. The feet should be tied together with a figure-of-eight bandage. Tie the knees together and put bandages around both legs and the splints above and below the levels of the fractures. If two long splints are being used additional bandages should be put around the hips and chest.

*Fractures of the jaw*: Bandaging is unnecessary. If both sides of the jaw are fractured passage of air into the lungs may be affected. An unconscious casualty should be put in the unconscious position. A conscious casualty should be in a sitting position with the head tilted slightly forward. The casualty must be taken to hospital.

*Fracture of the hip bone or pelvis*: This can be a serious injury depending on the amount of damage that is done inside the body. The casualty must be put on his back on a stretcher. Put padding between his knees and ankles. Tie his feet together with a figure-of-eight bandage. Warn the casualty not to pass water on his way to hospital.

*Fracture of the spine*: This can be a very serious injury and be both life-threatening and the cause of paralysis below the site of the fracture. Send for help, a stretcher and an ambulance.

*No attempt* should be made to move the casualty until at least four and preferably five people are present. The movement of the casualty on to a stretcher is a job for an expert because the position of the spine must not be changed at any time during the manoeuvre. Minor flexion or bending forward of the spine is the most dangerous change of position because it can compress the spinal cord and cause irreversible damage to the nerves below the level of the fracture.

*Dislocations*: Any dislocation is a very painful and frightening injury and the casualty needs reassurance and calm treatment.

No attempt must be made to restore the joint to its normal position. The injured area must be supported in the position which is most comfortable for the casualty. The casualty must be taken to hospital.

## Poisoning

Poisoning is a hazard that should be prevented rather than treated. There are so many poisonous substances now in general use that it is impracticable to give the treatment of each one. A general outline will be given. In the United Kingdom there are poison reference centres to which an urgent telephone call can be made for information. The numbers are as follows:

TELEPHONE NUMBERS OF POISON REFERENCE CENTRES

| | | | |
|---|---|---|---|
| *Belfast* | 0232 40503 | *London* | 01 407 7600 |
| *Cardiff* | 0222 33101 | *Manchester* | 061 740 2254 |
| *Edinburgh* | 031 229 2477 | *Newcastle* | 0632 25131 |
| *Leeds* | 0532 32799 | | |

ALWAYS KEEP A CONTAINER FROM WHICH THE POISON IS BELIEVED TO HAVE BEEN TAKEN AND SEND IT TO HOSPITAL WITH THE PATIENT.

If the patient is not breathing artificial respiration must be given. When the patient starts breathing put him in the unconscious position. Send him to hospital.

If the casualty is conscious but shows signs of burning in or around the mouth send him urgently to hospital and do not make him vomit.

If the casualty is conscious and shows no signs of burning in or around his mouth make him vomit. This can usually be achieved by giving him two tablespoons of salt in a cup of warm water or putting your finger down the back of his throat. If you are trying to make a child vomit put a spoon handle down the back of his throat and not your finger. After he has vomited give him at least a litre of water, milk, weak tea or coffee while waiting for him to be taken to hospital, or on the way.

## Miscellaneous mishaps

### FOREIGN BODIES IN THE EYE

A loose foreign body in the eye may be removed by rapid blinking of the eye or by pulling the upper lid outwards and downwards over the lower lid. No attempt should be made to remove a foreign body forcibly even if it can be clearly seen. A pad should be put over the eye and medical help obtained.

### FOREIGN BODIES IN THE NOSE AND EAR

These are usually self-inflicted accidents by small children. The presence of the foreign body may only be suspected by the observation of a one-sided blood or pus-stained discharge. No attempt should be made to remove the object and medical advice should be obtained.

### NOSE BLEEDS

A nose bleed may follow an injury to the nose and is sometimes associated with a fracture. More often a nose bleed occurs spontaneously. The casualty should then be made to sit leaning slightly forwards and hold a pad of handkerchief or soft paper firmly around the end of his nose. Sniffing must be discouraged and the pad should be held in place for 10 minutes after the bleeding has stopped.

### SNAKE BITES

In the United Kingdom the only poisonous snake is the adder. Its bite is seldom dangerous or fatal but the anxiety it produces is very great. The casualty should be lain down and the bitten limb raised. No attempt should be made to cut or suck the bite. The casualty should be taken to hospital.

In parts of the world where snake bites can be fatal the same initial treatment should be given and transport to hospital arranged as speedily as possible. It may be helpful if the species of the snake can be identified so that appropriate treatment can be given.

# APPENDIX 6

## Abbreviations of some Degrees, Diplomas, other Titles and Organizations

| | |
|---|---|
| AIMSW | Associate of the Institute of Medical Social Workers |
| ARRC | Associate of the Royal Red Cross |
| ARSH | Associate of the Royal Society of Health |
| BA | Bachelor of Arts |
| BCh, BS, BChir | Bachelor of Surgery |
| BChD, BDS | Bachelor of Dental Surgery |
| BM | Bachelor of Medicine |
| BSc | Bachelor of Science |
| CHC | Community Health Council |
| CM, ChM | Master in Surgery |
| CNAA | Council for National Academic Awards |
| CQSW | Certificate of Qualification in Social Work |
| DA | Diploma in Anaesthetics |
| DCH | Diploma in Child Health |
| DCP | District Community Physician |
| DDS | Doctor of Dental Surgery |
| DHSS | Department of Health and Social Security |
| DM | Doctor of Medicine |
| DMR(D) | Diploma in Medical Radiology: Diagnostic |
| DMR(T) | Diploma in Medical Radiology: Therapy |
| DMT | District Management Team |
| DN, DipN | Diploma in Nursing |

| | |
|---|---|
| DNE | Director of Nurse Education |
| DNO | District Nursing Officer |
| DO | Diploma in Ophthalmology |
| DObstRCOG | Diploma in Obstetrics of the Royal College of Obstetricians and Gynaecologists |
| DON | Diploma in Orthopaedic Nursing |
| DPH | Diploma in Public Health |
| DPM | Diploma in Psychological Medicine |
| DipPhysMed | Diploma of Physical Medicine |
| DSc | Doctor of Science |
| DTM&H | Diploma in Tropical Medicine and Hygiene |
| DivNO | Divisional Nursing Officer |
| ENB | English National Board |
| FCSP | Fellow of the Chartered Society of Physiotherapy |
| FChS | Fellow of the Society of Chiropodists |
| FFARCS | Fellow of the Faculty of Anaesthetists of the Royal College of Surgeons |
| FPS | Fellow of the Pharmaceutical Society |
| FRCGP | Fellow of the Royal College of General Practitioners |
| FRCN | Fellow of the Royal College of Nursing |
| FRCOG | Fellow of the Royal College of Obstetricians and Gynaecologists |
| FRCP | Fellow of the Royal College of Physicians |
| FRCPath | Fellow of the Royal College of Pathologists |
| FRCPE, FRCP(Ed) | Fellow of the Royal College of Physicians, Edinburgh |
| FRCPI | Fellow of the Royal College of Physicians of Ireland |
| FRCPsych | Fellow of the Royal College of Psychiatrists |
| FRCR | Fellow of the Royal College of Radiologists |
| FRCS | Fellow of the Royal College of Surgeons |

| FRCSE, FRCS(Ed) | Fellow of the Royal College of Surgeons, Edinburgh |
| FRCSI | Fellow of the Royal College of Surgeons of Ireland |
| FRFPSG | Fellow of the Royal Faculty of Physicians and Surgeons, Glasgow |
| FRS | Fellow of the Royal Society |
| FRSE | Fellow of the Royal Society, Edinburgh |
| HV | Health Visitor |
| LDS | Licentiate in Dental Surgery |
| LMSSA | Licentiate in Medicine and Surgery, Society of Apothecaries, London |
| LRCP | Licentiate of the Royal College of Physicians |
| LSA | Licentiate of the Society of Apothecaries, London |
| MA | Master of Arts |
| MAO | Master of the Art of Obstetrics |
| MB | Bachelor of Medicine |
| MBAOT | Member of the British Association of Occupational Therapy |
| MC, MS, MCh, MChir | Master of Surgery |
| MChD, MDS | Master of Dental Surgery |
| MChS | Member of the Society of Chiropodists |
| MCSP | Member of the Chartered Society of Physiotherapy |
| MD | Doctor of Medicine |
| MPS | Member of the Pharmaceutical Society |
| MRCGP | Member of the Royal College of General Practitioners |
| MRCOG | Member of the Royal College of Obstetricians and Gynaecologists |
| MRCP | Member of the Royal College of Physicians |
| MRCPath | Member of the Royal College of Pathologists |
| MRCS | Member of the Royal College of Surgeons |
| MS | Master of Surgery |